The
Daily Nugget
366 Tips for a Healthier You

Subscribe to
The Daily Nugget
for free and receive one nugget
a day direct to your inbox!

Dr. Kim Makoi

This book is written as a source of information only. The information contained in this book should not be considered a substitute for the advice of a qualified medical professional, who should be consulted before beginning any new diet, exercise, or other health program.

All efforts have been made to ensure the accuracy of the information contained in this book as of the date published. The author expressly disclaims responsibility for any adverse effects arising from the use or application of the information contained herein.

This book is dedicated to my very first round of Nuggeteers!
Were you receiving The Daily Nugget between July 2022 – July 2023?
Then that's you! 😊 ♡ 🙏
Thank you for keeping me on track!

* Special Thanks to Honorary Editor Nolana Daoust,
who patiently sent me many edits along the way. 😊 🙏

The Daily Nugget is best enjoyed in its original form:
one nugget at a time,

direct to your e-mail box,

at 4 in the morning, *every morning!*

Sign up at **www.dailyhealthnugget.com**

Table of Contents

Introduction

Note for the TL;DR ("too long; didn't read") crew:

If you don't or didn't receive The Daily Nugget e-mails, then the best way to use this book is to get a bookmark and read just one page each day first thing in the morning or each night right before bed. Honestly, you should get the e-mails. They're free and they're magical! Sign up at www.dailyhealthnugget.com. If you have received the e-mails and are looking for a specific one, then use the index in the back of the book! I know, the table of contents is crazy. And apparently, this is "a great bathroom book."

Books are funny. Until I wrote one, I thought that they were an "end product." The end of a process, a final creation, a thing with a vibe, or an energy, but still a thing, like a rock. I never dreamed that a book was really an alive thing – a creature with a life of its own and even perhaps a will of its own! I learned that with my first book, *The Issues are in the Tissues*. And despite learning that lesson, here I am, surprised again, that this book, *The Daily Nugget: 366 Simple Tips for a Healthier You*, has gone off and is living a life of *its* own with its own ideas about what it is!

In the beginning, it seemed simple enough. I thought, "Wouldn't it be great to have a book of daily health tips? People could read just one a day and learn a lot and feel better after a year!" But how to create such a book? It's not easy to sit down and just knock it out. Life gets in the way. But what if I built in an accountability system? Like, what if I created a series of daily e-mails that people subscribed to? And then I would "have to" create one a day or else the subscribers would be disappointed! And then, at the end of the year, I would have a book!

But how could I create a daily e-mail that people wouldn't be sick of? That they would actually *welcome* into their crowded inbox? Stick figures! Nobody does stick figures anymore. If I started each e-mail with a stick figure drawing and a simple caption, then maybe they wouldn't even have to read the whole e-mail to get the message. I could do that! And thus, the Daily Nugget e-mails were born. A simple stick figure type of drawing along with a simple health tip

Over time, it became clear that people were really enjoying the Daily Nuggets *as e-mails*. And when it came time to put together a book at the end of the year, it was way too long! I had imagined a standard 6x9" paperback. But at those dimensions, keeping the drawings intact and formatting the text properly, the book was over 600 pages long! 666 pages to be exact. 😠 I'm no George R.R. Martin. Nobody wants a 600+ page book from me. So finally, I settled on an 8x10 sized book and squished the text together as best I could and ended up with around 400 pages. It's still a big book. I don't know how many people will really want this big of a book. Time will tell.

The searchable .PDF version was the first to come out. Some people have requested card decks (which I'm excited to try, but... yeah, that's a lot of cards!) or desk calendars. I'm turning the nuggets into YouTube videos in the hopes of attracting more Nuggeteers, and it turns out there are some people who really enjoy them as quirky videos! The original intention was just to create a *book*. And the e-mails were my road to getting the book done. But now, it looks like the book may well exist mainly to support the e-mails! 🫣 Go figure. I'm just happy that people are excited about the Daily Nuggets and are eager to continue to see them in their lives!

My intention is that they will continue to evolve. I'm replacing the less awesome ones with better ones over time. I've already replaced the "2-Ingredient Healthy Cookie" with "Just Dance." The 2-ingredient healthy cookie may have been "healthy," but it was a godawful "cookie!" For those of you who actually tried it out... I'm sorry.

I have included that awful recipe in the "duds" section at the end of the book.

So, to the Nuggeteers who really wanted a physical book with all the nuggets inside of it, here you go! 😊 And to those of you who don't – or never have – received the Daily Nugget by daily e-mail, what are you waiting for?! Sign up at www.dailyhealthnugget.com ! (Or, if I haven't set up that link correctly, you can also find it at www.drkimsf.com/dailynugget) Or scan that QR code that I keep putting all over the place because subtlety is not always my strong suit! 😑

Thank you for your continuing love and support!

-DK
San Francisco, 20 September 2023

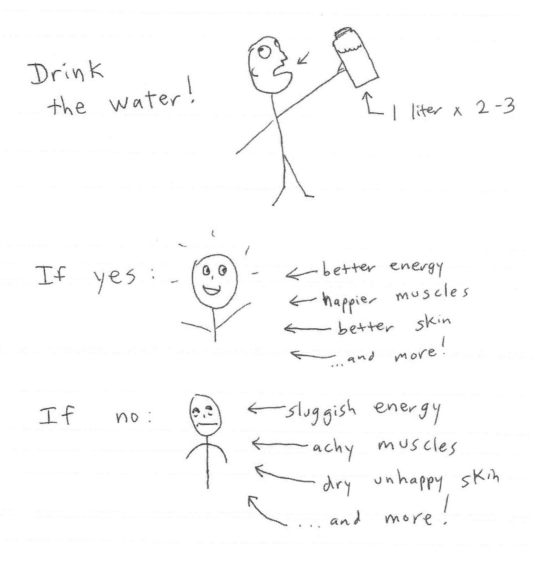

Drink the water!

↳ 1 liter x 2-3

If yes : ← better energy
← happier muscles
← better skin
← ...and more!

If no : ← sluggish energy
← achy muscles
← dry unhappy skin
← ...and more!

Drinking more water is a basic that we can all do good to remember every single day!
Sure, there are nuances and all that, but here's the basic basics.
Aim to drink about one liter or quart of water for each 50 pounds of body weight that you
have. On average, this means about 3 quarts a day. Drink more water if you are doing things
that dehydrate your body, such as consuming caffeine and alcohol. You can drink less water
if you are consuming things that naturally add hydration, such as smoothies containing chia
seeds. Bonus nugget: if you get that first liter or quart down by noon, you can avoid that early
afternoon energy crash!

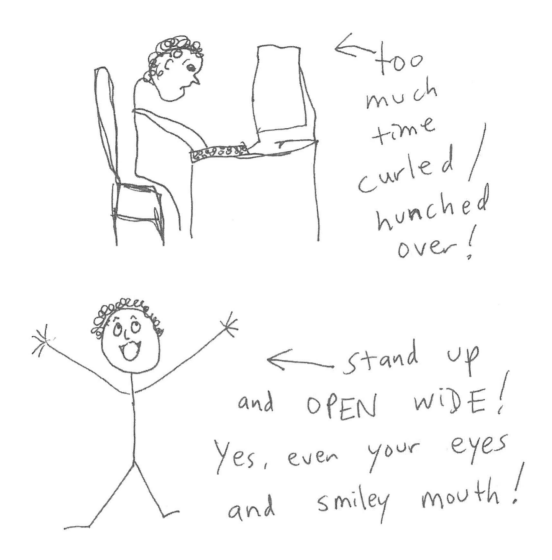

If you're reading this, chances are good that you are in something of a hunched or curled over posture! This is fine sometimes. Heck, it can even be therapeutic! But for most of us, **we spend way too much time like this.**

So, if you can, go ahead and stand up and open wide! Open your arms wide, stand with your legs apart, arch your back and look up to the sky! Open your eyes wide (but don't stare into the sun) and your big mouth! (Open your mouth in a big happy way, not in an existential scream way.)

If you're sitting on a bus or in a boring meeting, at least open your hands or spread your toes wide and remind yourself to do it with your whole body when you get a chance!

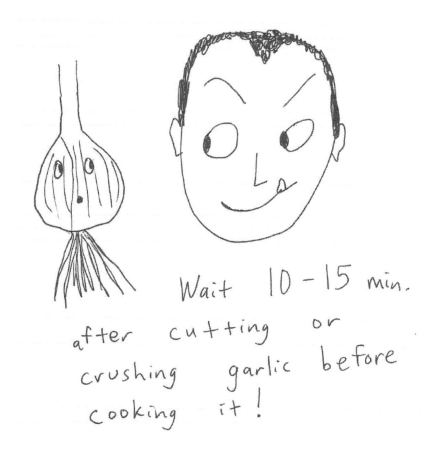

Wait 10 - 15 min.
after cutting or
crushing garlic before
cooking it!

Everyone knows that garlic is good for you and helps to make for a strong immune system, amiright? One of the powerful components within garlic is a compound called allicin. When you cut or crush the garlic cells, enzymes are released which then react with the oxygen in the air, forming sulfide compounds such as allicin! It takes about 10-15 minutes after cutting or crushing for the maximum amount of allicin to form. Allicin can survive cooking, but the enzymes that help to form it do not. So, next time you are crushing garlic for cooking, let it sit for about 10-15 minutes before putting it on the heat!

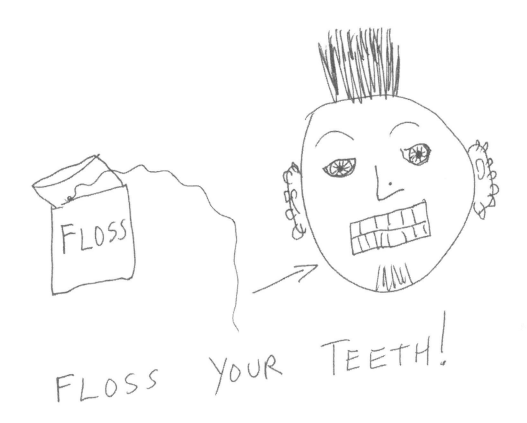

FLOSS

FLOSS YOUR TEETH!

For the **L**ove **O**f **S**weet **S**miles! Yes, FLOSS!

I can hear the groans all the way from over here!

You hear it from your dentist every time. And yes, it's so important for your teeth and gums! But... did you know that it's also so important for your heart?!

Research shows that the presence of gum disease can triple the risk of heart disease! The theory is that inflammation in the gums can allow bacteria to enter the bloodstream and make its way to the heart. It sounds crazy, but it actually happened to one of my mentors! While he ended up needing surgery, he did live to tell the tale!

I floss after every meal and use a waterpik when I am at home!

Am I such a goody-two-shoes dentist-pleaser? Maybe, maybe not, but I am freaked out by the high cost of dental care, and my dental bills have been much lower since I became a champion flosser!!! 😁

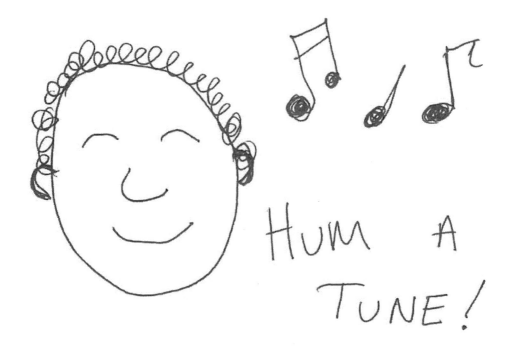

What kind of tune? Anything hummable, I guess. Preferably something you enjoy!

What does humming have to do with health?

Humming is one of the activities that stimulates the vagus nerve.

The vagus nerve is one of the most important nerves in your whole body!

It's one of the 12 cranial nerves - meaning, nerves that emerge directly out of your brain, without having to travel first via the spinal cord - and it connects to most of your vital organs!

It's the main part of the parasympathetic nervous system, which is the counterbalance to the sympathetic or "fight/flight" nervous system.

You don't need me to tell you that you are probably spending more time in the "fight/flight" nervous system than the relaxation and recovery system!

Stimulating the vagus nerve is a great way to help tone the parasympathetic nervous system.

And humming is one of the simplest things you can do to strengthen your vagus nerve.

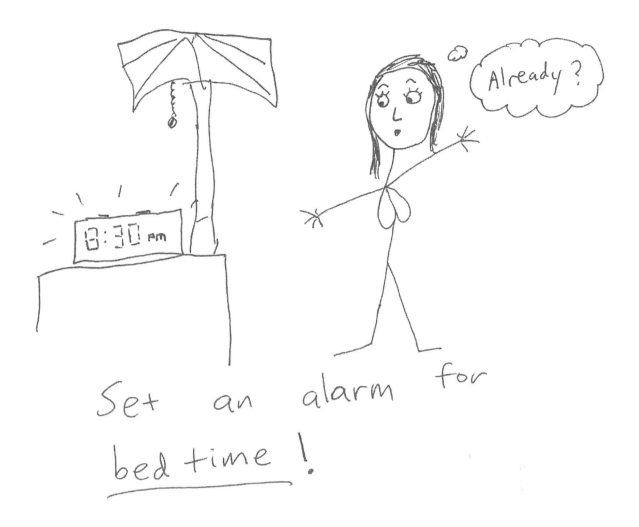

Set an alarm for bed time !

Most people set an alarm for when it's time to get OUT of bed.

But what about when it's time to go TO bed?

Personally, I think it's more important to set an alarm for the latter!

Getting a good night's sleep is one of the most powerful things you can do for your health!

And the most rejuvenating hours of sleep happen between around 9pm-2am. This is where you get the most restoration bang for your sleep buck!

So set your alarm for when it's time to get ready for bed.

Aim to be **in** bed by around 9pm and hopefully asleep by 10!

You may find that you naturally wake up a lot earlier than usual, but you will also feel more refreshed and ready to take on the day.

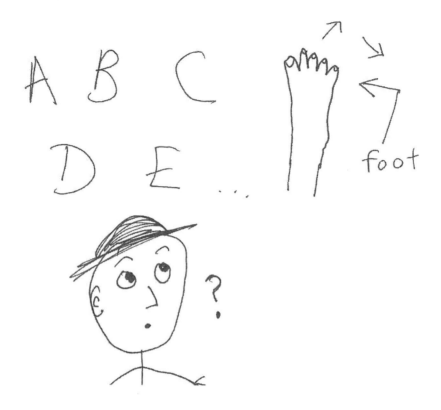

tl;dr: make the shape of the alphabet with your foot!

The first time I heard that making the letters of the alphabet with your feet was a great foot and ankle exercise, I was around 23 years old. Still just a kid in chiropractic school! I remember moving my youthful feet through the exercise with ease, thinking, "OK, what's the big deal? Anyone can do this. [shrug]" But as I repeat the exercise with my almost-50-year-old feet, it's not so smooth or easy anymore! D'oh! Anyway, the point is... Every part of your body needs some love and attention! Making the alphabet with your feet really is a good exercise for your feet and ankles, and you can do it almost anywhere, any time. At home, on the plane, at work, during a boring meeting, on the bus, at the beach...
For the over-achievers out there, try it with the Russian alphabet! Or another alphabet!

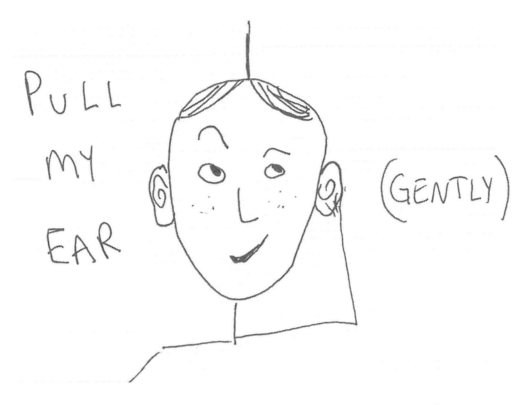

PULL MY EAR (GENTLY)

Are you pulling my ear? 😁 Sorry-not-sorry - I can't resist a corny joke. 🐛
Did you know that your ears are full of tiny nerve endings that connect to almost all parts of your body?! You might think that they are just traditional acupuncture meridian points, since some acupuncturists work extensively on the ears. However, auriculotherapy in neurology is also an evidence-based treatment for pain. But you don't need needles or electrodes to get some benefit for yourself! You can simply massage and gently pull on your ears in different directions. Some directions will feel really good! Some spots of your ears may be very tender and could use some extra love. (I've added a basic auriculotherapy chart in the appendix of this book. You can find it on pages 406-407.)

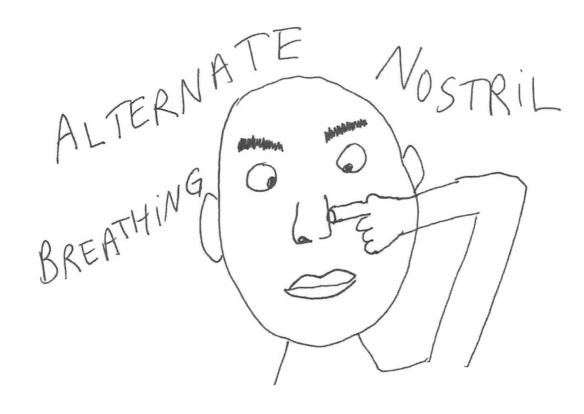

ALTERNATE NOSTRIL BREATHING

I know, this person looks like they are picking their nose. But they're not! They are trying out alternate nostril breathing! This is pretty much what it sounds like. You block off one side of your nose, and take a nice deep breath in and out. And then you switch sides. Breathe in and out. And switch again. Back and forth, nice slow deep breaths with one nostril blocked off. What is the point of this?? Well, for one thing, it has been shown to improve heart rate variability and to lower blood pressure. It is good for the autonomic nervous system, balances the brain hemispheres and helps to relieve anxiety. Even just 5 minutes is enough to have positive measurable effects on the heart! This is a good before-bed practice after a long stressful day.

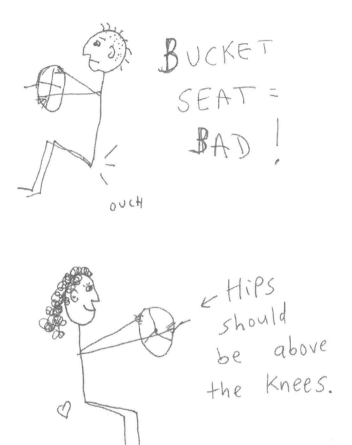

I'm not hating on cute cars with bucket seats!

Buuut...

if you're having back or hip pain, and you drive one of those cars... those seats ain't helping. When it comes to sitting down, your hips are happiest if your knees are below them - even if only a little bit! Once the knees go higher than the hips, it starts to put more pressure on the pelvis and hip flexors. Pay attention to the relative position of your hips and knees. Old couches where the cushions have lost their spring and your butt sinks deeper and deeper into the couch can also cause this same problem.

If you're stuck with bucket seats, you can buy a wedge to sit on - or even try sitting on a big, folded towel. Work with what you've got!

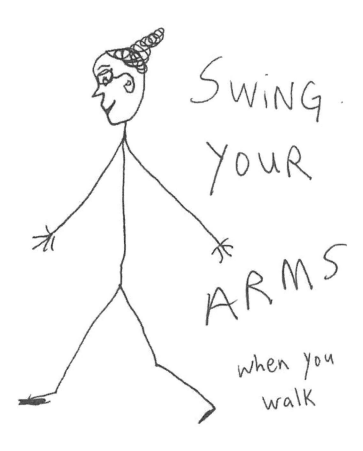

SWING YOUR ARMS when you walk

Yes, swing your arms when you walk! This should be a natural movement, but a lot of people don't do it. Why not? Could be stress, could be biomechanical problems, could be habit. I used to walk with my left arm very rigid for some reason. 👤

Swinging your arms while you walk (in a cross-crawl pattern, meaning opposite side of the body working together: left arm moves with right leg, and right arm moves with left leg) is great for your brain!

Cross-crawl exercises are used for helping to improve communication between the left and right brain hemispheres.

So pay attention the next time you are walking!

Make sure you are swinging your arms!

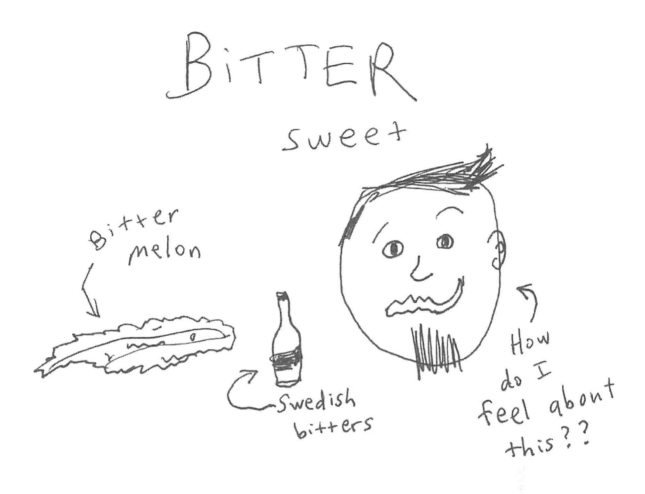

BITTER
sweet

Bitter melon

Swedish bitters

How do I feel about this??

That's my attempt at drawing an "ambivalent face." That person doesn't know how they feel about this news. Why? Because the truth is, we need more bitter foods! The American diet is heavy - way, way too heavy - on the sweets and the salties! We would do good to add more bitter flavors into our diets.

Why?

Because bitter foods have those powerful antioxidants and nutrients that help to balance things like blood sugar, improved liver function and so on and so forth.

So, you can go FULL BITTER and eat some bitter melon, which I sometimes do with a splash of ketchup to cut the taste.

Or you can go easy and add a splash of liquid bitters into your water.

Start where you can!

But keep it in mind when you are offered some bitter food.

Just say yes and know that life will be sweeter... if you incorporate more bitter into your diet!

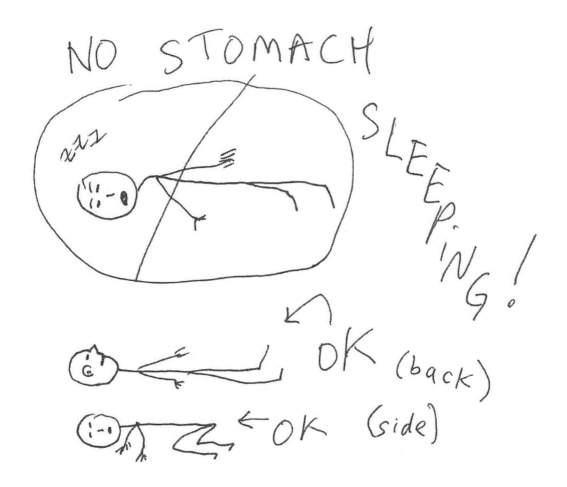

Stomach sleeping? Just NO!

It's bad for your back, and it's **terrible** for your neck!

(See what I did there? I used a terrible font - **Comic Sans** - for "terrible." That's how bad it is!)

If you are sleeping on your stomach, I don't even know why you bother to see a chiropractor about your neck! One side of your neck will always be too tight, and one side will always be too loose. It won't hold a good adjustment.

But it feels so good on your tummy? Well, invest in a good body pillow!

Don't hate.

I'm just the messenger!

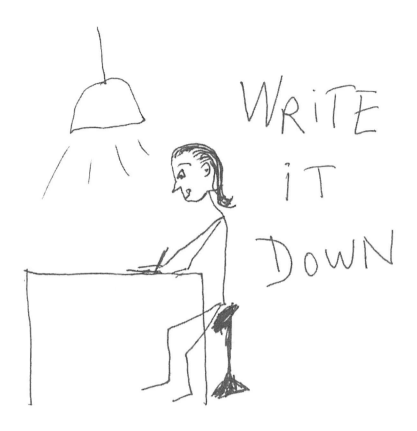

Write what down?

Basically, the thing you're trying to change.

There's something about writing things down that makes it process in a different way. ✎
For example, there are studies that show that people tend to lose weight if they simply write down everything they eat. Even with no particular dietary guidance, people just eat less (and even a bit healthier) if they have to write everything down.

They become their own accountability buddy!

We always do better when there are eyes on us - even our own eyes! 👀

Same with your schedule and that story that you simply HAVE NO TIME for the things that you "have to" do in your life! 🕐

For 2 weeks - yes, 2 whole weeks - write down everything you do all day long. Write it down in 15-minute increments. Everything! This exercise needs to be a couple of weeks long, because anyone can fool themselves or modify some habits to look good on paper for a couple of days. But 2 weeks will capture the true picture.

EPSOM SALT BATH *

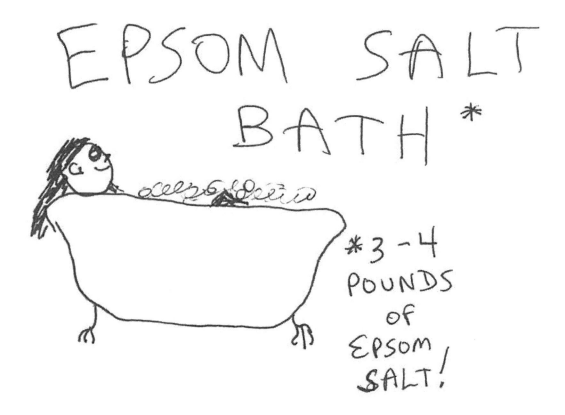

*3 - 4 POUNDS of EPSOM SALT!

I know, I know, not everyone hath a bathtub. (And it's a guilty activity during times of drought!) But... for tight and sore muscles, a nice Epsom salt bath is sooooooo good! Epsom salts (magnesium sulfate) are a great way to get magnesium into your muscles. Can you take magnesium supplements? Sure, but you can't really get a high therapeutic dose by way of supplements. If you've ever taken too much magnesium, you know why: it will give you diarrhea! 💩 💥

But if you absorb it through the skin - as in a nice warm Epsom salt bath - then it will not have to go through your guts!

Just make sure that you are using a therapeutic dose, which means 3 to 4 **pounds** (not scoops!) of Epsom salts into the bath. You can throw in a couple of pounds (2 boxes) of baking soda into the water as well, for extra therapeutic benefits. Do this, and you will feel like you just had a mini spa day.

Did you know that people make "bath time spa music" on YouTube??? Yes, you can look it up! Of course, when **I** think of "bath time music," I still think of Ernie from Sesame Street and his Rubber Duckie song.

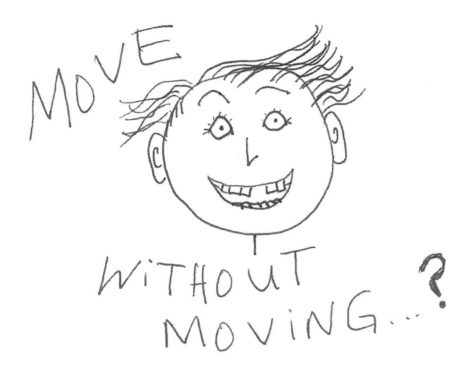

What is this person even doing? 😳

Somewhere, below their neck, they are doing isometric exercises. But I don't know how to draw that, because when you do isometric exercises, it looks like you are doing a bunch of nothing. Isometric exercises are when you engage a muscle, but the muscle doesn't appear to move. For example, here is an isometric exercise that we could **all** use. Put your hand behind your head. Then, press your head backwards into your hand, but don't let your head actually move anywhere! Block the motion with your hand. (Or your pillow or headboard or wall or whatever.) What is happening here? You are engaging the extensor muscles in your neck, which are weaker than they should be since we spend so much time looking down. While doing this exercise, you can feel the extensors engage and also feel the relief as those tired flexors get a break! 😌 Another easy urban isometric exercise is to press downward while holding the pole if you are standing on the bus. When you do this, you will feel your abs and core engage. And we all know that a good strong core is good for your back! Isometrics are also a great way to get some exercise in when you are recovering from injury or find that "normal" exercises are too painful. This is because you can choose the level of muscle engagement while keeping the joint nice and steady.

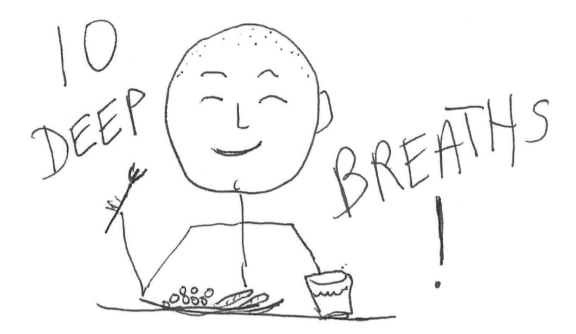

You know how when you're stressed out, the "fight/flight" system gets activated, and blood flows to your muscles and all that?

Well did you know that when that happens, blood is flowing away from your digestive system? If we have to get away, then that's no time to waste energy on digesting breakfast! (or anything!)

So, when you're running around like crazy and decide to stop and shove some food into your pie hole, guess what? Your body probably thinks that it's not a good time for eating! No wonder so many people have trouble with digestion!

Well, you can't magically eliminate the stress of life, but you can help your body to know that it really is OK to slow down when it's time for food.

One very simple way to do that is to take 10 slow deep breaths before you eat a meal.

I know, I know, 10 slow deep breaths??? Who the hell has time for that???

Hey, I'm just the messenger.

Seriously, though, do it! The 10 slow deep breaths help to activate the parasympathetic nervous system, bringing more blood to the digestive system (and away from the skeletal muscles).

The benefit of slowing down before a meal may well be the origins of saying grace before meals!

Give it a try. Your tummy will thank you. 😊 🙏

p.s. I got turned on to the 10-breaths before eating idea by Marc David, the author of *The Slow-Down Diet.*

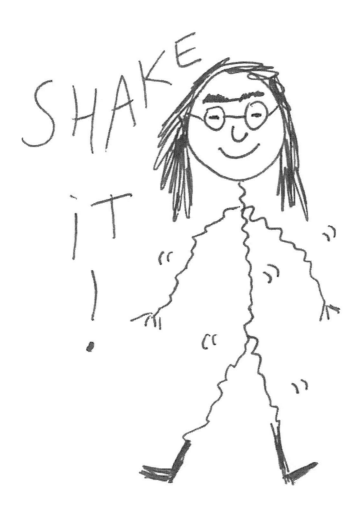

Shake what? 😲

Uh, everything? 🫤

Yeah, pretty much! Shaking your body (gently - don't give yourself a concussion or anything like that) is good for your lymph system. The lymphatic system doesn't have any pumping mechanism of its own, and it relies on muscular movement to move its fluids around. Seeing as most of us are sadly deficient in the muscular movement department, it means that we need to do more to help our lymphatic system.

You can do a nice simple full body shake by standing up, knees about shoulder width apart, soft bend in the knees, and just start bouncing very gently. Let your arms hang loose and jiggle your hands around. Just get all loosey goosey and shake for a little while.

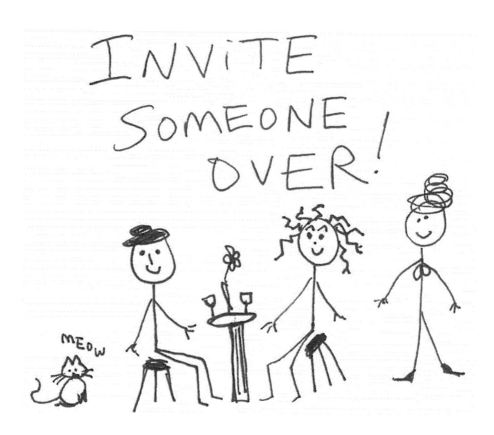

INVITE SOMEONE OVER!

Invite who over? Where? To my house? Why??!

I know, I know, this sounds like CRAZY TALK, especially coming from an Olympic Class Introvert. But... we can't escape it: being connected with other people is a part of being healthy. There are many hidden benefits to inviting someone over.

For one thing, there is really nothing that quite opens your eyes to the state of your home or gets you to suddenly tidy up like knowing that guests are going to show up! 🙄

If the inside of your home is just beyond the beyond, then maybe invite them for a walk.

You can invite a friend you haven't seen for a while, a family member, or even just a random neighbor or someone who you barely know. The point is just to do it. No real reason other than to spend some in-person time with another human being, with no ulterior motive or agenda.

Personally, I am socially indecisive, so I like to make a game of it. I mark a date and time on the calendar. Then, I put names of people I wouldn't mind spending some time with on little pieces of paper and put them in a jar. Then, randomly pick out a name and invite them. If they can't make it, pick out a different name. And so on and so forth! It's kind of fun.

If they are suspicious, just say, "My chiropractor told me to do it. It's for my health. Honestly, it'll probably help your health, too."

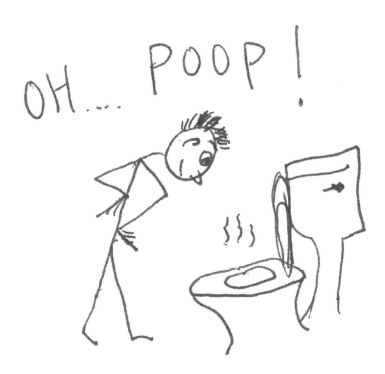

Are we really going to talk about poop? 💩 First thing in the morning? 📺

Yes, we are! (Most of you poop in the morning anyway, so if not now, when??)

You can learn a lot from your poop, and you should know what it basically should look like and when it's looking dangerously wrong! Can poop look dangerously wrong??

Yes. In fact, just this year, 3 patients discovered dangerous conditions thanks to some telltale signs in their poop. These signs were (in 2 cases): BLACK POOP. Sure, this can happen if you eat something loaded with charcoal coloring, like that time during some Halloween season when Burger King was selling **black hamburgers** (the buns were black- it was supposed to be spooky... it was spooky alright)! But in the absence of black food, black tarry poop means that you might be bleeding somewhere in your upper GI tract!

Another suspicious poop is if it is pencil thin or has sharp edges to it, like it came out of a Play-Doh fun factory or something. One patient noticed this, and it turned out that she had polyps in her colon! Fortunately, they were removed with no problem, and she is a-ok.

Healthy poo should be well-formed and basic boring brown. You should (generally) not recognize any of your meal(s) in there. (Corn is an exception.)

If it's pale or clay-colored (yes, that's a thing!) it means that there is a problem with the liver (not enough bile).

If there's obvious and recognizable food in there, it means that you are not chewing your food very well and also that you may need some help in the enzyme department!

OK, this was an exceptionally long message for a Daily Nugget. And yet there's so much more to say! Maybe I will write a book... 💩

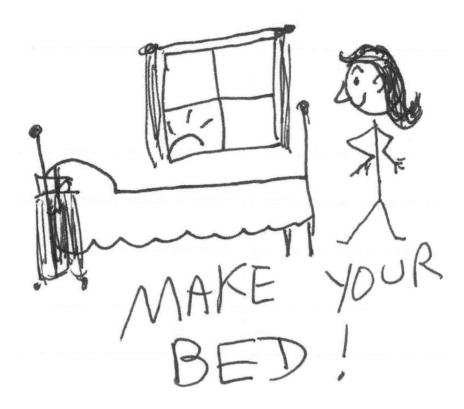

Yes, you read that right. Make your bed!

It is a mental health thing as well as a productivity and focus thing!

Making your bed gives you one simple "win" for the day and one completed task. Even if you think that an unmade bed doesn't bother you, you will notice a net positive feeling if you do make your bed and see it nice and tidy.

If you think this is stupid, and you find yourself sleeping in a little nest surrounded by (mostly) clean laundry and random items, well... you might be depressed... which is a whole 'nother thing. Hey, no judgement - I've slept in that nest before! I've felt like a human squishy-centered bon-bon nestled in my own slot in the box! So... I have been on both sides of the experience. And I can say with confidence that making your bed in the morning will have a positive effect on your health!

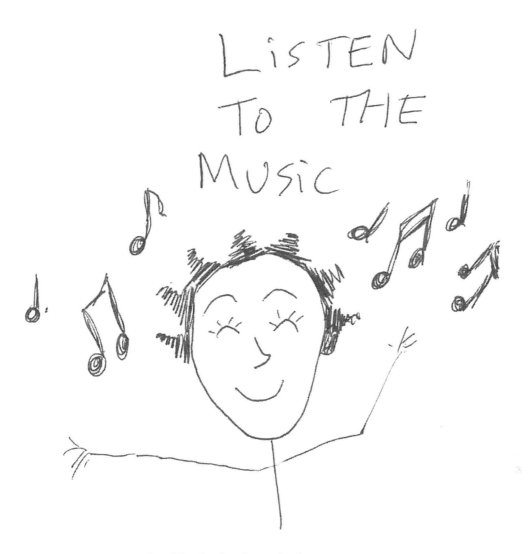

Music evokes memories. No doubt about that!

So if want your body to focus on healing and feeling good (again), one thing that can help is to listen to the music that you were listening to when you felt the best!

Was there a time in your life when you were eating well, exercising and feeling healthy and fit? Then listen to that music again, to remind your body! (I was listening to an awful lot of Bjork during my healthy heyday -- which probably inspired today's nugget hairdo!)

You can use this musical memory tool to help promote other states as well.

For example, if you choose a certain piece of music that you ONLY listen to while writing, then it will be easier to write if you turn on that music.

What is my writing music? Right now, it's a German military marching band CD from my dad's collection. 😵

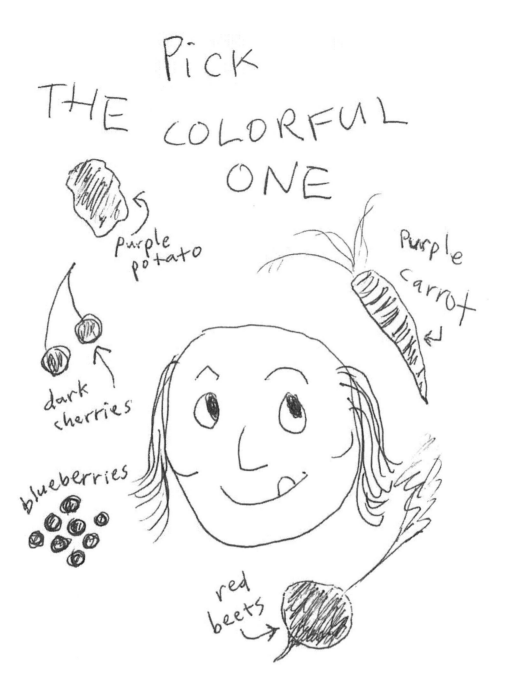

Those extra colorful fruits and veggies, such as the purple carrots and purple potatoes, have bonus nutrients! For example, anthocyanin, which is the cause of the purple color, is known to reduce inflammation and boost mood. 💜 So, while pale foods might look cool, such as the "white cherries" (which have been bred to look that way), they have fewer nutrients. So, if they taste basically the same anyway, then go for the more colorful variety! 🌈
You will benefit from the bonus nutrients!

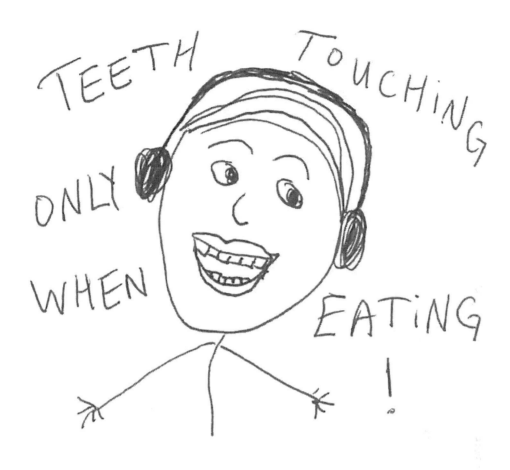

Your teeth should only be touching if you are eating or chewing! Otherwise, they should be resting with a little space in your mouth. If you are just sitting around doing nothing and your teeth are touching, it means that you are holding too much tension in your jaw. This is a sign of stress, and it can also cause damage to your teeth. Check in with yourself throughout the day and ask, are my teeth touching? And if so, focus on relaxing your jaw.

(There is a cool YouTube video that I link to in the e-mail and PDF versions of this nugget. Have I mentioned that it's free to get the e-mails? www.dailyhealthnugget.com)

SLEEP NAKED

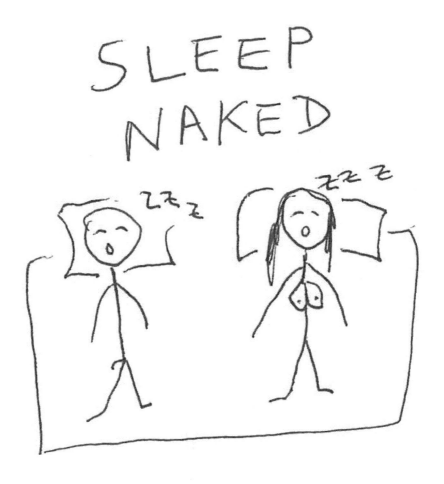

Did you know that your body sleeps better if the ambient temperature is about 5 degrees cooler than it is during your waking hours? You can achieve this by turning down your thermostat at night, or you can sleep naked. (I don't know how many degrees pajamas add - I'm just saying!) It's also good for your circulation to be unencumbered by tight elastic bands or bunchy sleep clothes. Personally, I also think it's good to spend some cozy time with your own naked self. Like RuPaul says, **we're born naked, and the rest is drag!**

I dunno why, but this post made me think of that Queen song, Bicycle Race, and the video with the naked girls racing on bicycles. Did you know that video was banned in some countries?!

EAT ½

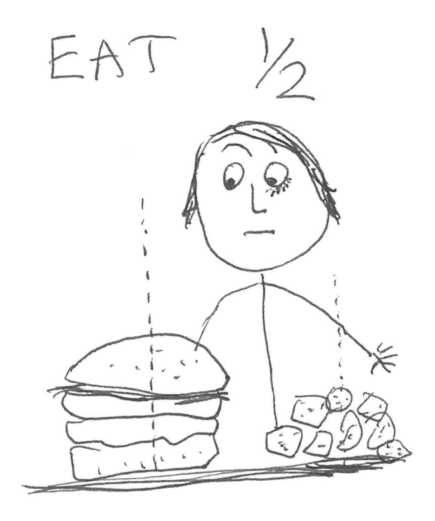

I know, that Clockwork-Orange-looking guy looks like he is about to eat a pile of rocks and a big cake shaped like a burger. 🐵

Eat 1/2 of what? Well, 1/2 of what you would normally eat. Unless you are one of the rare people who is trying to *gain* weight, you are probably eating more than you need to. This is an American thing. We habitually eat much larger portions than anyone else in the world! In my book, *The Issues are in the Tissues*, I talked about my "Russian diet," which I embarked on after a short visit from some Russian friends. They ate about 1/2 of what I considered normal portions, and I decided to give it a go. Turns out... I felt fine - maybe even better than usual - and lost a little weight, saved some money, and had totally normal energy throughout the days!

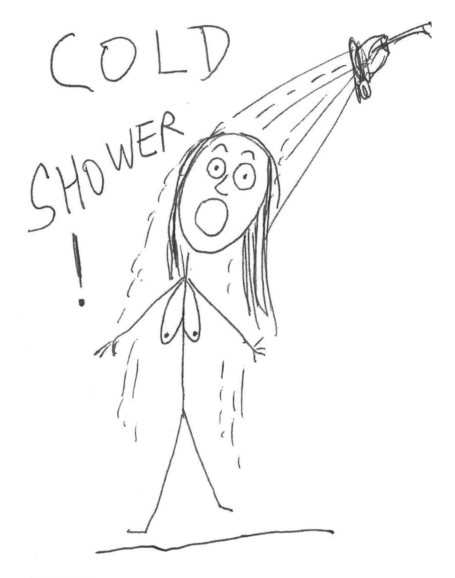

I know, I know.... **WHY?????!**

Hey, don't shoot the messenger!

It turns out that cold showers are *really good for the vagus nerve*. It helps with vagal tone, thus improving the parasympathetic nervous system.

This means better digestion, better mood, and better sleep.

More good news (and I'm not even being sarcastic here): you can get this benefit with as little as 30 seconds worth of cold shower at the very end of your regular shower!

As an alternative, you can also jump into the cold ocean for a few minutes, but the 30-seconds-at-the-end-of-the-shower method is the simplest for most of us!

Hey! Go to YouTube and search for Daily Nugget Cold Shower. It's my 2nd Nugget video ever.

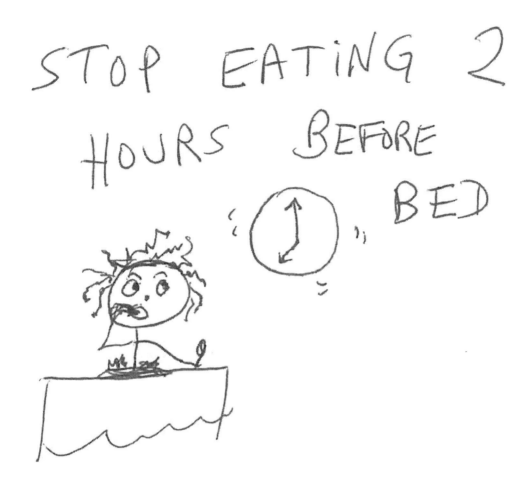

This is a classic tip from Traditional Chinese Medicine, but I've also heard it recommended by plenty of other practitioners as well! STOP EATING (at least) 2 HOURS BEFORE BED. This will give your body some time to get the digestion process started comfortably! If you eat too close to bedtime, then you will have less restful sleep, and you may also experience things like heartburn and indigestion. Good sleep is one of the best things you can do for your health, and this habit is one of the best things you can do for your sleep! Here's a tip that can help: brush and floss 2 hours before bedtime so you don't want to eat again! (Nobody likes that toothpastey taste on food!)

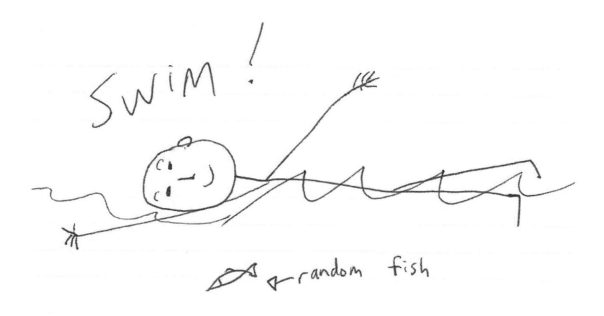

I know, it's not convenient or easy for most people, but... if you can... go for a swim! Swimming is great for your back, brain and body in general. It's easy on the joints - low impact - and it forces you to be very present. You just have to keep moving and find a way to breathe! You can't multitask or stare at your screen/device while you're swimming, and nobody can interrupt you with calls, texts, etc. Swimmers tend to stay in good spinal alignment, so, over the years, I rarely saw swimmers in the office. Snowboarders on the other hand... oof...

(and yeah, I drew that fish before I realized that it would be more disturbing than relaxing to find a random fish in the pool!)

DO THE "POOR MAN'S FOOD ALLERGY TEST"

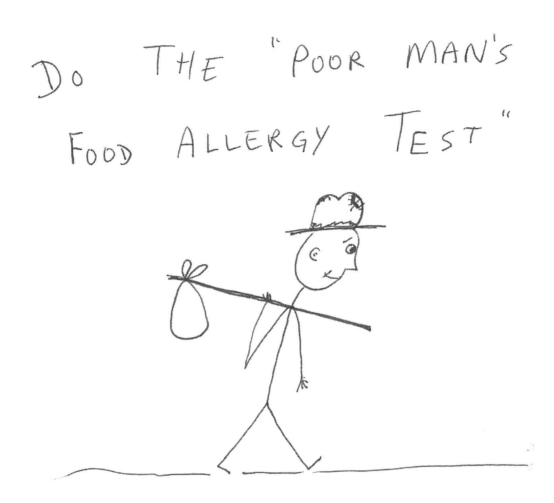

First off, in case you're wondering what the rich person's food allergy* test is, I think it's the Alcat super-duper food sensitivity test. It runs around $1000. This sort of test is still not generally covered by many health insurances (shocker!) but it's still much more useful than the skin prick tests that often are. 🐵

*yes, I know, we're not talking about true allergies here - not the anaphylactic reaction! We are more accurately talking about "food sensitivities." And yeah, yeah, it's for **PEOPLE**, not just **MAN**s.

Anyway... 👀

I learned about the "Poor Man's Food Allergy Test" from an old-timer clinical nutritionist years ago. Here's how it works:

(1) Take a piece of paper.
(2) Write down numbers 1-10 in a column.
(3) List the top 10 foods that you eat, in the order of the foods that you eat the most often **and** like the most.
(4) Starting at the top of the list, remove each food from your diet for 2 weeks.
(5) Pay attention to how you feel.

In most cases, if your health is not so great, then you are probably sensitive to one of the foods in your top 10 --- almost always something in the top 3!
If you remove one of these foods, you may experience terrible withdrawal symptoms in the first few days - headache, increased body pain, nausea, bad mood, fatigue, etc. - but then you feel much better by the end of the 2 weeks - increased energy and focus, decreased pain, etc.

Also, I shouldn't have to say this, but there's always *someone* who needs to hear it...
If your list looks something like, 1. bagels, 2. pasta, 3. pizza, 4. cereal, etc. then... I'm sorry, but it means that the first line should actually say, **1. wheat.**
Sorrynotsorry.

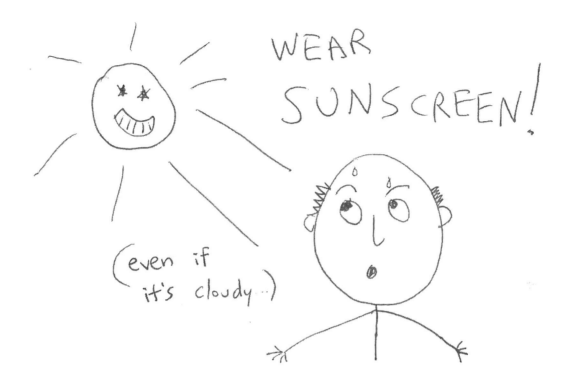

Yeah, I know, vitamin D is one of the most important nutrients ever, and we make it naturally by way of exposure to the sun! *However...* none of us at this latitude get enough sunlight to make enough vitamin D anyway (as evidenced by the epidemic of vitamin D deficiency) but we do get enough to suffer from the harmful effects of the UV rays! Womp womp.

A good clean sunscreen will help to protect your skin. But wait! There's more!

Moisturizing your skin - especially as you get older - may add an extra layer of protection against dementia! What?! It sounds like BS, but it's true. The mechanism is that some forms of dementia have been linked to increased inflammatory responses in the body. And since the skin is one of the biggest organs, anything that helps to reduce skin inflammation can have a significant effect on systemic inflammation!

BTW... as a goth kid, I never had any problem with being even more pasty looking, so, I was not aware that my darker-skinned friends did not enjoy the chalky look that most sunblocks conferred! If you are a darker hued human looking for a really clean product for moisturizing and sunscreen, I recommend Beautycounter's tinted line.

p.s. and yes! even if it's cloudy! My Gramma Blanche used to always tell the story of how she got the worst sunburn of her entire life on a cloudy day! She was just a baby and they did not bother to put her in the shade because it was so cloudy, but she burned so bad that they had to cut the clothes off of her! ☠ It's true, you don't have baby thin skin, but... skin does get thinner as you get older, too, sooooo........ I'm just sayin!

35

BRUSH YOUR "AURA"

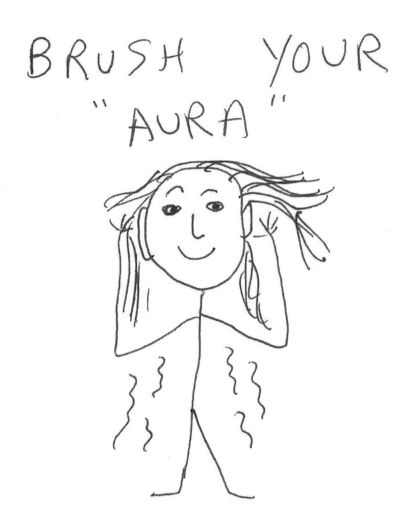

I try not to sound *too* "woo" around here.

And/but... this aura brushing thing feels really good!

I learned it from Dr. Hae Min Cho years and years ago when I used to take her chi-gong in the park class!

Basically, what you do is, you stand up, feet about shoulder width apart, soft knees, and you imagine that you are Cousin Itt from the Addams Family. Starting at the top of your head, you hold your arms just a little bit away from your body and run them down as if you are brushing your hair - your full body cousin Itt hair! Do this all the way from your head to your toes! Just imagine you are brushing that long silky hair. Keep your hands a few inches away from your body and focus on the energy.

You will be surprised at how much better you really do feel after even just a minute of "aura brushing."

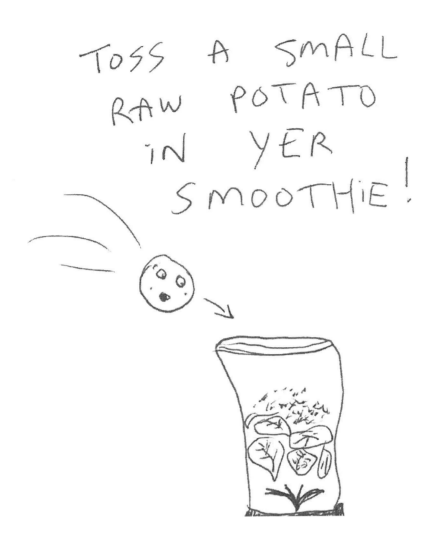

TOSS A SMALL RAW POTATO IN YER SMOOTHIE!

Wot! 😳
Can you even eat raw potatoes? Aye, ye can. (At first, it just sounded crazy to me.... so crazy that I thought of Groundskeeper Willie, from The Simpsons.)

But why? Why would you do it?

Well, raw potatoes have a high resistant starch content, which becomes food for beneficial gut bacteria, and which also prevent the unhealthy spike in blood sugar that cooked potatoes can cause!

But just as you wouldn't want to eat TOO MUCH probiotic or prebiotic at any given time, you don't want to put a gigantic raw potato into your smoothie.

Just a small one. Peel it if you are concerned about extra toxins, and slice or cut it up to make it easier to blend. And don't use a green potato! Green on a potato is a sign of fungus.

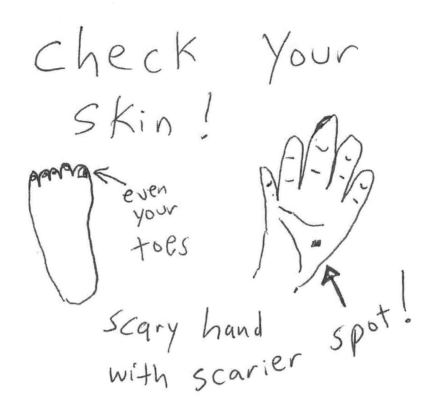

check your skin !

even your toes

scary hand with scarier spot!

Why did I draw a little black patch on that toenail up there?

Because that's how Bob Marley died, at the tender age of 36!

He saw a little black spot under his toenail, and he thought that maybe it was a little bruise from playing soccer.

Nope, it was melanoma. Melanoma is THE WORST.

It often starts as a little black spot with blurry edges.

Melanoma can happen anywhere on the body, but the most common place for it to appear varies by ethnicity.

White men tend to get it on the trunk - usually on the back. White women usually get it on the chest or legs. Black, Asian and Hispanic people tend to get it on their hands and feet.

It's a good idea to check your skin regularly, and have a friend check your back for you once in a while!

Get any suspicious spots looked at, especially if they have weird colors or blurry borders!

Anyway, Bob might have survived the cancer, but after it was diagnosed, he refused to have the toe amputated, for religious reasons. 😒 So it spread, and he died 4 years later.

PiCKLE PACKS FOR CRAMPS!

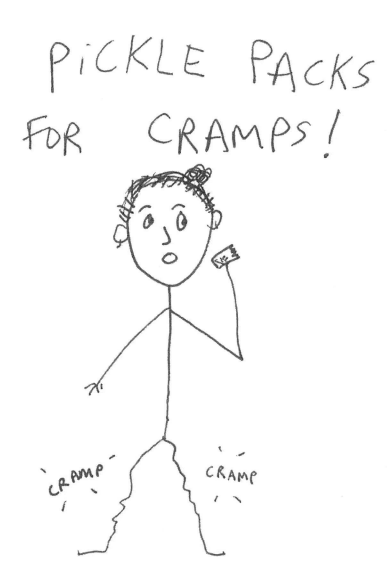

I know, I know. What the hell are pickle packs? 🫨

I guess we're talking about relish packs but hear me out! Pickle juice is a classic home remedy that can stop leg cramps very quickly. Just a couple of tablespoons will do the trick! But who carries pickle juice around with them? Well, ever hear of those grannies who carry relish and/or mustard packets in their purses for just such an occasion??

Yep, in a pinch, a couple of packets of relish or mustard will do the trick! Why???

Honestly, science hasn't figured it out exactly, except to note that there's something to it, because it performs better than placebo and is widely used in the athletic world!

The effect is too fast to be attributed to nutritional factors, so there is likely some sort of neurological reflex at play.

STIR THE POT!

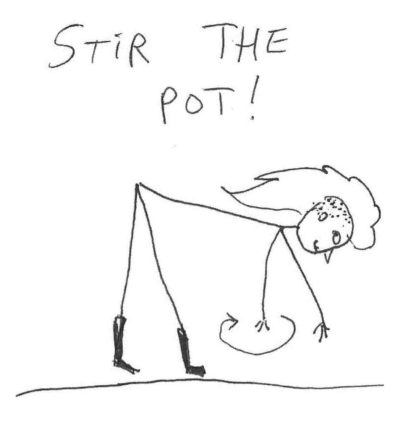

Before I explain what we're talking about here with stirring the pot, let me first say that yes I know this picture looks really weird and maybe oddly suggestive, butt, BUT! but... seriously, for the life of me, I cannot draw this move. This is like my 3rd try. Every one just comes out looking very very strange.

Anyhoo...

"Stirring the pot" is an easy and excellent shoulder exercise that I learned from my friend and trainer, Ace Morgan.

Here's what you do. You stand up, bend over at the waist, and let your arms just hang there. Then. you start moving one arm in a circular direction, as if you're stirring a pot. The movement comes loosely from the shoulder joint, while the rest of the arm just hangs limp. After a few good circles, go ahead and switch directions.

And don't forget to do the other arm!

This is an incredibly gentle exercise, and it is great for helping to loosen up tight shoulders!

MAIL A POSTCARD!

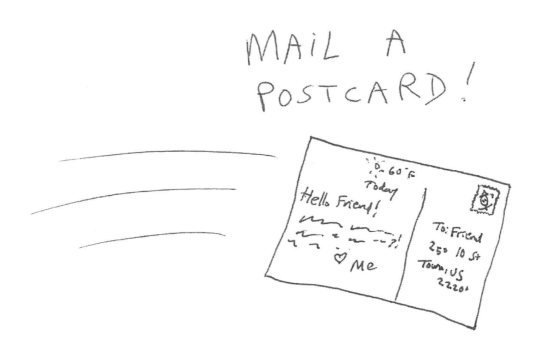

Not many people receive random postcards these days... so it can really brighten someone's day! You may not have time to write a full letter - or even know what to say - but you can say in a few lines that you're thinking of someone.

It's fun to see someone's real handwriting and not just the digital text from an e-mail!

Where does one acquire postcards?

Just keep your eyes out, and you will start to see them!

Obviously, tourist gift shops will have them, but so do bookstores, some drugstores, thrift shops, and estate sales.

I have a **ton** of them, so if you are **truly** hard up for postcards and sincerely want to send some but have NO POSTCARDS, then fine, I will share.

You can send me your mailing address and I will send you some blank postcards to get started with.

(But you better send them for realsies!)

And if you really want to get into it, I recommend Postcrossing.com.

Send and receive postcards to/from random people around the world!

Introvert heaven.

COMPRESSION SOCKS!

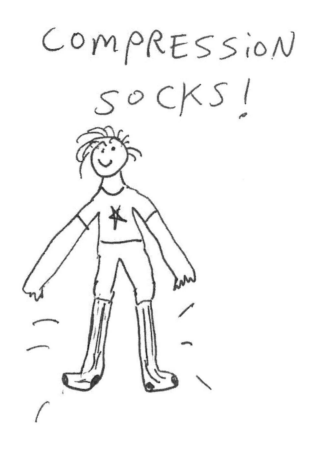

Compression socks! They're not just for old people! Or... am I old? Meh. Doesn't matter. Compression socks are great for helping to improve your circulation. Yes, they are indeed recommended for older people who have circulation problems. But you know who else could use some improved circulation? People who sit a lot. Do you sit a lot? Also people who stand a lot. Do you stand a lot? I can't remember why I first tried out compression socks, but I was really surprised at how much more energy I felt! I had no idea that I was leaking energy due to sluggish circulation while sitting or standing in place for a long time. Now, I always wear compression socks when I fly anywhere - especially long flights - and I feel sooooo much better when I land. ✈ I even wear them to the movies and find that it's easier for me to stay awake during the film! (Otherwise, I tend to fall asleep... awkward, because I also snore!) And I definitely wear them if it looks like I have a packed schedule for my day! Give them a try; you might be surprised at how much better you feel.
(And luckily for me, I even found some with a skeleton design.)
p.s. yes, I'm aware that the person in the drawing appears to need compression socks for their arms as well. Don't judge!

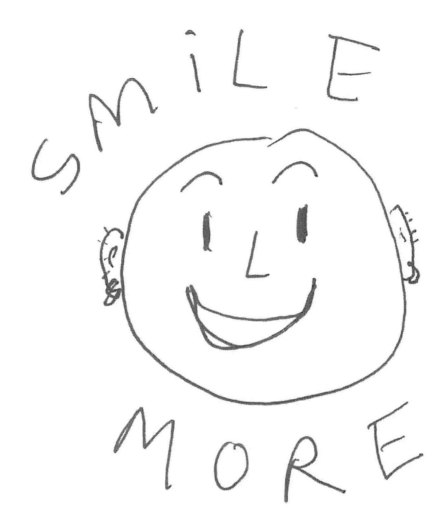

This cranky old metal goth is telling other people to "SMILE MORE" ??? Yep. 😁

If you feel weird doing it too much in public, then do it in private!

But do more smiling. 😊

It doesn't just convey information to other people. It conveys information to **yourself**.

Smiling signals to your brain that something is good and enjoyable.

If you want to "want" more healthy foods - such as those dark leafy greens we talk about - then smile before and after you eat them!

Eventually, this will associate a happy feeling with those foods.

(You can do the opposite, too, and make a disgusted face when you are eating something that you wish you could cut back on, such as sugary snacks!)

Smiling releases endorphins, which are the "feel good chemicals."

HOT WATER BOTTLE

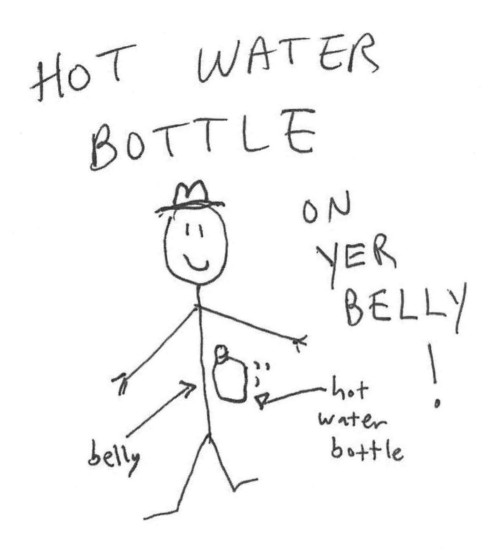

ON YER BELLY !

belly

hot water bottle

The humble old-fashioned hot water bottle is a handy tool that everyone should have at home!

It's another one of our vagal toners! Putting a warm water bottle on your belly can soothe that vagus nerve and help you to feel relaxed. It's the antidote to that pesky fight-or-flight mode!

It also helps with various types of abdominal pain, including menstrual cramps and intestinal pain. I love the low-tech easy-peasy nature of the hot water bottle! And it really does feel so good and relaxing.

Just remember to use a towel between the hot water bottle against your skin so that you don't accidentally burn yourself!

PINCH OF
(RAW) SALT BEFORE
BED

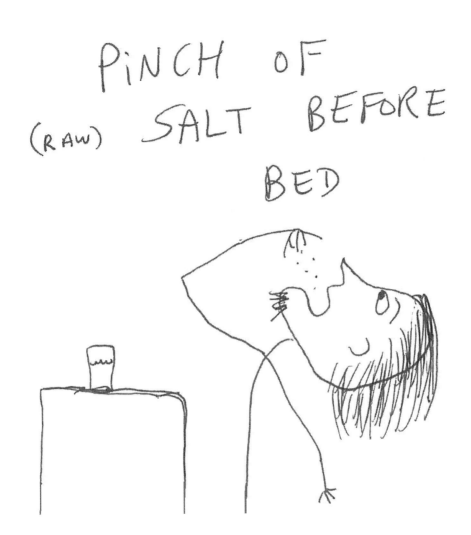

Are you getting up too many times at night to pee?

How many times SHOULD you be getting up to pee? Well, zero. Maybe zero to one? Certainly not 3, 4, 5 and beyond! Unfortunately, lots of people - especially men over 40 - are taught to "just expect to" get up more and more frequently at night to pee!

For a lot of people, the real problem is an electrolyte imbalance that can be remedied with raw sea salt. (Not the white refined stuff. No umbrella girl salt!)

I prefer the grey Celtic sea salt, but I know some people do just as well with the pink Himalayan salt. (Himalayan salt contains more potassium; Celtic sea salt has less sodium, and more calcium and magnesium.) Just take a couple of pinches of the raw salt and chase it with a little bit of water right before bed.

I have had many cases where guys were getting up 5 and 6 times a night and then after using this tip, their nighttime frequency drops down to 1-2.

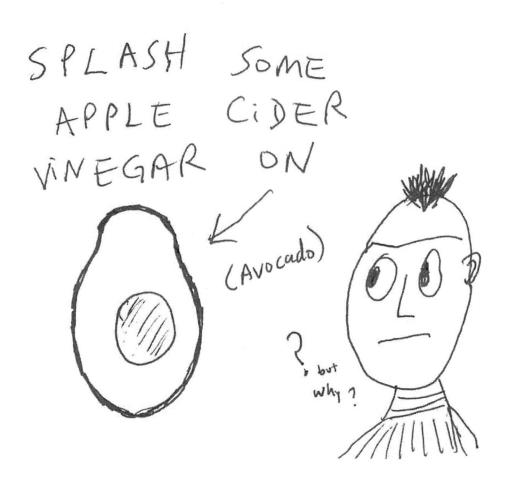

Avocados are pretty great all on their own, amiright? 🥑

You can add a little of this or a little of that to spice up a thing, but it's even better when the addition has a bonus health function!

Apple cider vinegar helps to facilitate magnesium absorption!

So, even though you're already getting a healthy dose of magnesium from that avocado, if you add a splash of apple cider vinegar, then you will absorb even more of that good stuff,

Magnesium is a very important mineral, and yes, most of us are deficient.

Are your muscles tight and painful? You probably need more magnesium.

Are you cranky? You probably need more magnesium.

And while we're on the avocado topic, if you sprinkle some turmeric on it, then that will add some anti-inflammatory action to the mix! Turmeric absorbs best when it is ingested with some kind of fat. And avocados have plenty of fat, too!

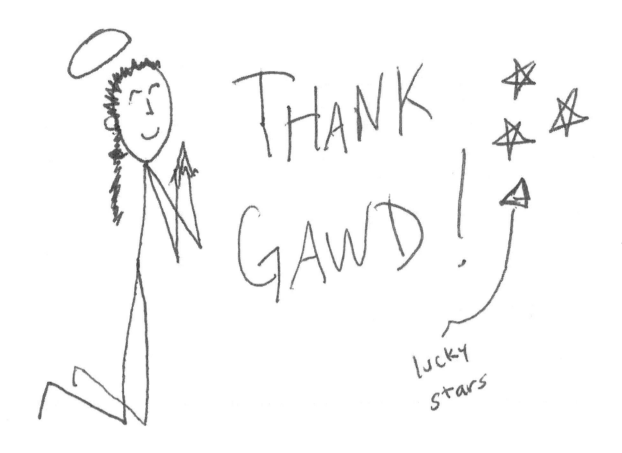

I thought that people might be getting sick of hearing "attitude of gratitude," so, I thought, what's another way of saying that without sounding too religious?

"Thank Gawd!" was the first thing that came to mind!

Thank Gawd for what?

For anything! <--- if you can do so without sarcasm.

If you've taken my 30-day Liver Detox Challenge or read my *Liver Lover* book (first published under my nom de plume Al Kimmy), then you know that **gratitude** is the liver-healthy opposite of anger.

(Chronic anger damages the heart as well as the liver!)

Take a few minutes and just think about things that you are grateful for.

Write them down in your journal.

They can be big or small, serious or ridiculous - as long as you can muster a true feeling of gratitude.

You don't even need to direct the gratitude towards an entity.

Just feel the feeling!

I am grateful every single day for hot showers and flushing toilets.

I don't care who's responsible for that - I'm just grateful to have them!

WATER FIRST!

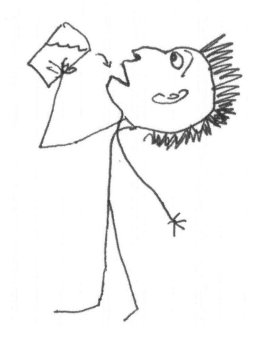

Water first what? Well water first before anything potentially sketchy!

Drink a glass of water before you have your caffeinated beverage. ☕

Drink a glass of water before you have an alcoholic beverage. 🍷

Drink a glass of water before you eat your questionable snacks or lunch. 🍔

Drink a glass of water before you go out and exert yourself. 🏋

By the time you are aware that you "need" water, it's usually way past when your body first started craving it!

A lot of our "hunger" signals are, in fact, "thirsty" signals. 💦

Sometimes, if you just drink a glass of water, you'll feel better and you won't want as much of the other thing after all.

Why do we need so much water?! 💧

Partly because so many of the things we eat, drink, breathe and do have a dehydrating effect on the body!

Yeah, yeah, I know, we already had a water nugget. But water is reeeeally important!

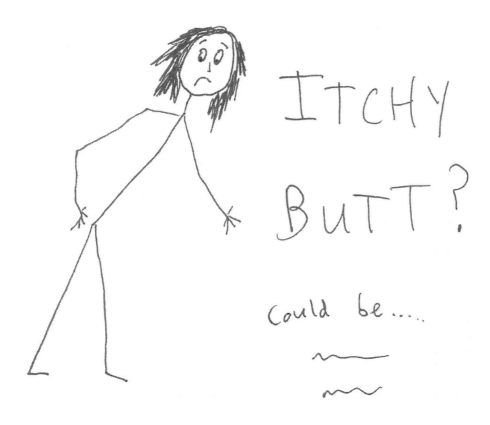

ITCHY
BUTT?

could be....

Well, since the poop nugget was so popular, I thought I would make another one for butts.
For little kids, itchy butts are usually from either not wiping well enough or parasites, such as pinworms!
For adults, the most common culprits are hemorrhoids, anal fissures, yeast infections and parasites/worms.
While some problems can come from sexual activity (you usually know which ones came from that), the others mostly come from food habits!
Hemorrhoids and anal fissures often result from a lack of fiber and water.
Yeast infections are often from too much sugar in the diet.
Some parasite/worm infections need to be treated medically, but many of them respond well to a simple remedy: oregano oil! You can buy oregano oil in capsules or in emulsified tablet form, such as in the Biotics product ADP.
Also, a great herbal remedy for hemorrhoids is Collinsonia root.

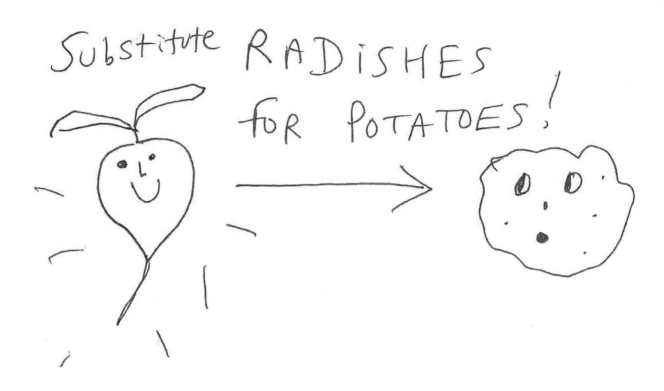

Substitute RADISHES fOR POTATOES!

Really? Radishes for potatoes?

I know, it sounds so wrong, but... it tastes so right!
You will be pleasantly surprised to see that roasted radishes taste great and can be used in many dishes that would ordinarily call for roasted potatoes!
This is **great news** when it comes to helping to balance your blood sugar or reduce overall simple-carb intake. Radishes are low carb and keto-friendly.

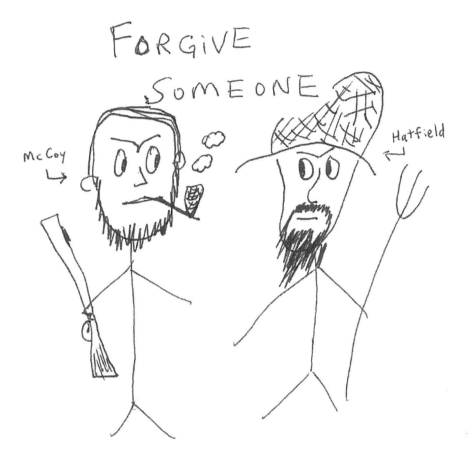

FORGIVE SOMEONE

McCoy

Hatfield

It's true: forgiveness is good for your health! It doesn't mean you have to become a doormat and let people walk all over you, abuse you, etc... It means letting go of anger, resentment and vengeance. When you hold on to anger and resentment, guess who it's hurting? It's hurting YOU! It doesn't bother the other person at all. So let it go! Just start with one person who you've been resenting for a while. You can use your own way of forgiving them or you can use this little prayer that I just made up:

"I forgive and release you [name of the jerk].
For you are just a little scamp like the rest of us,
getting through this short life the best you can.
I bless you on your journey.
And I joyfully move forward on my own.
For ain't nobody got time for that.
Also, bless your heart.
Amen."

NO COUCH SLEEPING!

We've already gone over "no stomach sleeping." Well... also, **no couch sleeping!**

Couch sleeping is a great way to mess up your neck.

Every few weeks, I always get clients who come in, unable to turn their neck in one direction, and I can tell from touching them what the cause was.

Couch neck! 🛋️💀

When you fall asleep in a bad position like this, you go limp, and your body moves even further into the bad direction.

Then, you wake up, and your body tries to suddenly self-correct and it's too late!

I guess I'm not a fan of couches in general.

They also throw people's backs out (remember the bad bucket seat nugget?).

If you have a terrible old couch, just get rid of it!

If you won't get rid of that thing, then at least move your sleepy self to bed if you want to fall asleep. Your neck will thank you!

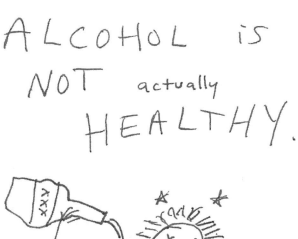

ALCOHOL is NOT actually HEALTHY.

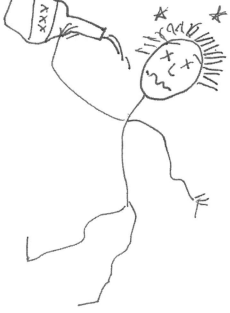

I know, I know! Call me a party pooper... but... I'm just sayin'... 🧌
but, but... but what about the fact that people used to basically ONLY drink alcohol? They lived on beer and wine! Well, yes, there was a time when the water was so filthy and dangerous (because people were pooping in it, tossing dead bodies in it, etc.) that alcohol *was* the safest thing to drink! (aaaand people also tended to live to around the ripe old age of.. what, 35?) and... but...but... what about all those studies that show that a glass of wine a day is actually healthy for you? What about that science? Wellllll... sorry to say, new science seems to be indicating that the real reason that drinking a little alcohol regularly seemed healthy is the *social* aspect of the drinking! Once they separated the solo drinkers away from the social drinkers, it became more evident that the alcohol itself was not healthy at all. Socializing is the healthy thing.
Womp womp.
So, can you never drink a drink again?

You can do what you want!

I mean, people ingest various poisons all the time recreationally, amiright?

The main reason I bring it up is so that you can do it or don't do it with a clear head. Don't do it if you think there's a health benefit to drinking alcohol!

It's not a health tonic!

The "health benefit" is from the social part.

Go invite someone out for a drink -- of tea!

p.s. There's been a big rise in the development of tasty "mocktails" lately. It's still fun to have a fancy little umbrella drink even if you're skipping the alcohol.

Here's a simple mocktail recipe to try:

3/4 ounce freshly squeezed lemon juice

3/4 ounce maple syrup

1 teaspoon soy sauce

3 ounces cola

Freshly grated cinnamon, for garnish

Combine the lemon juice, maple syrup, and soy sauce in a cocktail shaker.

Fill with ice. Seal the shaker and shake to combine (just for a few seconds). Add the cola, then double strain into a cocktail glass filled with crushed ice. Grate cinnamon over the top for a garnish.

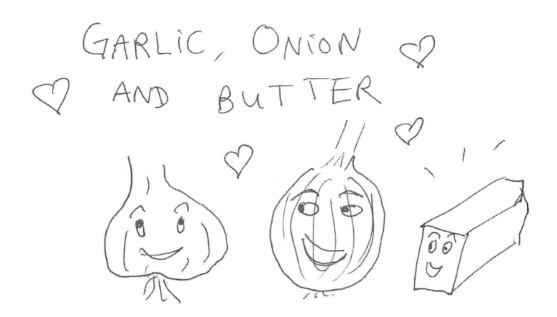

GARLIC, ONION AND BUTTER

Garlic, onion and butter: the trifecta of awesome!

Butter sometimes has a bad rap, but it's innocent and generally healthy!

Garlic and onions are **very** healthy.

And did you know that **all** onions are edible? If you come across a wild onion - and you know it's an onion because it smells like an onion - then you can eat it. There is no poisonous plant that smells like onion! Only onions smell like onions. And you can eat them. In fact, the more wild it is, the healthier it is.

The trifecta of awesome comes to your rescue if you're not sure how to cook some "healthy thing."

What do I do with this big mushroom?

Garlic, onion and butter.

What do I do with these greens?

Garlic, onion and butter.

What do I do with this meat?

Garlic, onion, and butter.

(In fact, if you just start cooking the garlic, onion and butter, people will probably say, "What are you cooking? That smells amazing!")

(apologies for the folx who are, sadly, allergic to the trifecta... 😵)

Oh, and did you know that the poet Pablo Neruda wrote an *Ode to the Onion*? It's a beautiful poem!

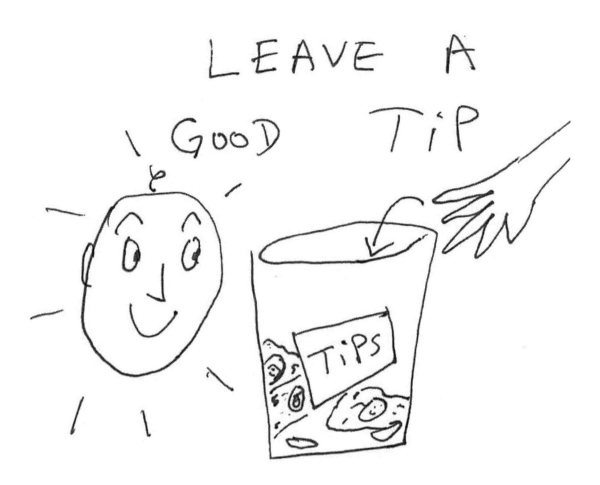

What does leaving a good tip have to do with health? 🫣

It's an opportunity to show kindness and extra appreciation to another human being.

My old minister, the late great Dr. J Kennedy Shultz, said in one of his lectures that two of the best practices that a person could do to improve their money health was to (1) donate to their church and (2) tip waiters and service people generously. He said that the reason those were both good practices was that those were 2 things that nobody could force you to do. You had to do it on your own volition, with your own free will.

Yeah, yeah, there's some politics tied up in American "tipping culture" so there's that.

But if you've ever worked in a tipping job, then you know what a difference it can make when people leave a good tip versus a bad tip versus no tip.

Exercise your generous heart where you can, and it will add to your health!

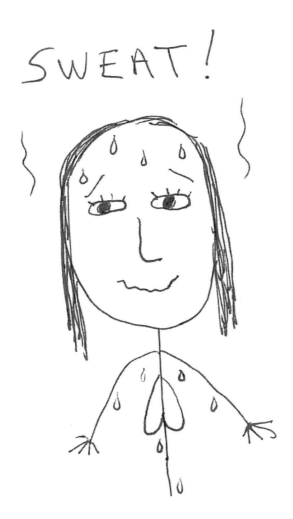

SWEAT!

Ew, who wants to sweat??? 😖
Sweating is inconvenient a lot of the time, but it's healthy to break a good sweat regularly!
Sweating helps to improve circulation, boosts endorphins, boost immunity, helps to eliminate some toxins through the skin, and has even been shown to help prevent kidney stones!
So even though we are often looking to avoid getting sweaty or telling each other "don't sweat it!"... once in a while, just go ahead and DO sweat it!

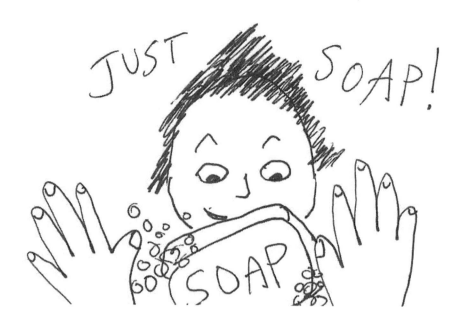

When you go to wash your hands, just use regular ol' soap and water!

It washes away just as much dirt and bad bacteria, etc. as "antibacterial" soaps, and it does not harm the natural good bacteria that live on your skin!

Why is that?

Because dirt and bad bacteria that are new to the scene are just at the surface, and they do not cling as strongly to your skin as the good bacteria that naturally live there.

However... when you use harsh antibacterial hand-sanitizers and antibacterial soaps, they will kill the good as well as the bad bacteria! This can also lead to dry cracked skin that is even more susceptible to bad bacteria getting in.

So use plain soap and water when you have the option, and save the hand sanitizer for when you don't!

MAGIC SNORING POINT!

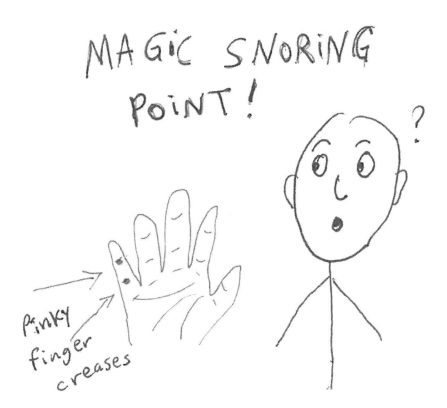

pinky finger creases

What is the Magic Snoring Point?! 😊 👀

To be honest, I don't remember. I know it's on one of the pinky finger creases. Which crease, not sure. Which hand? Not sure.

And so, whenever I have used it, I always use both pinky creases and both hands!

Because I am a beast of a snorer, too!

So how does one "use" the points? Easy.

Right before you go to bed, tape a rice grain (or something tiny and poky like that) right onto the center of the creases on the pinky finger!

And then go to sleep.

You will be surprised that it really does reduce the intensity of snoring!

For mild snorers, it can eliminate it all together.

Heavy duty snorers may still need to get checked and treated for sleep apnea, etc. but in a pinch, this is a surprisingly effective trick!

WHY does it work?

Honestly, I don't know. I was told that it's related to meridians that help people get into deeper levels of sleep. 😴

There's lots of stuff that seems to work but we don't know why!

And... whoa, I *just this moment* learned... that there is such a thing as an anti-snoring ring for the pinky finger! It doesn't use exactly the points that I show in today's nugget, but... whatdya know!

FUNGUS PROBLEMS = SUGAR PROBLEMS

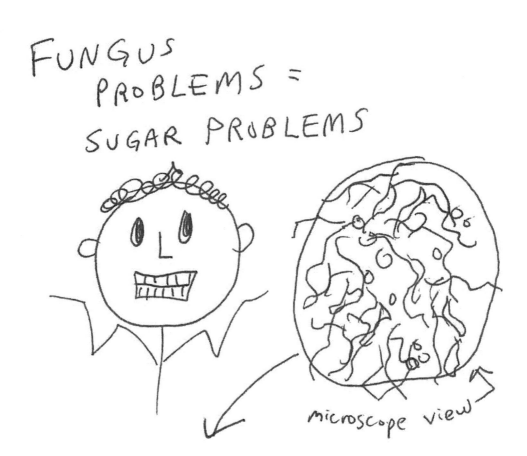

microscope view

Don't shoot the messenger!

I'm just sayin'... that if you have a fungus problem, then you have a sugar* problem.

(* means it could also be a bread problem, but it still basically comes down to sugar.)

Excessive sugar consumption causes the body chemistry to shift to an environment that is ripe for fungal overgrowth! What kind of fungus? Could be anything from athlete's foot to toenail fungus, ringworm, jock itch, etc.

Even if you think you "don't eat much sugar," it doesn't matter. I have seen more than one terrible case of fungus on the hands of people whose "only" sugar consumption was their daily Starbucks habit. Once they quit those syrupy beverages and crappy pastries, their fungus cleared up! I also had a case where a patient had terrible persistent toenail fungus for 20 years. They didn't think they ate much sugar, but they did feel addicted to their heavy duty morning breakfast bread item. Once they eliminated that for about a month, the toenails started to heal! It was pretty amazing.

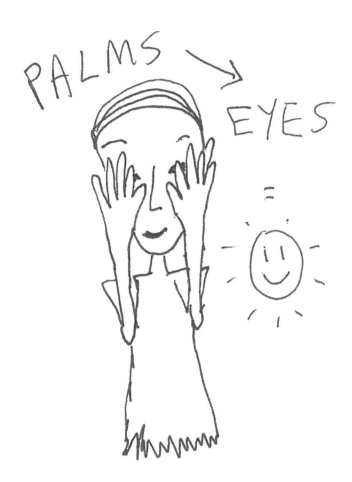

Everyone has tired eyes these days, because everyone is looking at screens all the time! (And as much as I appreciate that you are looking at the Daily Nugget, it does mean that you are looking at a screen right now!)

So here's an easy thing to help your eyeballs feel better, at least for a little while!

Sit back and rub your palms together quickly, building up some heat. Imagine that you are revving up your magical chi machine right there between your hands! Visualize a big fat healing ball of light as you rub your hands together faster and faster.

Then, whenever you are ready, gently hold your palms against your (closed) eyes and bask in the warmth and the healing self-lovey energy!

TRY BOX BREATHING!

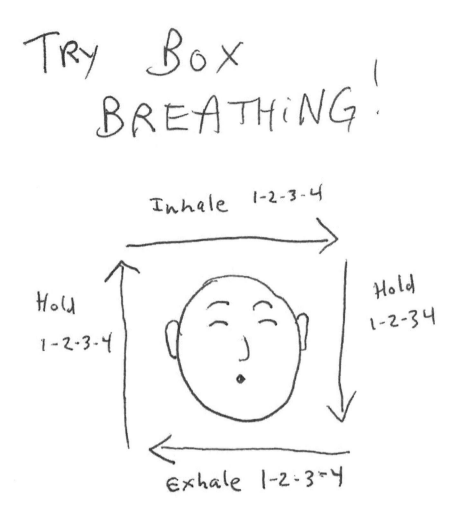

Inhale 1-2-3-4

Hold 1-2-3-4

Hold 1-2-34

Exhale 1-2-3-4

Well, we're not really breathing **out** of a box... but we're breathing kind of like a box... it's called Box Breathing! Box Breathing is helpful for stress reduction and for meditating. The picture shows why it's called "box breathing."

You just breathe in for a slow count of 4, then hold your breath for the same pace of 4, then exhale for the same slow 4 count, and hold again for a count of 4.

And repeat.

You can do this for as long or as short as you like!

It's also a good exercise for people with lung diseases such as COPD.

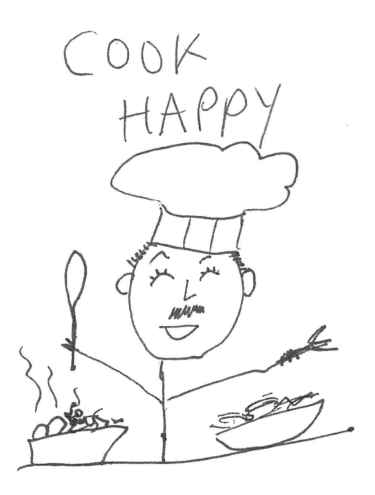

If you're gonna cook, cook happy.

One of my old neighbors was a chef at a fancy restaurant, and he said that he always tried to maintain a positive attitude while cooking! Early in his career, he noticed that whenever he was happy while he was cooking, the plates would come back empty, and people would be saying. "My compliments to the chef!" all night long! But if he was angry or negative while cooking - even though the food was technically fine - plates would often come back with the food just pushed around or partly eaten, and there would be more complaints than praise! That was when he realized the power of how food can absorb the energy of the cook!

So whatever you're cooking, you can make it "healthier" simply by cooking it with a light heart and a positive attitude!

(If you just can't muster it, then maybe that's the time to order in, from someone who hopefully feels less bad than you!)

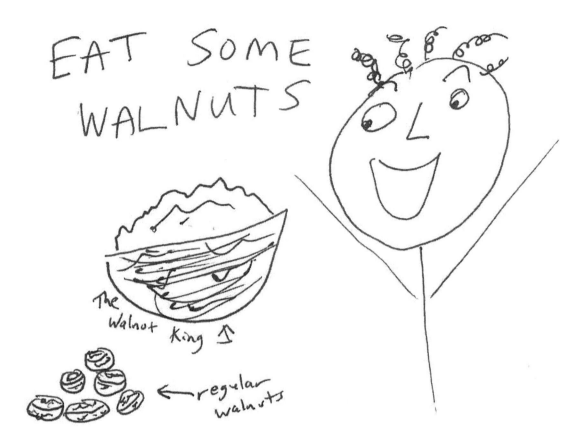

EAT SOME WALNUTS

The Walnut King ⬆

← regular walnuts

This nugget is not actually about Paulie Walnuts. Sorry - I just used that to lure you in.
(I guess I thought about him today because of a radio piece I heard about how all the classic TV and movie mobsters are dying lately!)
But walnuts really **are** healthy! They are one of the healthiest nut choices. They have been shown to have positive effects on cardiovascular health (specifically on blood lipids), blood sugar, gut health and more!
While many nuts are healthy, walnuts have a special place. If you don't like to eat them on their own, throw in a few walnuts into your favorite nut or snack mix!

OPEN A WINDOW!

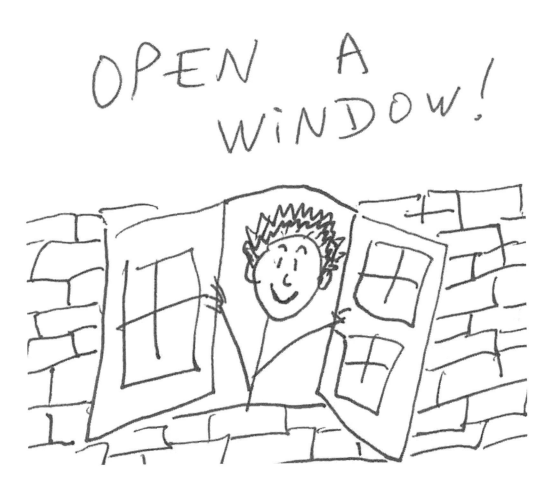

Now, this is assuming it's not "fire season" and the air quality is awful or you've got mosquitos and no screen, or some other sad factor!

But... otherwise... if the air is relatively good out there, then open a window!

Some cultures keep a window open in the bedroom all year 'round, and studies show that fresh air can help improve the quality of sleep!

If the outside is too noisy at night (due to traffic, screaming people, etc.) or if you're having bad allergies to seasonal pollen, then consider a small fan in your bedroom to keep the air moving.

No Aluminum Deodorants!

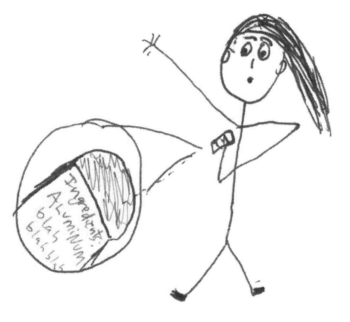

Choose deodorant **without** aluminum!!!

I know, I know, you don't want to stink, and you think that only the ones with aluminum really work! Not true.

After many years of hunting, I finally found one that really does work. The one that I have been using for years is the Soapwalla organic deodorant cream. Yes, it's expensive, but it really really works and has no aluminum! (But warning: their "sensitive skin" formula does *not* work as well!)

What's so bad about aluminum anyway? Well, it shouldn't be inside your body, and inside is where it's going to get if you put it all over your armpits.

That's why those aluminum deodorants all have a warning on the label that says it should not be used by anyone with kidney disease!

I also know that it gets inside your body because once upon a time, back in my 20s, I got a startling mineral analysis test that showed that my body had high levels of aluminum! I immediately cut out the offending deodorant and have never tested in the high zone since. Aluminum is bad news for bones, brain and blood, so use it for industrial things (like bike frames) but avoid it for things that soak into your body!

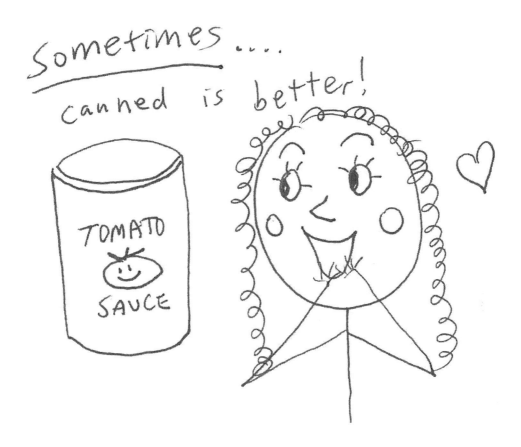

Did you think this nugget was going to be about home canning of foods?
Well, I'm sure that would be healthy, but...
quite a bit more complicated than I aim for with the Daily Nugget!
No, I'm talking about **canned tomatoes**.
The strange but truly truth of the matter is... that processed tomatoes, whether canned or cooked into a paste or sauce, are the richest known source of lycopene!
You can read more about how and why in Jo Robinson's excellent book, *Living on the Wild Side.*
So, while fresh food is usually best, canned tomatoes are a solid choice when it comes to nutritional value. (Obviously look for the ones without added sugar, etc.!)

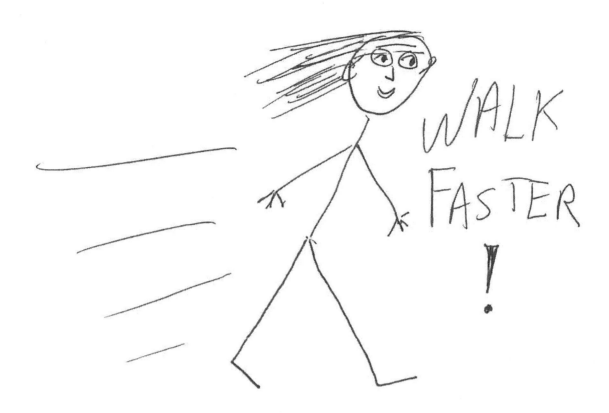

I know, I know, the usual healthy thing to say is, "Slow down!"

Well... today... walk faster!

According to a new study from the UK:

People between the ages of 40 and 79 who took 9,826 steps per day were 50% less likely to develop dementia within seven years. Furthermore, people who walked with "purpose" – at a pace over 40 steps a minute – were able to cut their risk of dementia by 57% with just 6,315 steps a day

But the largest reduction in dementia risk – 62% – was achieved by people who walked at a very brisk pace of 112 steps per minute for 30 minutes a day, the study found.

So, walking helps to avoid dementia. Walking "with purpose" helps even more. Walking fast helps the most, and can even cut down on the total number of steps needed for the benefit!

How fast is 112 steps a minute, anyway?!

You can tell if you get a pedometer (or use your smartwatch or smartphone to track) or set a timer for 15 seconds, count your steps, and multiply that by 4!

You should aim for about 28 steps per 15 seconds.

Simple things to fight the odds of developing dementia? Yes, please!

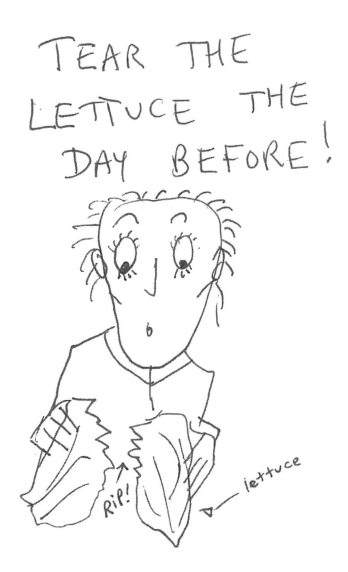

Here is another tip straight out of Jo Robinson's *Eating on the Wild Side.*
If you rip up your romaine or iceberg lettuce the day before you eat it, you will **quadruple** the antioxidant content! This is because the leaves are still alive at this point, and it starts the repairing process after being torn, which releases lots of antioxidants! Who knew?

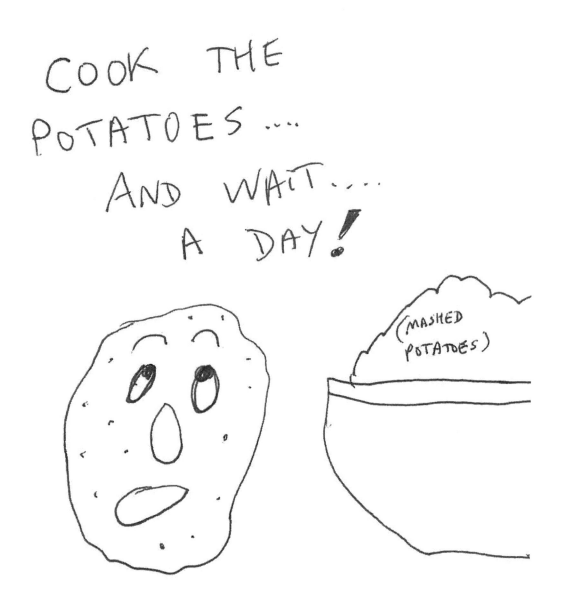

I couldn't resist... one more tip from Jo Robinson's *Eating on the Wild Side!*
I think we all know that white potatoes are so starchy that they have a glycemic index almost as high as straight up glucose. But! If you cook them and then chill them for about 24 hours before eating them, they magically become a low- to moderate-glycemic index food! Well, it's not magic. But it sounds like magic.
Anyway, the low- to moderate-glycemic index of the day-old potatoes holds true even if you re-heat them! So don't worry, you don't have to eat cold potatoes to get this benefit!

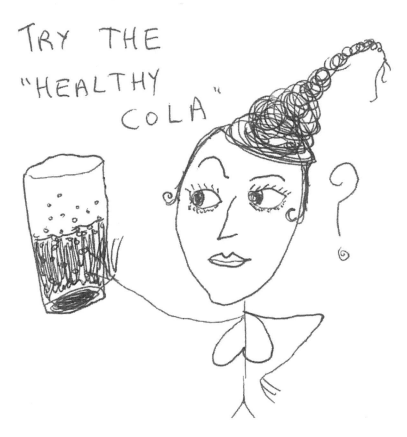

TRY THE "HEALTHY" COLA

I know, I know, "healthy cola??" No such thing! But... the less bad thing? You kids in the audience have probably already heard of this, but it's new to the old fogies like me! Here's what you do. You take one of those berry-flavored (but "no sugar added") sparkling waters, and you mix it with a splash of... balsamic vinegar! Mix and enjoy. The first time I heard this, I thought ☻. I'm not that crazy about balsamic vinegar (even though I know it's healthy)! But you know what? This beverage tastes good! It looks and feels like cola, so I can't tell whether or not it really tastes like it or if my brain just wants it to taste like it...

Doesn't matter! Because it might be "good for you" thanks to the healthy properties of balsamic vinegar! Good for your heart, blood lipids and blood sugar. Sometimes when you are craving something "bad" (like a Coke), it's not REALLY the syrup water it's craving. It's the whole experience. So, sometimes, substituting a lookalike can satisfy the urge and even help you come out ahead! The acidity of this beverage not good for your teeth, so beware of that and drink some water afterwards (as you would when drinking any other soda or acidic beverage). I wouldn't add this beverage to the category of "dietary supplement," but I would certainly consider it a good alternative to the corn syrupy stuff!

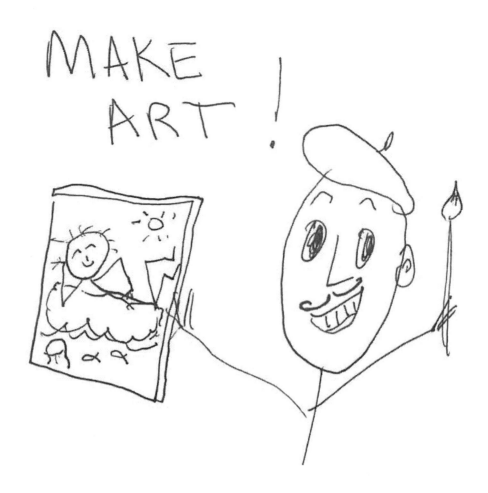

Making art (which includes music, creative writing, collage, knitting, LEGO sculptures, Shrinky Dinks...) can help you to feel (and be) more healthy!

It's good for your brain, and it's good for your soul!

Everyone has something to express, and you don't need to be a "good artist" to express it.

(*Trust me.* I know from whenceforth I speak! 😃)

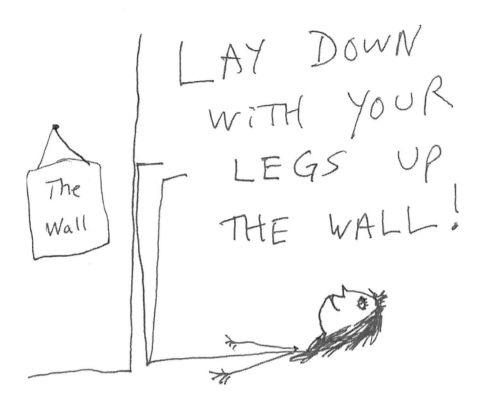

Not saying that I'm lazy... but... I do love me some lazy yoga... 😄

Putting your legs up the wall for a few minutes a day is a great way to help relieve swollen ankles, varicose veins, and help bring more blood flow to your core. This can help with digestion and certain types of headaches! It's a relaxing pose that eases stress, calms nerves and can even help you sleep!

Putting blankets under your head and hips can help maximize the benefits of this pose. This pose even has a proper name: Viparita Karani.

READ A GOOD BOOK!

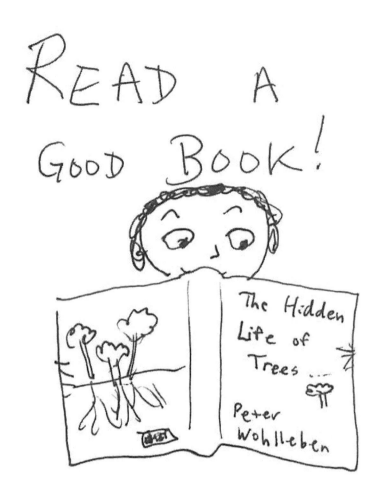

Reading is good for your brain, and therefore it's good for your health!

Sometimes we (OK... me?) get caught up with lots of "serious" reading (for work, projects, etc.) but not enough relaxing and fun reading!

Pick something that you'd love to just read and enjoy, and read it!

(Audio books count, too!)

(And yes, I heartily endorse the book in the drawing - *The Hidden Life of Trees,* by Peter Wohlleben!)

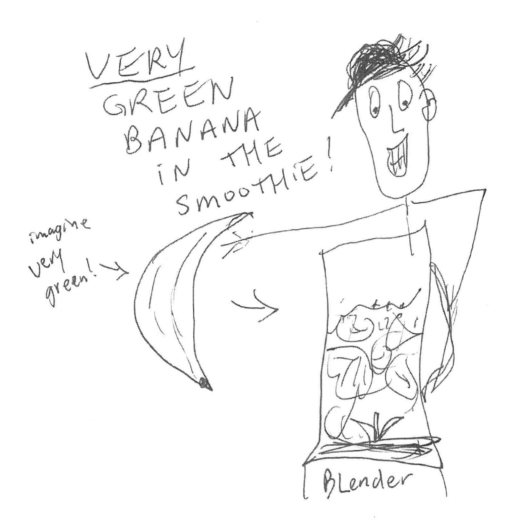

This is essentially the same as the little white potato into the smoothie.

If you put a very green banana - like, so green it's hard to peel and it is kind of hard like a potato! - into a smoothie, then it will not be sweet, but it will provide excellent prebiotics to help support your gut biome! Also, since it's mostly starch and pectin (which are the prebiotic components), it won't mess with your blood sugar. Mix it into your favorite smoothie!

PRETTY UP YOUR MEAL SPACE

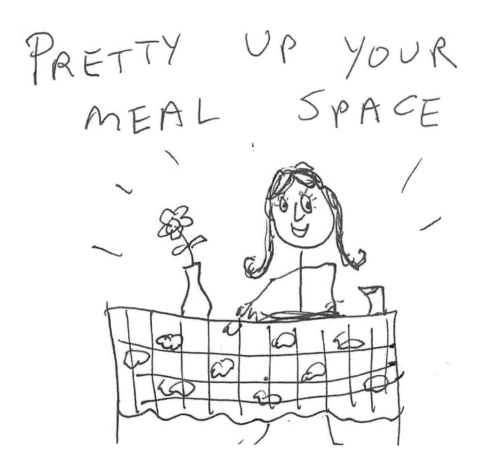

This does not have to be complicated.

It can be as simple as putting a flower - even a fake one! - in a little vase or a candle in the middle of the table.

Just something to give your mind the feeling of "nice" or even "fancy" or "special."

This helps bring positive neurochemistry to the act of eating.

Contrast this with eating in a depressing dingy pile of clutter with some faint sticky spots from quickie meals past. 😖

(This is one of the ideas I got from Marc David's audiobook, *Mind/Body Nutrition*.)

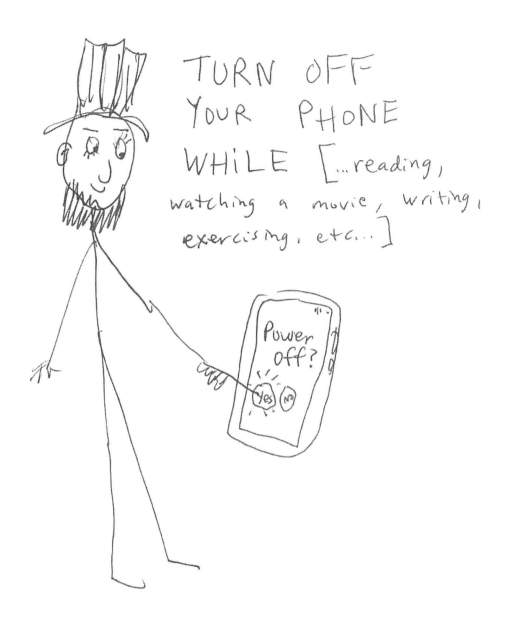

TURN OFF YOUR PHONE WHILE [...reading, watching a movie, writing, exercising, etc...]

Power off?

Yes   No

For some people, "airplane mode" is good enough, but... why not just like... TURN THE PHONE OFF? Turn it off while you are reading, watching a movie, writing, etc. "But what if someone needs me?" Unless you are a firefighter, ER doctor, etc., it's rare that someone would *really need you* during your precious few minutes or 1-2 hours of recharge time! Just think of it like the old days, when phones were tethered to the wall, and if you weren't within earshot of it then people just couldn't get a hold of you! The world kept turning and things were (generally) fine. It's fine. Relax and enjoy the peace and quiet!

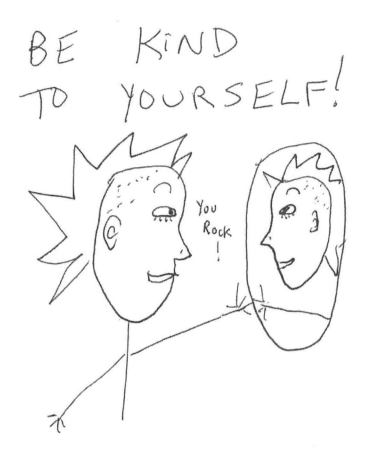

One of the biggest sources of bad health is self-sabotage!

And one of the biggest sources of self-sabotage is stinkin' thinkin' - or - self-defeating thoughts.

The human condition is rough.

Whatever else you may be, you are for sure **a human being**.

This means that you come with quirks and flaws and also amazingness... just like everyone else!

Don't beat yourself up for the quirks and flaws!

Just breathe deep, accept them for the moment, and have compassion for yourself.

All good stories, movies, books, etc. need to have points of friction, challenges, etc. to be a good story. Otherwise, it's boring as hell!

Think of your issues as part of what's going to make your story a good one!

The ending is still unwritten.

Have compassion for yourself! Warts and all.

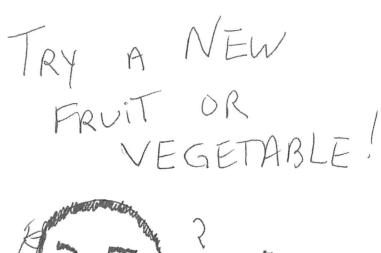

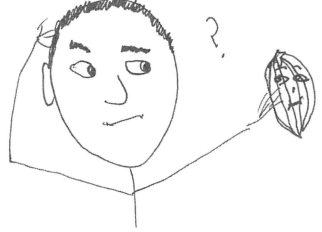

They say variety is the spice of life.

Well, variety is also part of a healthy diet!

It's easy to get into the rut of always eating the same things.

This week, try something totally new!

Just pick something in the produce aisle that you have never tried before.

Don't know what to do with it? Just look it up right there on your phone!

You will easily find tips and recipes.

Picked one that only seems to have complicated preparation instructions?

Pick something else!

RELAXING SIGH

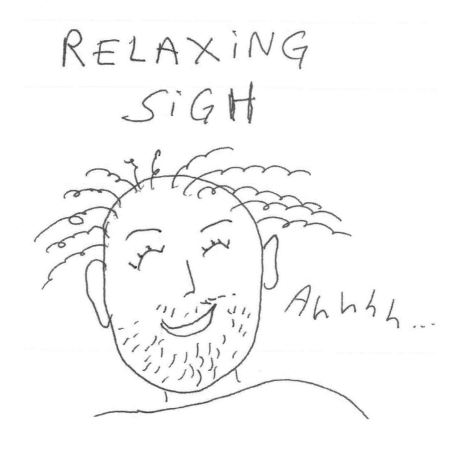

Ahhhh...

There is a huge and growing body of research that shows that mindfulness is a powerful tool for stress reduction and improved quality of life!

Mindfulness is all about focusing on the present, without judgement, and simply being with the sensations in your body.

Exercises don't get much simpler than The Relaxing Sigh!

Step 1: Breathe in through your nose.

Step 2: Breathe out through your mouth, making a gentle sighing sound.

Step 3: Repeat as desired.

A good way to see if/how this helps you is to first check in with your body and ask yourself, "How am I feeling right now?"

How is your body feeling? Your mood? Your mind?

Then, do a few relaxing sighs, and check in again.

Does your body feel different? Your mood? Your mind?

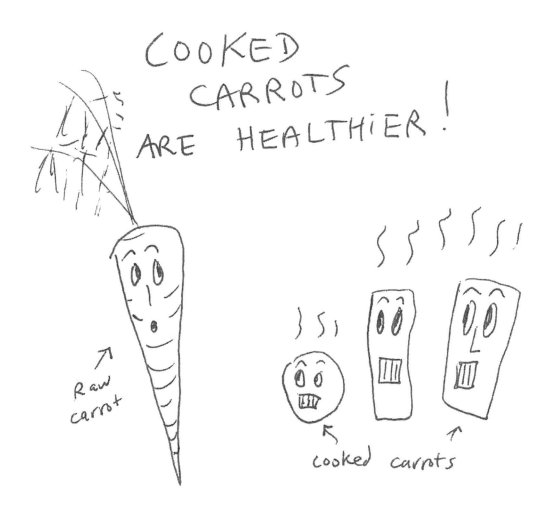

While there's nothing wrong with eating raw carrots, 🥕 the fact is...

Cooked carrots are healthier!

It's true! You can only use about 3% of the beta carotene from a raw carrot, but you can get closer to 40% with cooked carrots!

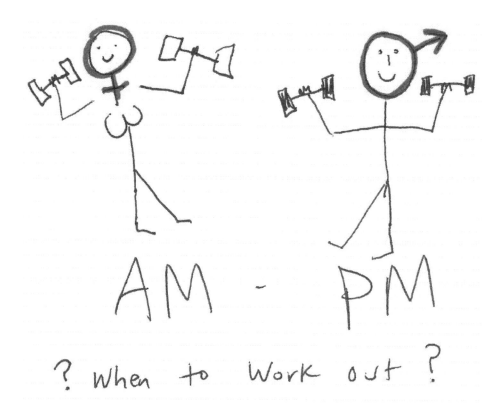

AM - PM

? when to Work out ?

Unpopular opinion (but supported by science): the best time to exercise depends on whether you are running on estrogen or testosterone! It turns out that exercising at specific times of day are more beneficial for specific outcomes. For women, morning workouts deliver more results when it comes to getting rid of belly fat and improving blood pressure! But for men, evening or late-day workouts are better for fat burning and blood pressure control. Evening exercising also increased benefits for strength straining, but more so for women. I know that I'm just a data point of 1, but I did notice that after transitioning hormonally to male, evening workouts did lead to better blood pressure control and fat reduction. 🤯

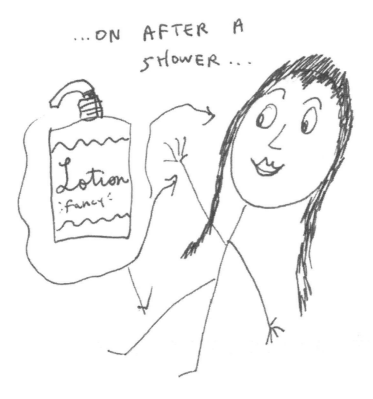

Lotion: it's not just for old people and serial killers! <--- dunno if I am marking *myself* as an old person with the serial killer reference???

This topic was kind of covered in the sunblock nugget, but someone asked that I mention it separately. Using lotion on your skin regularly is a great and simple way to help retain hydration and reduce inflammation! The best time to put on lotion is right after your shower, which helps to lock in some of that extra moisture!

And don't forget to keep drinking your water! Stay hydrated inside and out!

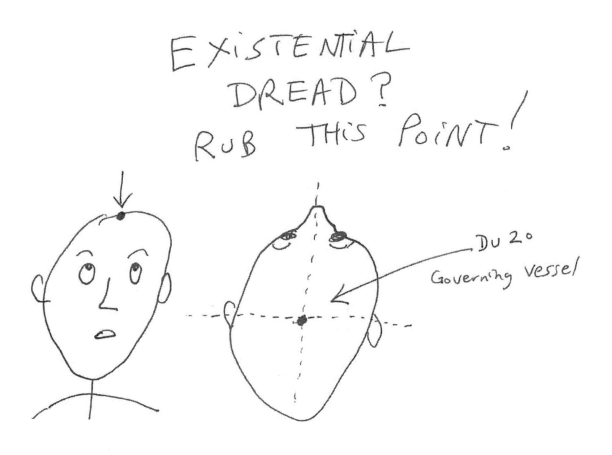

EXISTENTIAL DREAD? RUB THIS POINT!

DU 20°
Governing vessel

Here is an acupressure point that is used for reducing anxiety. One of the specific types of anxiety it is said to help alleviate is "existential anxiety." Well, there's plenty of that to go around, so get rubbin'!

How do you know if you're on the right point? You can usually feel a slight indentation when you are on this point. And it might be tender when you press it if it's in need of some attention. You can massage it for a few seconds or a couple of minutes. Some of you may recognize this point from the NIS treatment for electromagnetic stress! This also helps for jaw clenching.

Keep breathin'!

CHECK YOUR PILLOW!

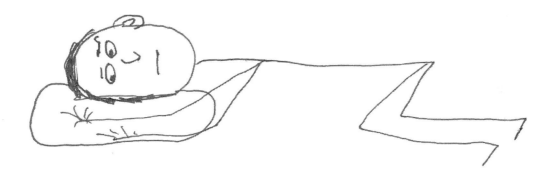

If your head or neck bothers you the most first thing in the morning, it may be your crappy pillow! Unfortunately, there is no universally perfect pillow. Womp womp. It has to be the best pillow for your head/body and your mattress situation. A soft mattress may warrant a flatter pillow, since your shoulders will sink more deeply. A firm mattress may require a taller pillow since your shoulders don't sink as much! That's for side-sleepers. Back sleepers may do best with a cervical pillow (one with a little dip) that gives a gentle tractioning to the neck. If you do sleep on your side, ask a friend to help you evaluate your pillow height. Have your friend stand behind you while you are laying on your side with your pillow. From the back, it should look like your neck is basically in line with your spine. If the pillow is too flat, your neck will appear to be tilting downward towards the bed. If it's too big, your neck will appear to be tilting up.

Notice that I don't recommend special pillows for stomach sleepers. There's no such thing! Don't sleep on your stomach! It's not good for your neck **or** your back!

p.s. make sure your pillow and pillowcase are clean, too! Sometimes a dirty pillow can trigger allergies!

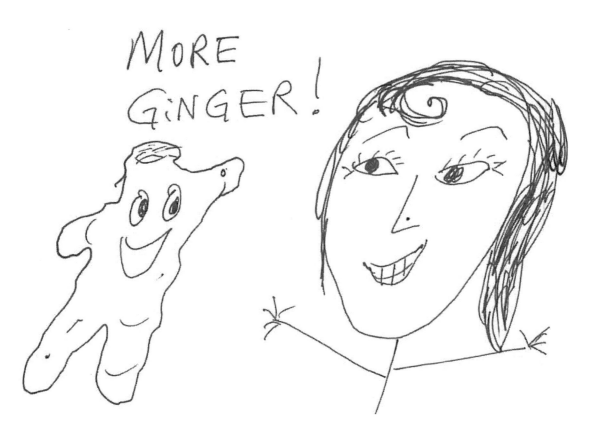

MORE GINGER!

More ginger in what? More ginger everywhere! Why not? It's jam packed with antioxidants and is one of the healthiest spices on earth! It can help with blood sugar, blood pressure, cholesterol levels and immune function and more! Here is a simple fruit salad recipe with some ginger mint glaze.

Ingredients: 2 pears, cubed
2 nectarines, cubed
2 cups strawberries, hulled and sliced
½ cup blackberries
¼ cup raspberries

Ginger mint glaze
¼ cup organic maple syrup
4 fresh mint leaves, chopped [1 tablespoon chopped]
2 tablespoon lemon juice
1 tablespoon grated fresh ginger root
1 tiny pinch of cayenne pepper

Instructions
Place all salad ingredients in a large bowl.
Combine glaze ingredients in a small bowl, and drizzle over the salad.
Enjoy!

FISH FRIDAY!

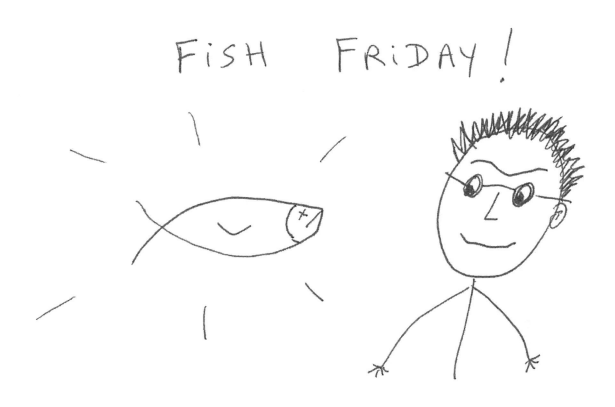

I grew up in a very Catholic family... which followed all the old traditions, including fish Fridays! I did not like fish. 😣 So I did not like Friday dinners!

But now I realize that it was because we didn't eat good fish - not like we were going out for sushi! (I didn't have sushi until I was 27 years old!)

The idea is not so much that you should eat fish on Fridays - although most Americans COULD stand to eat more fish and less red meat in their diets! The idea is to set aside a day (or days) when you don't indulge in all the heavy or rich foods that you crave.

After my Catholic years, I spent a few years practicing Russian Orthodoxy, and they had even more restrictive food days. I think that we avoided meat on Wednesdays AND Fridays and then certain entire weeks of the year that preceded big feasts like Christmas and Easter! Although the rationale for restricting the diet on certain days was spiritual, I noticed that it improved my physical health as well! My family was physically leaner and more energetic in those Orthodox years when we spent almost half the year as vegetarians!

Consider choosing one or two days a week when you just don't eat meat or heavy rich foods. It's a small thing that can make a big difference in the long run!

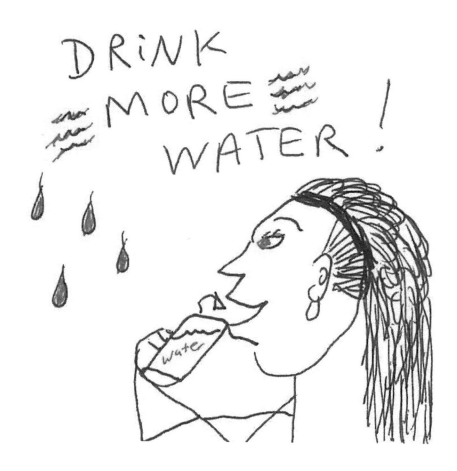

I know, we already had a nugget about drinking water!

But you know what? Drinking water is so important that if I made 50 water nuggets (out of the 366 I'm aiming for), it would still be legit! You can survive for about 3 weeks without food. But you will only last about 3 days without water. (Technically, yes, some very fit and young people can last longer, but 3 days is the generally accepted number.)

Feeling sick? Drink more water.

Feeling tired? Drink more water.

Feeling anxious? Drink more water.

Have a headache? Drink more water.

Feeling angry? Yes, drink more water!

Staying hydrated won't solve the problems of the world (or even all the problems of you), but it will help **YOUR BODY** to weather the storms and fight the good fight!

A well-hydrated body is more **resilient**, flexible and let's face it, also more cute. 😵 🤖

A rough guideline for water intake is: about 3 quarts or liters a day for women, and about 4 quarts or liters a day for men.

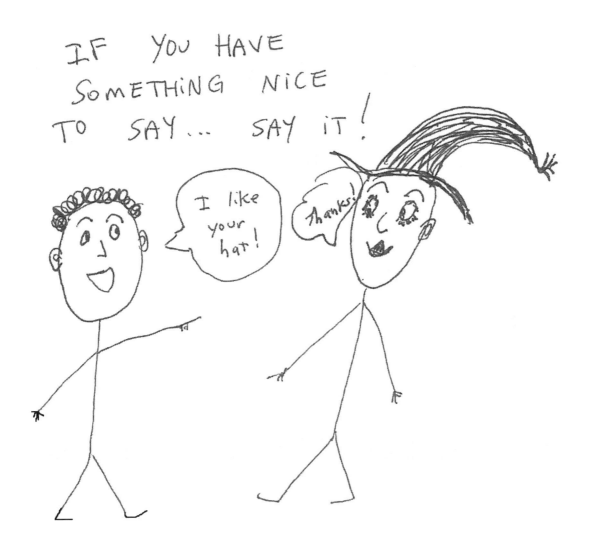

Today's nugget is pretty simple. If you have something nice to say, then say it! Sometimes, you may feel shy or weird to just say a random nice thing - especially if it's to a stranger - but you would be surprised at how much it can brighten a person's day. We have all sorts of biases towards negativity, and one of them is to have a negative bias towards the positive impact that we can have on others. There are even studies that demonstrate that people who perform random acts of kindness underestimate the positive impact of those acts! We all know how stress and stress hormones hurt our health. Well, the opposite is true, too. The chemistry that lifts our mood also lifts our health! People expect crappy things from other people. Angry drivers, rude weirdos, indifferent strangers...

But they don't expect something nice.

EXERCISE YOUR EYEBALLS

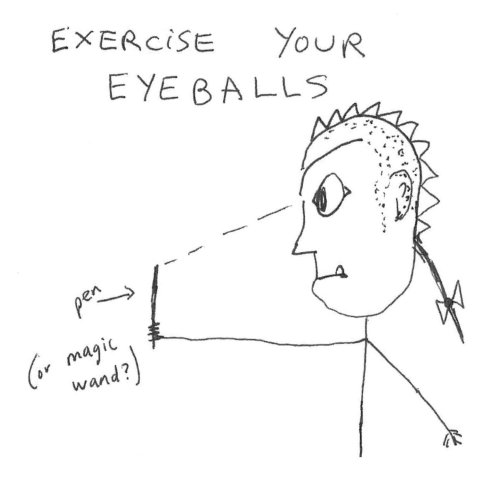

pen →

(or magic wand?)

When I am checking people's cranial nerves in the office, guess what comes up weak on almost everyone?? Cranial nerve 2, aka the optic nerve.

In other words, our eyes are stressed! 👀

The cranial nerves are the 12 nerves that come directly out of the brain and do not travel through the spinal cord at all.

The optic nerve is the sensory nerve controlling vision.

It also controls the eyes' ability to focus on objects near and far.

Since we now spend so much of our time focusing our eyes at a fixed distance (hello screen life!) this nerve loses some of its natural tone.

To exercise it, take a pen (or something like it) and hold it out at arm's length. Focus on the tip of the pen. Then, slowly bring the pen close to your face, keeping focus on the point. Do this about 5 times, taking about 5 seconds to move the pen from the far to near distance.

And that is the easy way to exercise your cranial nerve 2!

It's a good exercise to do periodically when you catch yourself staring at a screen for too long!

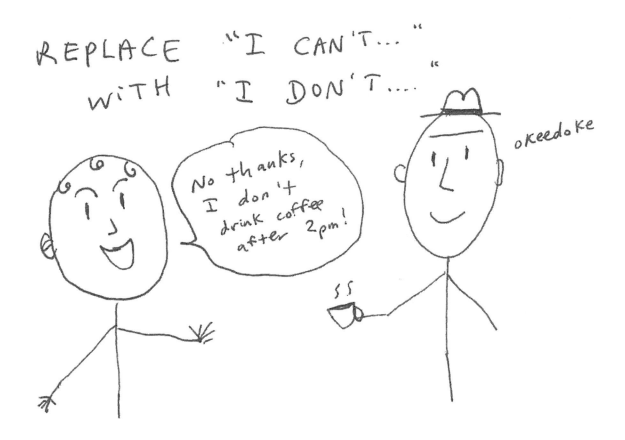

Sometimes, when we are trying to change a habit, we use words that set us up for failure. Like, when you're trying to avoid wheat and sugar, and someone offers you cake! And you say, "Oh... thanks, but... I can't have that cake." When you say you "can't," it implies a sort of longing... like... you wish you could, but... 😩

But what if you don't smoke, and someone offers you a cigarette? You don't say you "can't." You just say, "No thanks, I don't smoke."

And that's that! No emotion, no guilt, no biggie.

So if you shift your language, it can help ease the new habit.

"No thanks, I don't eat cake." or "No thanks, I don't drink caffeine after 2."

...or whatever it may be.

Well well well, when I looked for something to link in the e-mail for this nugget, I found a 2013 article from Forbes... and they talk about cake, too! I guess we all think about cake even when we don't want to think about cake. 😵 🍰 😵

STAND WITH "SOFT" KNEES
(don't lock your knees)

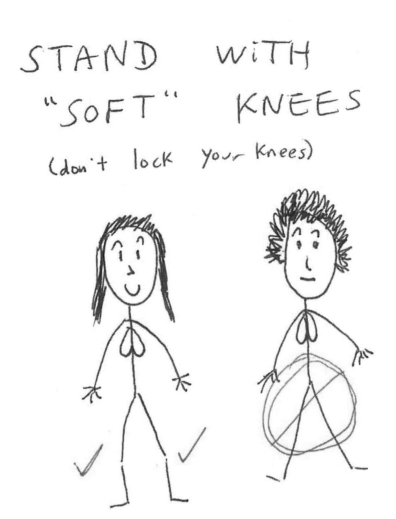

Here is a simple one.

When you are standing, don't lock your knees!

Keeping your knees a little "soft" (or very slightly bent) helps to keep your back and pelvis in a better position, and is much better for your posture!

Go ahead and pay attention to the difference that you feel in your posture when you stand up straight with knees locked versus with knees softened and slightly bent!

Your back will thank you for following this tip.

GENTLE PELVIC TILTS!

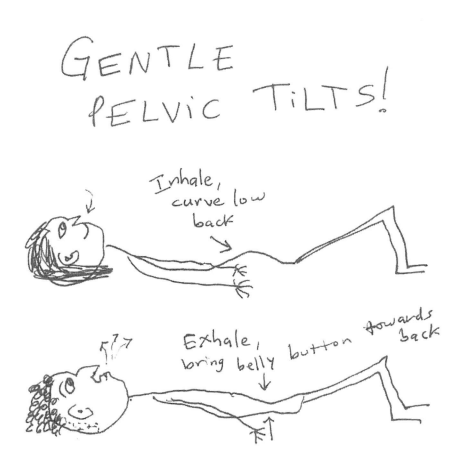

Inhale, curve low back

Exhale, bring belly button towards back

Have I mentioned lately how much I like exercises that you can do while lying down?? This one is really good for those postural muscles in your core - especially if you have the bad habit of locking your knees! It's pretty simple. You inhale and arch the lowest part of your back. Then you exhale and squeeze your belly button towards your flattening spine. (In the e-mails I have a link to a video of Diane Waye demonstrating this move, so, look her up or grab the searchable .pdf version of this book for all the links!)

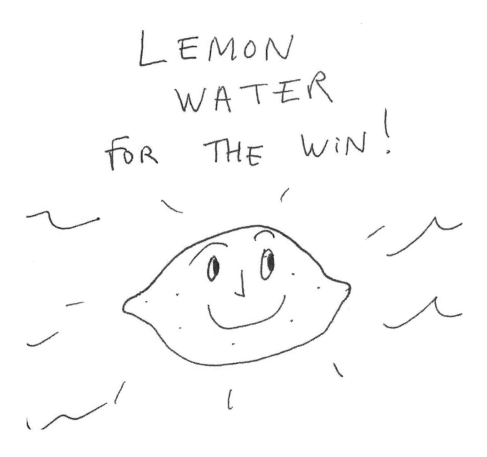

LEMON WATER FOR THE WIN!

Can't believe it took me almost 100 nuggets to bring up the easy peasy lemon squeezy! 🍋
Lemons are packed with all kinds of goodness, and lemon water is an easy way to get this into your body.

Plus, it's a great way to get more **water** into your body!

Lemons add electrolytes and vitamins into the water, which help to keep you hydrated.

Lemons are rich in antioxidants, vitamin C and potassium. And while they are acidic, they have a net alkalizing effect on the body, which is a plus, since most of us tend to run too acidic.

They are also anti-inflammatory, and chronic inflammation is enemy #1!

You can juice or blend the lemons and add them to a pitcher of water, or just slice them up and toss them in.

PROTEIN FOR BREAKFAST!

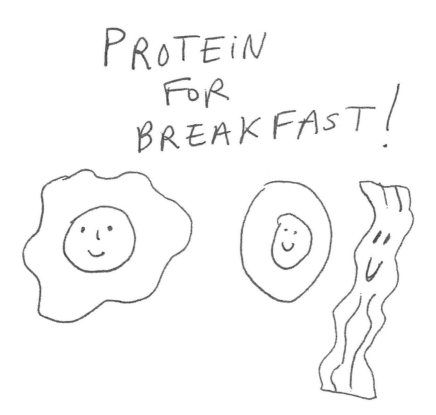

Marketing tells us that breakfast is carb time - cereal, bread, oatmeal, pastries, fruit juice, etc... BUT... protein for breakfast is best for your health! How much protein are we talking about here? Aim to get at least 40% of your breakfast calories from protein! If you're into gram counting, aim for about 20-30 grams of protein for breakfast. Studies show that eating more protein for breakfast leads to less overeating at dinnertime and also encourages weight loss. If you're not that hungry in the morning, eat something small but protein-dense, such as an egg or two. Protein includes things like eggs, meat, cheese, fish, nuts, legumes, protein powder shakes, etc.

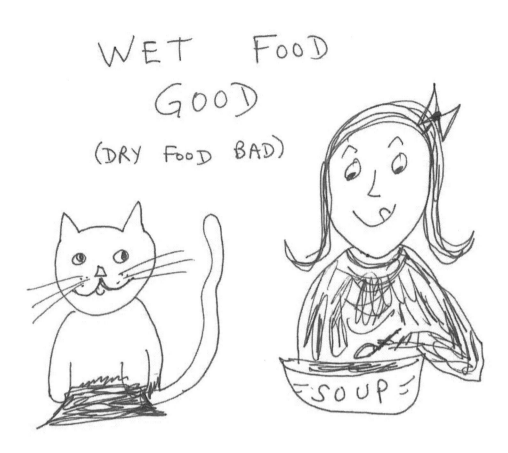

WET FOOD
GOOD
(DRY FOOD BAD)

It's true for cats and it's true for you, too!

Wet food is healthier because it helps with hydration, which is a big key to basic health! Wetness is another easy indicator that can help you make choices when it's just too hard to weigh out the other factors. Like, bread and oatmeal are both grains, but which is worse? Well, [wheat] bread is worse for a number of reasons, but the dryness makes it worse when it comes to simple hydration.

Starting a meal with wet foods such as soup can also help to prevent overeating (partly because we often mistake thirst for hunger).

Really dry food such as chips and various processed snack foods can deplete the body of water and contribute to constipation, among other unpleasant things.

Avoid them in general, but if you eat them, make sure to drinks LOTS of EXTRA water!

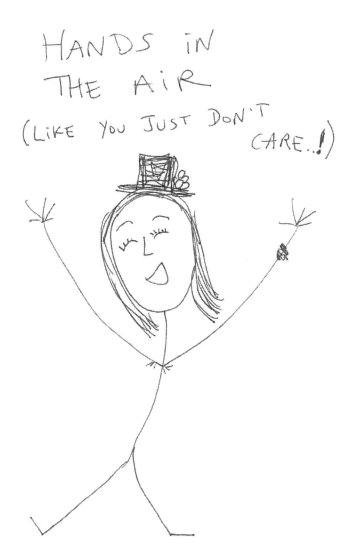

HANDS IN
THE AIR
(LiKE YOU JUST DON'T
CARE..!)

This nugget is basically just to say, don't forget to move your arms around, far and wide! Even people who kind of hate to exercise know that they should at LEAST walk around, get their 10,000 steps a day. That's good! Walking = good. But... it's not everything, and those arms need muscular movement, too, to move the lymph and all that! Tip-tapping on your phone or your keyboard doesn't cut it. You have to make big movements to get the big benefits! But you DON'T necessarily have to do big movements in the gym, with weights, etc. You can just wave your arms around like a gentle maniac! The idea is to get a variety of movements and move through your full natural range of motion - without straining yourself. And if you don't remember who was the first one to say wave your arms in the air like you just don't care, I think it was Cameo in Word Up. That is a fun video if you love the 80s... I did not remember that there was a quick Duran Duran meets Princess Di shot in there!

EXERCISE YOUR BALANCE!

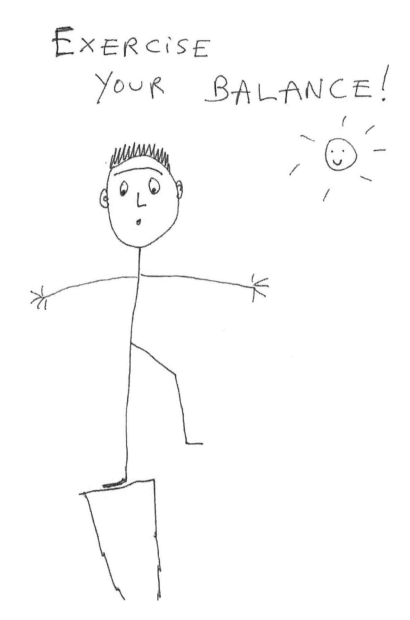

We usually think of strength and endurance when we think of "exercise," but don't forget balance!

Just as strength and endurance decline with age, so does balance.

Nobody wants to be the old person who keeps falling down!

There are gadgets (such as balance boards) that are designed to help improve balance.

But you know what else there is?

Your own body!

Practice standing on one leg (holding onto a chair or something with one hand if you need to steady yourself!).

WEAR CLOTHES THAT FIT.

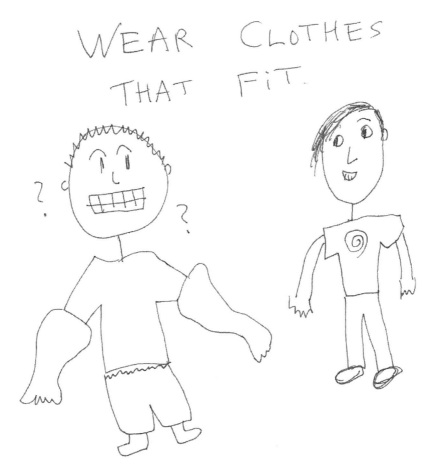

OK, I admit, I have no idea what is going on in today's drawing. 😀

And you might have no idea what I am talking about. Is this about fashion health or health health? (Gawd knows I should **not** be the one to give **anyone** fashion health tips! 🙄)

But this is a legit health nugget! I have treated many people over the years who have been injured by badly fitting clothes! The worst culprits - by far - are badly fitting bras. But badly fitting shoes, jackets, pants - and even underwear! - have also caused trouble.

(I'm not making up the part about the dangerous underwear, either! I'm not just a doctor... I **was a patient, too!** 🙄)

Aside from the structural/mechanical stuff, it's good for your mental health, too, to wear clothes that fit.

If your clothes are too big or too small, they probably just feel weird and uncomfortable. People might stare or offer you "advice."

Tight clothes might stress you out and make you continually feel bad about being "too fat."

Your body right now is your body right now. If you have to wear clothes at all, wear the ones that fit. 😊

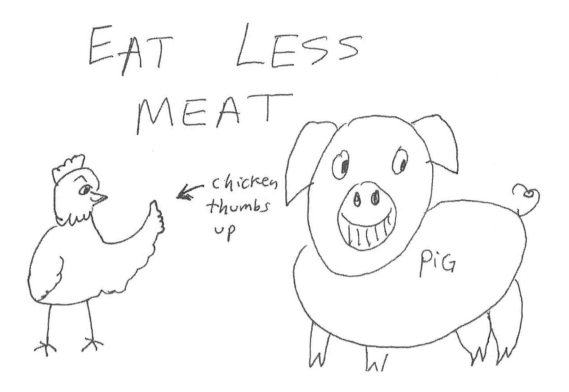

It is my personal belief that humans need **SOME** animal-based food to be optimally healthy, since we are, after all, designed as omnivores... 😑 👹

But even I have to admit, the evidence is pretty clear...

If you eat less meat, you will significantly reduce your odds of getting certain cancers.

A recently released huge epidemiological study from the UK (using data from 472,000 participants) showed the breakdown for "high meat-eaters" (people who ate meat more than 5 days a week), "low meat eaters" (people who are meat less than 5 days a week), fish eaters and vegetarians. The evidence is clear that less meat seems to equate with less cancer.

Interestingly, the most dramatic difference in subgroups was for colorectal cancer in men: the vegetarian men had 43% less incidence of colorectal cancer than the meat-eating men!

😲 (The difference in that group was not significant for women.) Some researchers point out that not **ALL** of the benefit of vegetarianism is likely from the diet itself. Vegetarians tend to be more health-conscious overall, and they are more likely to exercise, be married, and avoid tobacco and alcohol, which are all additional factors that tend towards positive health outcomes. But still, even if we are designed as omnivores, our ancestors did not eat meat every day. It was relatively hard to come by and was mostly for special occasions.

Yeah, yeah, every day is special...

but... it doesn't have to be **MEAT** special! Not every day is Taco Tuesday.

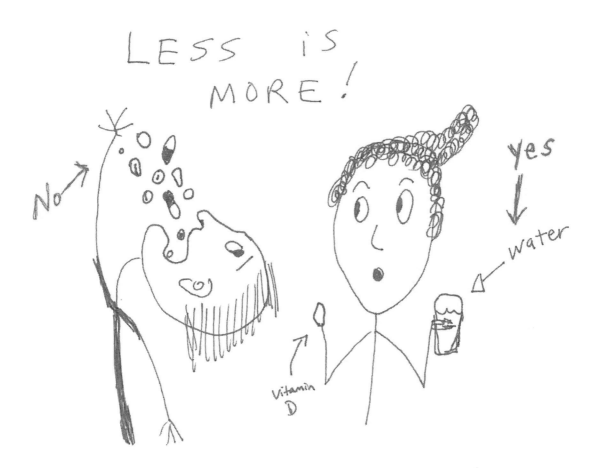

Throughout history, most health problems were problems of lack. We didn't have enough food, or the right kind of food, or water, or shelter, or [fill in the blank]. And so, deep in our DNA, we are programmed to seek **more**, and when there's a problem, we are naturally inclined to **add something**. We are inclined to take pills or supplements. It just makes sense! For us modern humans, the fact of the matter is that most of our health problems are due to **excess**. We'll feel a lot better if we STOP adding things and instead **remove** some stuff! What should we remove? It's different for everyone. (...but I'm sure you have some ideas already!) For now, it's a great step to just start shifting the mindset.

You're probably not missing as much as you think you are. You probably have too much of something. (But I drew the "yes" person in today's picture holding some vitamin D because that really is something that most of us are missing, since we no longer get enough sunlight to produce optimal levels of vitamin D!) The Wikipedia entry on Diseases of Affluence is an interesting read. Look it up! You may not think that you are "affluent," but... in this sense, yes you are.

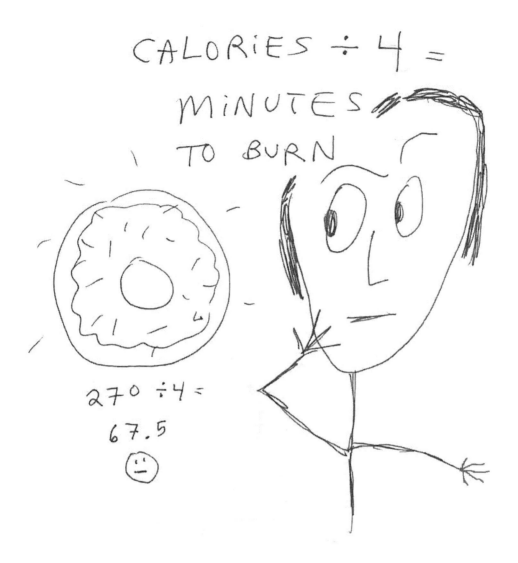

CALORIES ÷ 4 = MINUTES TO BURN

270 ÷ 4 = 67.5

This nugget is mainly for people who struggle to say "no" to tasties like donuts and such. It's a quickie trick that I learned today -- well, quick if you're good at math!

The trick is this.

If you take the number of calories within a food and then divide it by 4, that's how many minutes you have to exercise to burn it off!

So, our sprinkled donut friend there is about 270 calories. Divided by 4 is 67.5. So, if we eat the donut, we would have to exercise for a little over an hour to burn it off! Womp womp. Seems like a lot of work for a donut.

Sometimes that little womp womp is enough to get us to move along and let the urge pass!

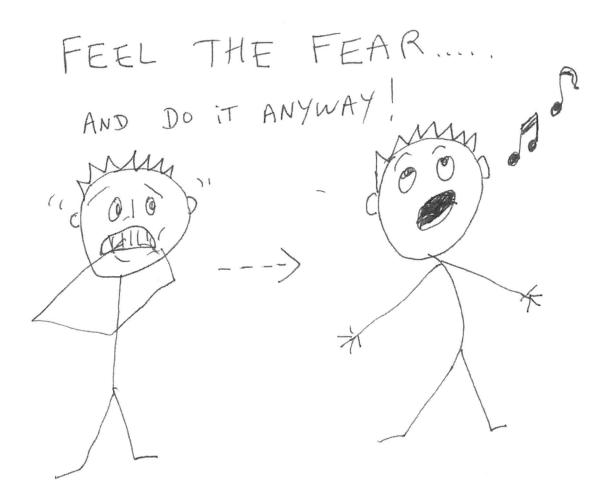

There is a book called *Feel the Fear and Do It Anyway.*

I read it a while ago, but I don't necessarily "recommend" it. Not that it doesn't have a good message. It does! Alls I'm saying is... it's one of those books where if you read the title, you have basically read the entire book.

The WHOLE THING is just FEEL THE FEAR AND DO IT ANYWAY.

It's OK to feel afraid! It's OK to feel the feeling. Just feel it.

And do it anyway.

What is "it?"

It's the thing that you are afraid to do!

Not the terrible thing that you are afraid to do. Stay scared and don't do **that!**

But it's the good thing that you want to do, but you're afraid.

You know, "putting yourself out there."

Stuff like that!

In my NET work, it's easy to imagine that NET totally "erases" the fear.

In my book, *The Issues are in the Tissues*, I tell the tale of how I used to get a killer migraine and barf every time I had more than 5 patients on the schedule. I used to also get at least a mild headache every single time I had to see a new patient.

As a 100% introvert, it's just never naturally exciting to meet new people.

NET saved my bacon, and I don't get those headaches anymore!

But... when I got my first smartwatch recently (yes, I'm late to the party) I saw something interesting.

In the 3 days leading up to a New Patient appointment (or any social event, such as a party), my resting heart rate climbs a few points! And then it drops back to normal the day after.

Even though I no longer have the debilitating headaches, my body still feels stress and anxiety about these things.

I'm not on a quest to "fix" it. That's just how I roll.

But if I let that feeling drive me and prevent me from taking the action that I know is going to be best for my life - and for others - then that would be a lose-lose situation, even if my animal brain doesn't know it!

Sometimes your fear is steering you to safety, and sometimes it's just old faulty programming.

Yes, for your health, *feel the fear, and do it anyway!*

STRETCH THOSE CALVES!

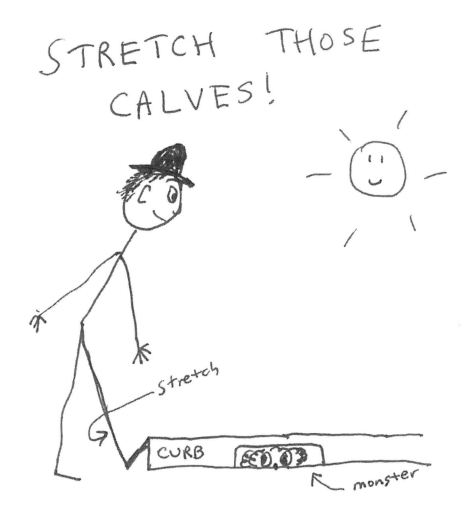

The muscles on the back of our legs get soooo tight, because we spend so much time sitting, and thus our legs are often in flexion.

If you have pain in your heels, that can also be a sign of tight calves!

There are lots of great calf stretches out there, but here is a really easy one.

Just flex your foot and put it up against the curb (or something like a curb) and lean down into the stretch!

(There may or may not be a monster nearby. I have been reading Stephen King again lately.)

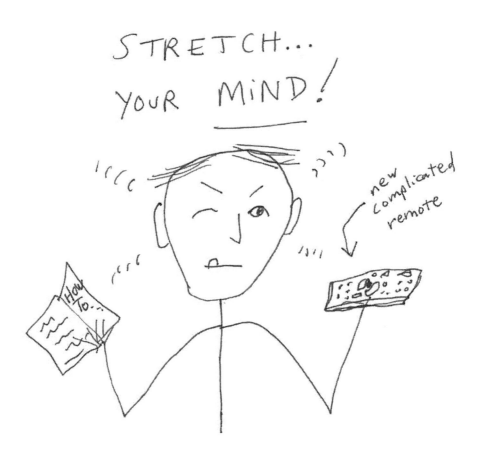

Did you ever notice... that one of the characteristics of getting old is both physical AND mental stiffening???

It's scary and sad but true.

I'm only 49, but I can already feel my mind stiffening up.

I used to learn new things so quickly!

I was the young "tech person" in the household who would program new gadgets and troubleshoot for the old people!

Now, when I look at a new gadget... I heave a heavy sigh... and think about whether I could get someone else to deal with it!

It just seems like so much... work...

Well, you know what? It's like a gym for your brain.

Learn new things - big and small - to help keep your mind flexible!

It's true that we start losing neurons after about age 25...

...but it's also true that the brain is capable of laying down new connections IF we work for it!

And we work for it by **physical exercise, paying attention and learning new things.**

(Read up on neuroplasticity if this is something you want to learn more about!)

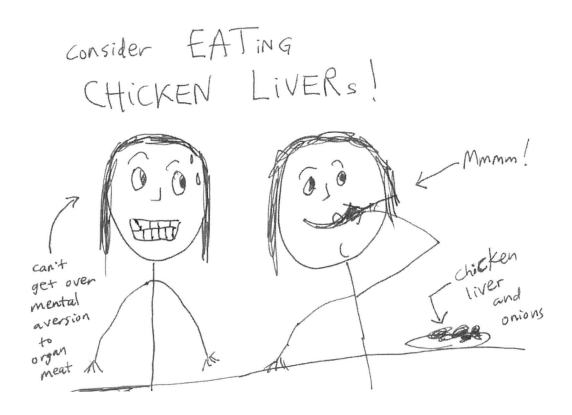

I know you feel suckered in because the picture has **NOTHING** to do with lily-livered varmints, but don't be mad - we will get to the lily-livers! But for now... I know people are all up in arms over the crazy rising cost of meat! Well aside from the fact that we shouldn't be eating so much meat anyway, consider this. You know what's one of the healthiest **and** cheapest things in the meat section? **Chicken livers.** And they will probably stay cheap, because Americans are just never going to go for them en masse! But they are recommended a lot in Chinese medicine for fortifying the blood, and even WebMD (which is pretty conservative) has a page on the health benefits of chicken liver! It's got a ton of vitamins and minerals, including iron, folate, niacin, vitamins B12, C, A (but too much A for pregnant women) and more.

OK so now for the lily-livers. What does that even mean?!

Well, it comes from the Middle Ages! Back then, they believed that the liver created blood and also controlled the emotions! It was thought that physical weakness and mental illness came from a badly functioning liver. Someone with a robust liver - full of blood and vigor - was considered to be very strong! But if your liver was (figuratively) white as a lily - thus empty of blood - then you were considered to be wimpy and a coward! Thus lily-livered.

As for the varmints, I was just thinking of Yosemite Sam for some reason. 👑

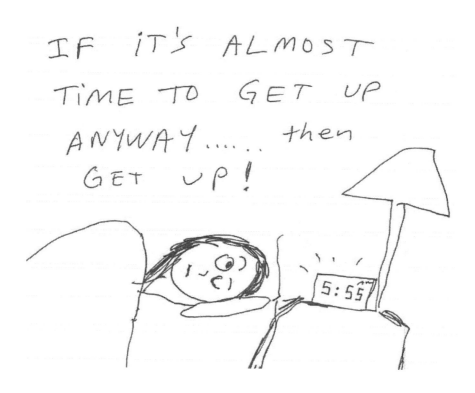

IF IT'S ALMOST TIME TO GET UP ANYWAY...... then GET UP!

Have you ever had that annoying thing happen where you wake up feeling pretty good and refreshed, but you look at the clock and it's not really "time to wake up" yet? You are still entitled to another 30 minutes or maybe even an hour of sleep! So instead of getting up, you decide to go back to sleep... and then you are jolted awake by your alarm, and you feel groggy - worse and more tired than you did when you woke up a little bit earlier! What kind of b.s. is that?!?! I'll tell you. Turns out, the body doesn't sleep in one big fat continuous chunk. It goes up and down through various stages of sleep. Under optimal conditions, the body sleeps in roughly 90-minute cycles. About 5 of these cycles equals just under 8 hours of sleep. Most people go through 4-6 cycles a night. When you naturally wake up, it's usually at the end of one of these cycles! But if you are forced to wake up by way of an alarm, depending on which part of the cycle you're in, you may feel awful. (This is also why those "smart alarms" will give you a range of time when it will wake you rather than an exact time, because it will try to avoid waking you during deep sleep and will aim to wake you during light sleep). So, if you naturally wake up, feel pretty good, and it's less than an 60-90 minutes from the time you'll have to wake up anyway, then just get up!

Get your exercise out of the way and feel no guilt for the rest of the day! 😄

Keeping in mind the 90-minute cycles can also help you to figure out a good bedtime for yourself.

IS BREATHING THE BEST PART OF YOGA?

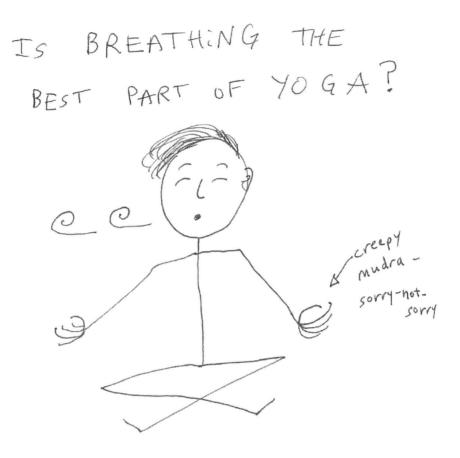

creepy mudra - sorry-not-sorry

I saw an article entitled The Most Important Part of Yoga? Breathing.

This tickled my lazy bone so hard.

LOL!, I thought, **YASS!!!** I can skip the hard part and just do the breathing part!!!

(My ears must be tuned to the topic, because about a week ago, I also heard some nerdy medical person say that "evidence shows that the main benefit of yoga might be from the breathing.")

Of course, [sadly] that wasn't really even the gist of the article.

And of course, the whole-body exercise part of yoga is plenty important!

Sorry, fellow lazy bones. ***But!***

It's true, that the breathing part is super important and beneficial for so many things.

Since you have to breathe all day anyway, here are some tips to practice:

* Your stomach should rise and fall more than your chest.
* Breathe in through your nose and out through your mouth.
* Breathe out twice as long as you breathe in.

If you follow just those few simple tips, you will calm your mind and strengthen your heart and lungs!

KEEP A LACROSSE BALL HANDY!

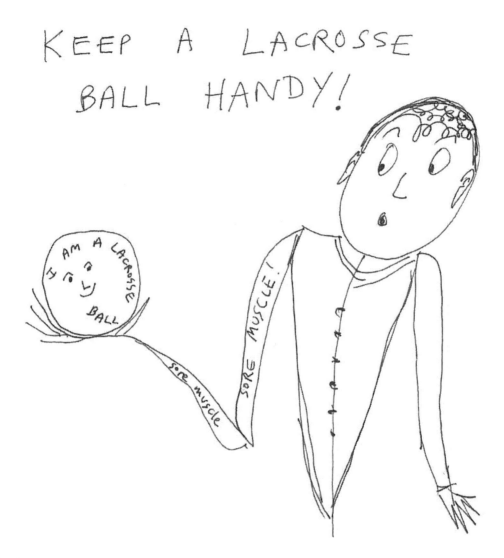

What's so great about a lacrosse ball? And why not a tennis ball? And what are we going to use it for?!

We're going to use it for self-massage! A tennis ball is "OK," but the lacrosse ball is much firmer and naturally grippy, making it perfect for doing targeted self-massage!

Keeping one handy in your desk also makes it easy to massage those achy arms and legs.

Don't think your arms and legs are achy?

Are you a human living in "the modern world?"

Then your arms and legs are achy.

So get the lacrosse ball and keep it handy!

"EXERCISE REGULARLY AND EAT MORE HEALTHILY."

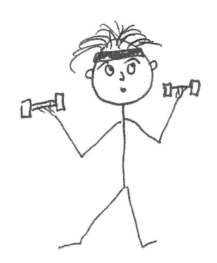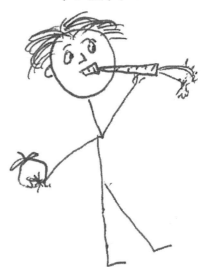

As you may recall, my main hobby is a thing called Postcrossing.

I recently sent a postcard to a young girl (college kid) in the UK. There's not much room on a postcard, so the messages tend to be short. Some people put writing prompts on their profiles to give people ideas about what to write.

(On my profile, I say that I enjoy reading people's spooky stories! 👻)

This person included several prompts, including "tell me what troubles you."

I have no idea what I wrote, but it must have been something about being worried about dying before my son is ready to be 100% independent of me! 😑

She replied that if my son is 19, then I am probably not **so** old yet to be worried about dying, and she gave me this advice for longevity:

"Maybe need some health supplements? And exercise regularly and eat more healthily."

I mean...yeah!

Everyone knows it.

But somehow, we also forget it! 🤭

Oh well. Just remember it again and most important of all, do it.

Exercise regularly and eat more healthily.

MAKE PEACE WITH "GOOD ENOUGH!"

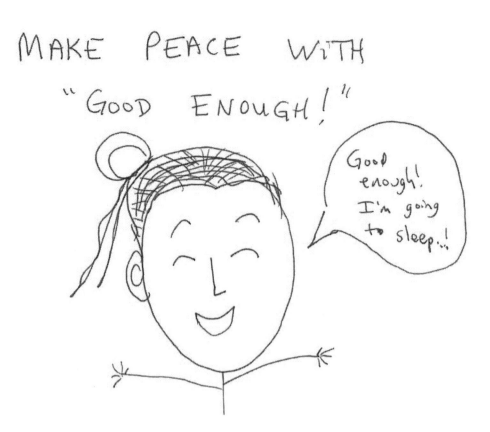

I know, a lot of you perfectionists are bristling at today's nugget.
I can hear you from all the way over here!
"*'Good enough'* is NOT good enough!!!"
Yes, it is.
Good enough is, literally, by definition, GOOD ENOUGH!
The world is crazy.
We were not designed for this level of crazy.
Nobody ever finishes everything they "should" be doing.
You cannot do it ALL.
So...
You've got to get OK with good enough.
Make peace with the fact that not everything can get done.
(This is not the same as saying go to town with the procrastinating! Priorities, people, priorities!)
But since one of the most important things you can do for your health is to get enough rest, you have to make peace with knowing when to call "good enough" and stop a thing, and move along.

EAT SOMETHING YOU PICKED YOURSELF!

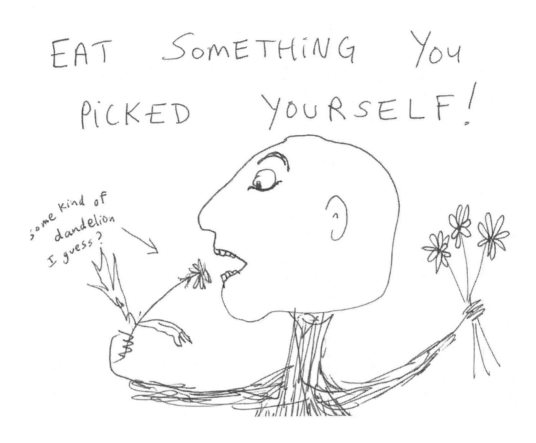

some kind of dandelion I guess?

Now... when I say, "eat something you picked yourself," I don't mean something you picked yourself off of the grocery store shelf.

I mean, something you picked fresh out of the ground! Or the sea. Or even (vegetarians close your eyes!) something you hunted yourself.

There is something so different about food that you ingest within moments or minutes (or even just hours) from when it was alive.

The energy is real!

And you gain a much greater appreciation for food, where it comes from, what it takes to harvest it and bring it to your mouth.

You naturally become more mindful about food!

As you may know, I'm a fan of backyard weed harvesting -- stuff like plantain weed (my fave!), dandelions, cleavers, wild onion, purslane, and on and on...

Wild foraging is where it's at if you have a black thumb, like me, and are incapable of deliberately cultivating any plant! 😳 🐒

TRY DELICATA SQUASH!

This is basically a plug for my favorite squash: delicata squash!

I love it because it is tasty, but maybe even more because it's **EASY**!

What's so easy about delicata squash?

You don't have to peel it!

The skin is so thin that you can eat it up!

You still have to scoop out the seeds, as with any other squash, but you can eat the skin.

Just make sure to completely cut off the hard stem and also the little hard dot opposite the stem. They are like rocks if you accidentally get one in your mouth!

Delicata squash is so great. I wish delicata squash had an ambassador like the corn kid.

TURMERIC INSTEAD OF NSAIDS!

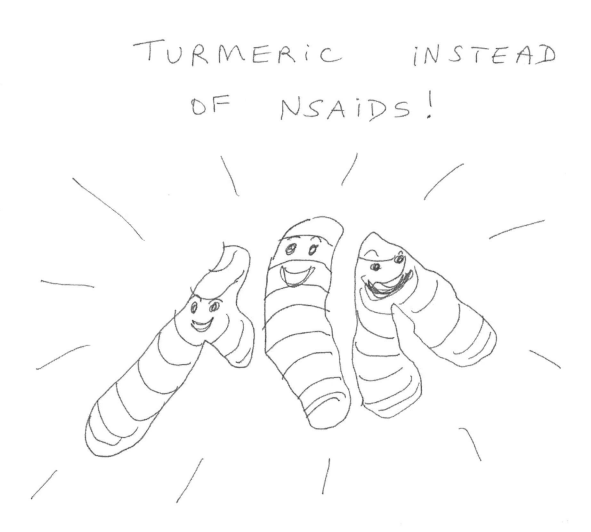

For many people, turmeric (taken with some kind of oil or fat) can be just as effective as NSAIDs (non-steroidal anti-inflammatory drugs) such as ibuprofen.

The therapeutic component of turmeric (curcumin) is hard to absorb on its own, and some people get gastrointestinal side-effects at high doses, so always take it with some kind of fat or oil, which makes it easier to digest. (For example, take it with some avocado, or with flax seed or fish oil supplements.)

You can eat turmeric in its natural form, which looks a lot like ginger root, but the orange/yellow will probably stain your teeth and hands.

Some people say there is no therapeutic value for taking curcumin alone (without anything to aid in its digestion) but even in that form, it is still beneficial. Curcumin in its undigestible form has been shown to have some antimicrobial properties that help with gut health!

Overuse of NSAIDs can lead to serious kidney damage, so, if you can get away with using turmeric instead, then do it!

BLUE - LIGHT BLOCKERS BEFORE BED!

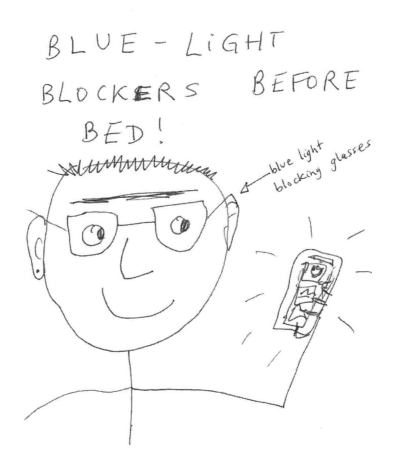

blue light blocking glasses

Artificial light has been messing with people's sleep ever since... well... the invention of artificial light! 💡

But the body's circadian rhythm is particularly thrown off by blue light, which is not supposed to be shining around bedtime!

Some smartphones now have a "night mode" feature that turns off most of the blue light coming from the screen.

You can also buy special "blue light filtering" glasses to wear around the house for the couple of hours before bedtime!

You can even get "blue light filtering" added to your prescription glasses nowadays, although there's no evidence that it's particularly helpful to block blue light **ALL** the time. It's mostly beneficial in the hours right before sleep.

So if you are having a hard time falling asleep, and you have a lot of screen time before bed, try blocking the blue light!

GROUND* YOUR BODY

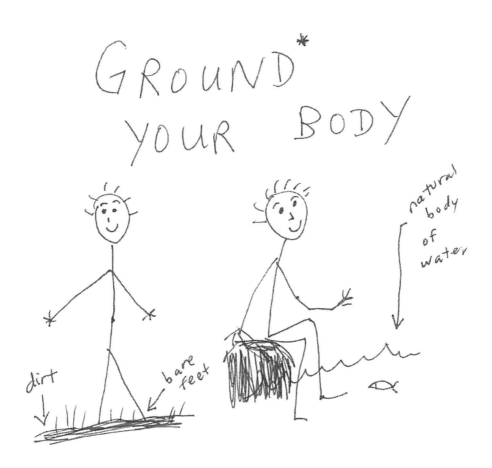

When I say, "ground your body," I am not speaking metaphorically today!

I mean, like, put your feet in the dirt!

(I put a * next to the word ground, though, because sand, rocks or a naturally occurring body of water count, too! I read that concrete also counts, due to its conductive properties, but... it doesn't sound as nice.)

Not to be overly hippy dippy or anything, but... touching your body directly to the earth is good for your health. It can help you feel calmer and more energized.

We tend to forget that our bodies run on electricity!

And electrical circuits need healthy grounding - connecting to the earth for healthy flow of electrons.

So, for at least a few minutes a day, be in physical touch with the earth! Walk barefoot around a nice patch of earth or stick your feet in the water for a few minutes!

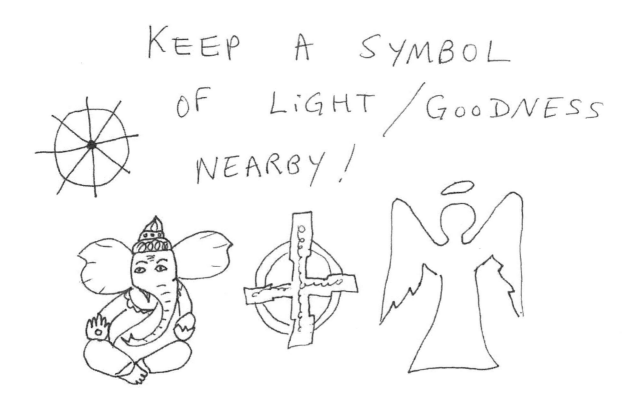

KEEP A SYMBOL OF LIGHT / GOODNESS NEARBY!

Now, I'm not necessarily advocating for "religion" here... because "religion" has been used to justify and cause all manner of ugliness over time! (And it still does!) But! Symbols have meanings. And over the course of generations upon generations upon generations, these symbols have very deep meanings that touch our core and can change the mood and the energy around us. A lot of people have experienced trauma under the banner of certain religions. If this happened to you, then obviously you may not want to keep those symbols around you! But if there is a symbol that (for you) evokes huge and powerful peace, love, healing, and deep goodness, then keep one in your home, office and maybe even on your person! There is a part of our brain (the nucleus accumbens) that lights up when we focus on "spiritual" ideas. If there's a part of our brain that's adapted for it, then it's probably something that we need to be healthy. There's so much gross stuff happening in the world, it sometimes seems like it must be "the forces of evil." Simple reminders of forces of good may not save the world. But they can help save **you** from getting pulled down that dark rabbit hole.

Oh, and if you're wondering how I drew such a nice Ganesha, it's because I watched a cool YouTube video on "How to Draw Ganesha from Number 5." 😄

118

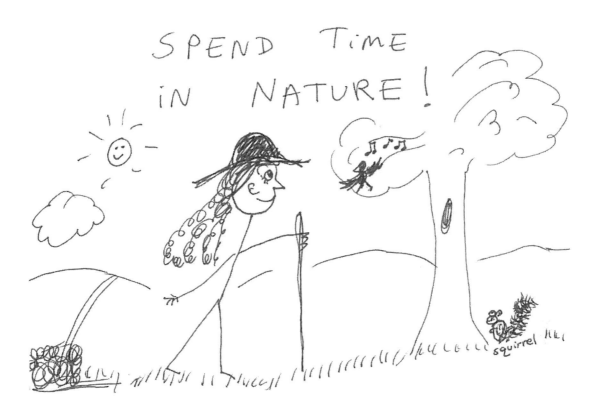

Spending time in nature might sound like a repeat of grounding, but... it's different! You may or may not be grounding while out in nature, but you get lots of other benefits, such as: reduced exposure to electromagnetic pollution, increased vitamin D production, improved focus, reduced anxiety, improved mood, relaxation, and even improved productivity! Even if you are stuck in a city, you can find pockets of nature where you can take a mini escape! Introvert pro-tip: aim to hit your local nature spot about 20 minutes before official sunrise, and you will be in for a treat. You will get to experience "the magic hour" of perfect light, the sunrise and the best chance to experience the peace of nature!

BENT KNEE LEG LIFTS INSTEAD OF CRUNCHES

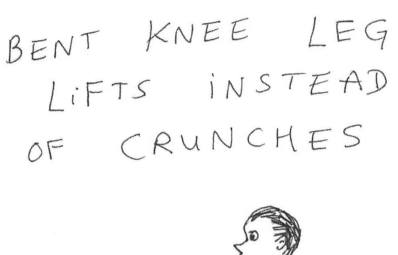

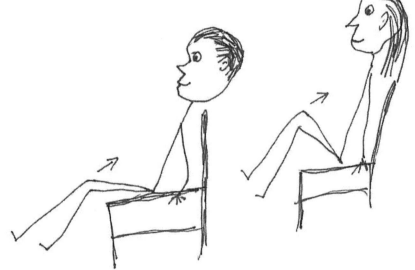

Crunches are the go-to exercise that most people use for abs.

But would you believe that every year, I take care of people who hurt their neck while doing crunches?!

If you're going to do crunches, pay attention to your neck.

Keep it neutral and in line with your spine!

The easier way to exercise your abs while keeping your neck and spine neutral is to sit for leverage, and then bend your knees and lift your legs. (Use you arms to stabilize your body by holding on to the seat.)

If your abs are weak, you will need to bend your knees a lot at first. As this gets easier and you want more of a challenge, extend your legs out further.

And remember, strong abs help to support a strong back!

WEAR A BRACE (SOMETIMES)...

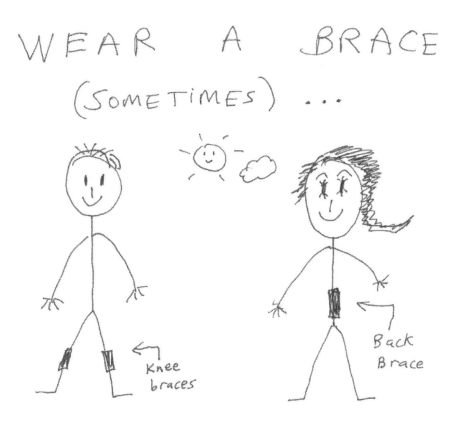

Knee braces

Back Brace

Should you wear a brace if you're not hurting or injured? Sometimes! By the time we reach middle age, we've all been through the wringer - even the non-sporty people! Everyone has old injuries or weak links. Cue that sad trombone! On top of all that, as we get older, it takes longer and longer to heal and recover. So if you want to stay active, you have to avoid injury and re-injury! Part of this means knowing yourself, your body, your history and your realistic risk of injury. Years ago, I really messed up my knees during the brief capoeira chapter of my life. They mostly don't hurt, and I don't wear a brace most days. BUT! I would never go to a gym or do anything sporty (other than swimming or riding a bike) without knee braces. I just know that my knees are easily injured with sudden lateral movements, and if I get injured, then I'm inflamed and unable to work out for a couple of weeks! The braces give me the extra stability I need to avoid (re)injury. Some of you have old back injuries that flare up every so often. Maybe you get warnings, little twinges that make you think, "Is my back going to go out on me?" Yes, this would be a good time to see your chiropractor. But these little warnings may also be signs that it's worth taking out your back brace and wearing it if you are doing physically intense work (lifting, etc.) You don't want to wear a brace *all* the time, because long-term use can weaken your muscles. But it's OK to use them short-term for stability when you need it! *And you don't have to wait until you're in a ton of pain to reach for it.* If you have an old back injury, I recommend having a good quality back brace at home "just in case." I like the ones that are kind of like corsets, with the little pulley string to tighten it.

121

JUMP FOR JOY

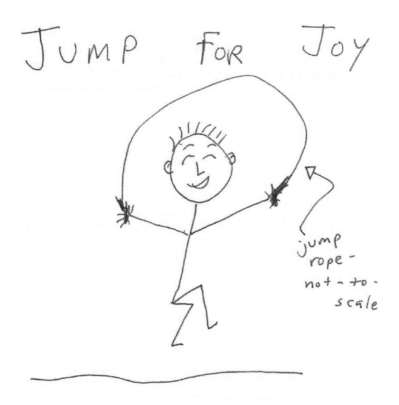

jump rope - not - to - scale

Actually, today's theme is more about weight-bearing exercises for your bones, but, sure, jump for joy - why not?! As we get older, we lose bone density. People tend to focus on calcium supplements for bone strengthening. But do you know what really does the most to strengthen bones? **Weight-bearing exercise!** You probably know that one of the hazards of astronaut life is the loss of bone density. Why do they lose so much bone so fast?! Because the body is highly efficient. It doesn't waste resources. In zero gravity, there's not much need for strong bones, so the body takes the calcium and uses it for something else. Conversely, if you are handling weights and carrying yourself around in gravity then the body needs strong bones, and it lays down more calcium.

High-impact weight bearing exercises (such as jumping rope, running, dancing, tennis, etc.) are the most effective at building bone, but you should be cautious with this type of exercise if you have joint issues. Other weight-bearing exercises include lifting weights, hiking, stair-climbing and even gardening! Swimming, while great for so many things, is **not** a weight-bearing exercise, so it is not that helpful for building and strengthening bones. If you already have osteoporosis, then jumping rope is not for you! 😵 Make sure to include weight-bearing exercises in your routine so that your aging body knows that you still need strong bones because you are still using them!

STRETCH YOUR ROAST CHICKEN INTO SOUP!

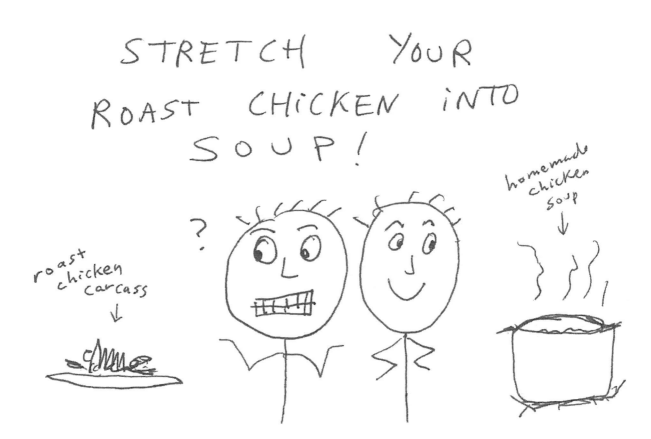

If you're like me, then you sometimes buy a rotisserie chicken, eat it as best you can, and then stare at the carcass guiltily thinking about all the meat that appears to still be on it, but that you don't really know "how" to eat. 🐵

Then someone says, "Just make a soup with it!" 💡

And then you say, "good idea!"

And then feel dumb because you suck at cooking and you're not sure how to "make a soup with it." 🧑‍🦰

Well, I'm here to tell you that I've climbed the mountain and discovered that the soup is easy, and it's good, and it saves you a lot of effort in coming up with the next meal (after the main chicken)! You can see how it's done in this video:

https://www.noreciperequired.com/recipe/homemade-chicken-soup-carcass

Also, if you go the extra mile and boil the chicken long enough that the cartilage comes off the bones, that is really good for your joints, too. Even though it sounds gross.

You can add or subtract veggies according to your taste.

And good ol' raw sea salt is your friend for tasting!

THROW OUT EXPIRED SUPPLEMENTS, etc.

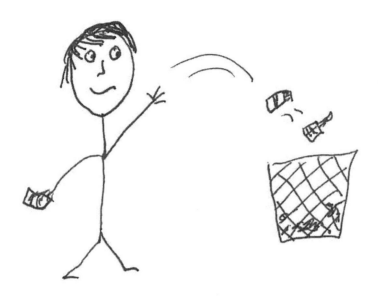

"Are these supplements still good?"

Let's just say NO and throw them away!!!

The real answer is "maybe" or "kinda" or "yes?" or "no!" depending on the brand, the ingredients, the conditions under which they've been stored, the universe that we are existing in at the moment, etc. etc.

And you know what? Ain't nobody got time for that.

Decision-making takes up energy and is stressful. What is the point of taking supplements anyway? To enhance your health! So, what if you are taking your old expired supplements and you still feel like crap, and then you wonder if it's because you're taking old expired supplements, or maybe they didn't work in the first place, or, or... ???

Just don't.

If you're taking something for your health, take the best, freshest most potent version.

Not your sad dusty expired bottle from your cluttered supplement closet!

If this inspires you to declutter other things, I heartily recommend this book: *Decluttering at the Speed of Life.* It is a SIMPLE method that does not require you to spark joy or dump your belongings into a big pile! 😄

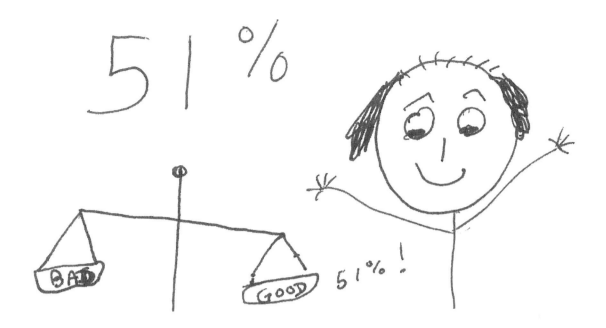

Nobody's perfect.

Nobody gets it "right" 100% of the time.

Probably not even 99% of the time.

97%?

What should we be aiming for anyway?!

I mean, some days, you can barely scrape yourself up off the floor.

On those days, are you even hitting 10%?

Most of us waste too much energy beating ourselves up for not being in that 99% or whatever club.

Today, can you be sure to get to 51% and find joy in that?

If you're at 51%, then the balance is starting to tip in favor of the positive!

From that point, you will find it easier to get some momentum.

If you're 51% on the good side, then your net profit is "good."

Good enough for today!

WORK ON YOUR RELATIONSHIPS!

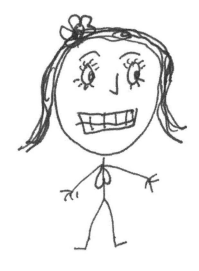
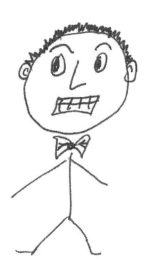

Hmm... Work on your relationships? For your health?

Yes!

Why do we want to be healthy in the first place?

In order to live a good and happy life!

Well, according to the Harvard Happiness Study - the longest running study ever - the key to a long and happy life is **warm and satisfying relationships!**

Conversely, loneliness "is as powerful as smoking or alcoholism!"

The world of "relationships" extends beyond romantic partners, so don't get all paranoid just because you're single!

It extends to friendships and family relationships as well.

The basic idea is that people who have community and feel supported tend to be healthier.

If you struggle with love and relationships, I recommend checking out Gary John Bishop's book, *Love Unf*cked: Getting Your Relationship Sh!t Together*. I like his no-nonsense, action-oriented approach!

(If you need a gentler touch, maybe find a good therapist!)

But anyway... whatever you do, if you care about your health, then make sure to nurture your relationships, too!

FAST

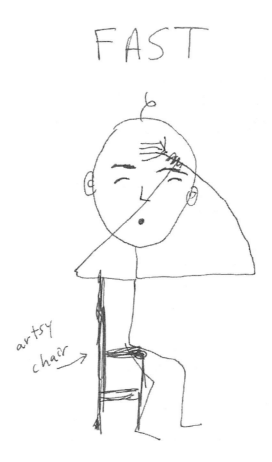

artsy chair →

I can't believe this is the first Daily Health Nugget about FAST!
(Honestly. it's because I can't draw hands, and hands are an important part of this technique.)

FAST is a simple yet powerful stress-relieving tool that you can use anywhere anytime! It's related to NET in that it uses the same pulse points and forehead emotional points that are used in NET, but there is no muscle-testing involved.

In a nutshell, here's how it's done.

First, identify an issue that is stressing you out. For example, the big tax bill that is coming due! It may be helpful to ask yourself how intense the stressful feeling is, on a scale of one to ten? Is it a seven? A ten? Next, put one of your wrists (palm up) into your other hand. Using three fingers of your bottom hand, gently wrap your fingers around your wrist as if to take a pulse. (You probably will feel a pulse, too.) Next, put the open palm against your forehead, centering it between the eyebrows and the hairline. Now, take a few deep breaths while focusing on the feeling of the stressful thing. After a few good deep breaths, switch hands and repeat. Check in again with the intensity of the stress. Where is it now on that one to ten scale? Did it drop down a notch? It probably dropped down several notches!

FAST helps the body to process the feelings and it helps them to move **through** your body without getting **stuck** in it.

In addition to the primary wrist pulse points shown on the diagram on the FAST webpage (www.firstaidstresstool.com), there is one more "bonus point" that is located in the fleshy area at the base of the thumb. This point corresponds to feelings of shame, bullied, confused, self-conscious, worthless, less than and mortified. If these feelings are present and intense, then use the FAST method but hold on to the point on that thenar pad. You can do this point on both hands. Sometimes one side will seem more helpful than the other side. This is a great technique to do at the end of a stressful day, and it's also great for kids!

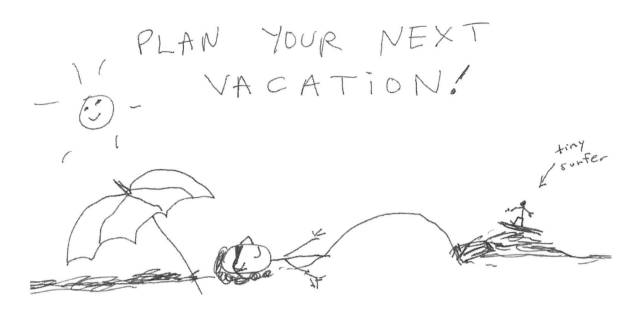

PLAN YOUR NEXT VACATION!

tiny surfer

I know, I know...

A lot of you out there in Daily Nugget Land are self-employed, like me!

You are saying, "Vacation?! I can't afford a vacation! I don't have the TIME! I don't have the money!"

Or maybe you're not self-employed, and you might even have a bunch of paid time-off but you just won't use it!

"I can't... they NEED me!"

So, but here's the weird thing.

What happens if/when you get sick - sick enough that you can't work - or some terrible emergency comes up that forces you to travel (to a funeral etc.) or miss work for some reason?

Somehow, the world keeps going, the people who usually count on your for whatever figure out how to make do while you're gone, and *somehow, **it always just works out.***

Well guess what? The same thing happens when you take some time off for yourself.

The world will keep turning, and somehow, it's going to work out.

Planning your next vacation doesn't have to mean flying away to some exotic location. But it could! And you'd be surprised... sometimes, it doesn't cost as much as you think it does.

When I went to Egypt a few years ago, I found a round-trip ticket for around $680! When I went to Iowa recently (for my "50 states by age 50" goal trip) I found a ticket for just $138! The important thing is to decide to do it and to make it happen.

Vacations are important not just because everyone needs time off and a chance to "get away." They are also important because you **need something to look forward to.** The feeling of happiness comes from the sense that you are getting closer to a meaningful goal. The excitement of getting closer to your vacation is often more exciting than the thing itself! (It's kind of like how the run-up to Christmas can feel so good and exciting, but then so many people feel sort of a let-down feeling by the end of the actual day!)

So plan your next vacation!

Here's how you do it.

Step 1: Mark your calendar. Decide when you're going.

Step 2: If you can't afford to buy a plane ticket yet, then go ahead and reserve a hotel room. You usually don't have to pay anything to reserve your room in advance, and you can usually cancel with no penalty within 72 hours of arrival if need be. But making the reservation gives your brain the feeling that this vacation is for real! It starts to build the energy!

Step 3: Start looking for good deals on plane fares. This can be tough! But there are websites where you can get an alert when your destination shows a good price.

Step 4: Book your flight as soon as you get that good deal!

Step 5: Everything will now fall into place. Once you booked your flight, which is probably non-refundable, you are GOING! And everything else is just going to have to work out. Oddly enough, it will.

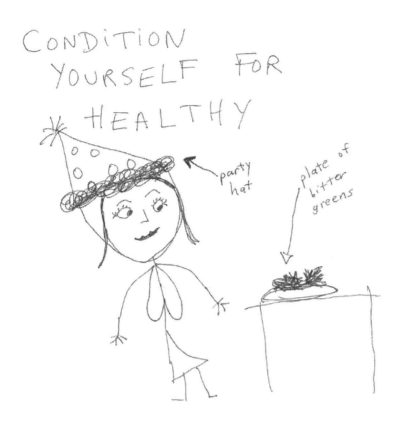

CONDITION YOURSELF FOR HEALTHY

party hat

plate of bitter greens

Will wearing a party hat while you eat bitter greens make you crave it like birthday cake? Maybe, maybe not. But hear me out! Part of why we crave things like cake and alcohol has to do with biochemistry and genetic programming. Sure. But also... part of why we crave things like that is because of the positive social associations that go with it! If we're lonely, we might want a glass of wine or a cocktail because it reminds us of relaxing with our friends in a nice place. Or we might pull towards cake if we're depressed because it reminds us of celebration times. But what do we associate with bitter veggies? ugh. "You eat those veggies, missy/mister or else you are not leaving this table!" 😖 😒 Well, guess what? You can create new programming. Chances are, bitter greens will never ever become the hot new dish at all the best parties! But **you** can condition **your** body to associate them with good times. How? Make it a point to eat them right before you head out to something fun. A party, a movie you've been looking forward to, a show, coffee with an old friend... Anything nice. Then, eventually, your body will associate those bitter healthy green foods with "something good is coming my way!" rather than "I'm being punished." or whatever else negative feeling currently goes with them. I think this might be what the kids these days are calling "brain hacking." Using your powers for good! 😇 Oh, and if you feel emotional resistance to this idea or practice, do FAST and breathe through the feeling, and see if you can shift it and take the positive action step!

POPCORN + FIBER ?

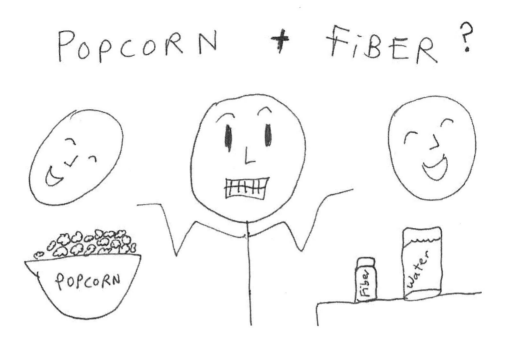

I know, this sounds like a weird one. But hear me out.

First of all, I'm not saying that popcorn is a "healthy" food.

It's not. 👾

But it's one of those things that we end up eating anyway!

Sometimes by the bucket! 🍿

So, if you're going to eat it, then at least know how to help your body handle it better!

Those annoying little skins get stuck in your teeth, so make sure to floss really well afterwards, and use a water pick if you have one! If you don't get them out, they can wedge in your gums and trap bacteria, leading to all sorts of trouble.

But you know where else they get stuck? Around your ileocecal valve!

The ileocecal valve is the connecting point between your large and small intestines. It occurs at a relatively sharp angle, and so that area is prone to things like parasites and irritation from stuck little bits of stuff like popcorn skins.

I have seen this many times over the years, and the ICV (ileocecal valve) dysfunction then often sends a referred pain signal to the low back (as well as abdominal discomfort).

One way to nip it in the bud is to take a good quality fiber supplement (such as Colon Plus, from Biotics) afterward with plenty of water. This can help the body to gently scrape away the trapped bits and move it along! Plain old psyllium husks will work, too, but always and only with lots and lots of water, otherwise you might make the problem worse!

CHOCOLATE CRAVING = MAGNESIUM CRAVING

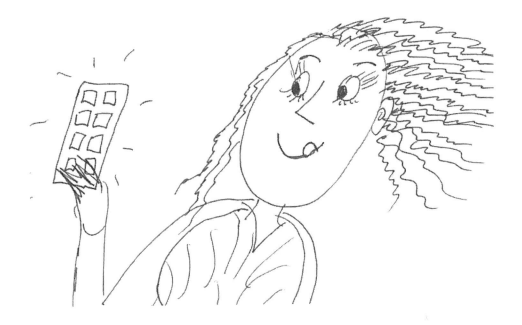

Do you crave chocolate? Like, really *really* crave it?? ◈◆

Then your body is probably really craving magnesium!

Chocolate is high in magnesium. ☺

A magnesium deficiency can manifest in many ways.

The most common symptoms are: migraines, muscle cramps and brain fog.

But they can also include ankle swelling, numbness, tingling and more!

I do realize that **good** chocolate is one of life's pleasures and joys. ♥

So I'm not trying to take away your chocolate!

I'm just sayin'... if you have intense chocolate cravings, add some more magnesium to your diet or add a good magnesium supplement.

You will feel a lot better in your body, and will be able to truly enjoy the full pleasure of your occasional chocolate! 🏃🏃

TIME FOR A TIME AUDIT!

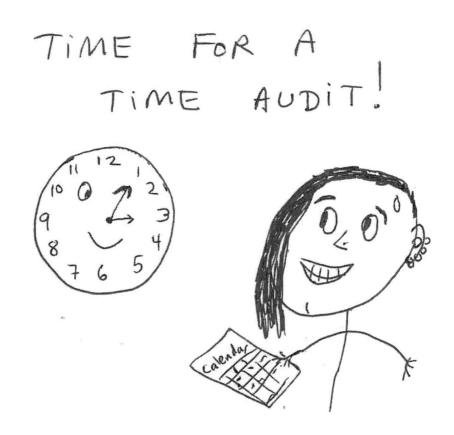

What the heck is a time audit, and why is it considered a health nugget?

How can anything with the word "audit" in it be healthy?! ☹

Well, if you've ever said the following phrase, then you need to do a time audit.

"I DON'T HAVE ENOUGH TIME!"

A good time audit takes about 2 weeks, but you can do it faster if you are really honest with yourself. At least 1 week is recommended.

What you do is, you write down everything you do during your waking hours, in 15 or 30 minute increments, then at the end of the 1 or 2 weeks, you evaluate it and see where your time is going!

You will be surprised to see that you have more time than you think you do...

How might your health improve if you found a few more hours in a day or a week?

More time to exercise? Or meditate? Or cook something nice? Or call an old friend?. You need to do it for more than 3 days, because your brain can fool you and fake "good behavior" for a couple of days. But you will see you true patterns if you do it for at least a week.

Get a better grip on your time, and you will have less stress, and that will help your health - a lot! ☺

MASSAGE YOUR FEET!

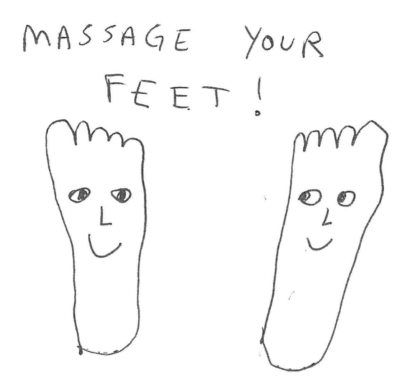

I really hate trying to draw feet... and I know that those feet are backwards... and I know that some of you think feet are so gross, so I tried to make them cute with happy faces, too... I tried! 😐 🐵

But anyway, it was an important nugget, because for some reason, foot reflexology has been coming up on my radar a lot lately! I keep running into people who have been getting great results with reflexology!

Reflexology is basically the art of massaging certain areas of the feet in order to improve the health of other parts of the body. You may already be familiar with foot reflexology charts such as the one on page 408.

One of the great things about reflexology is that it is one of the forms of massage that you can do for yourself! You will probably not dig in as hard as a seasoned reflexologist, but you can still help yourself to feel better.

Use a reflexology chart to help you figure out where to focus the pressure based on your own symptoms and challenges.

MUSHROOMS + SUN = MORE VITAMIN D!

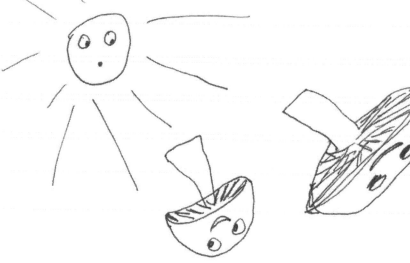

I know... it looks like those mushrooms are doing something naughty at the sun! 😳 👹
But they're not!
They are just making maximum vitamin D!
Gills up?? Yes, gills up.
You see... animals aren't the only things that create vitamin D by way of sunlight.
Mushrooms do it, too!
And some mushroom nerds discovered through experimentation that you can greatly increase the amount of vitamin D in a harvested mushroom by exposing it to sunlight!
If you expose them to the sun (or a UV light with UVB) with the gills facing up, that maximizes the vitamin D production.
If you have the time and inclination (and access to intense summertime sunlight) you can increase the vitamin D content so drastically that you could dry the mushrooms and store them for your own homemade vitamin D supplements!
Mushrooms are amazing. I am a fan! 🍄 👍

COVER YOUR NECK ON COLD / WINDY DAYS!

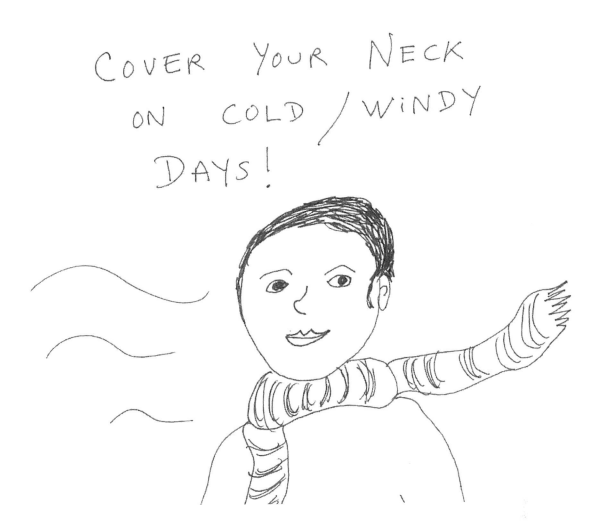

In Chinese medicine, there is a magic door in the back of the neck that is very vulnerable to wind and cold! I don't remember what it's called or if it even exists as such, but I can say that I do take care of people every year who manage to hurt themselves "while doing nothing" after spending time in the cold and wind with a bare neck!

Before I became a scarf user, my acupuncturist used to get on my case about being careless in the wind. She'd be like, "You got wind in your neck again!"

But seriously. Cold weather is not so great for joints and muscles. When muscles are cold, they are more likely to spasm or get injured.

So, if it's chilly or windy out there, grab a scarf!

Plus, they are cute and cozy!

Today's picture looks like Isabella Rossellini. She is awesome. And strange. Have you seen her bedbug seduction video?! It's amazeballs.

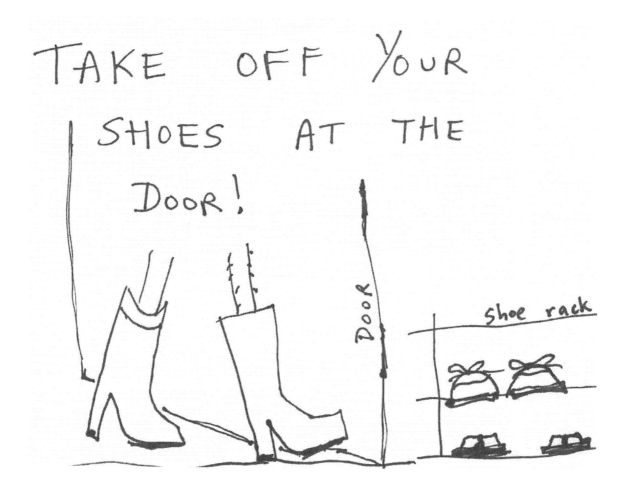

TAKE OFF YOUR SHOES AT THE DOOR!

Door

shoe rack

Man, it never even occurred to me that this was a health nugget until I heard it on a podcast today! I just thought "it's just what you do."

I grew up with a Korean mom, so, **NO SHOES INSIDE THE HOUSE** was just the way it was! We always left our shoes out on the back porch (it was a covered porch) or in the garage! Shoes were not allowed inside the house.

Now that I live in a smaller space with no porch OR garage, the shoes do make it inside the door, but not by more than a few feet!

There's so much gross stuff outside. Or, if you're in San Francisco, **THERE'S SO MUCH GROSS STUFF OUTSIDE!!!**

It's a no-brainer that you should wash your hands when you get home.

But also, take off your shoes and don't wear your outside shoes inside your home!

Aside from keeping dirt, chemicals and bacteria at bay, it's also healthy to spend time barefoot.

Get a nice cozy pair of house slippers or house shoes if you must.

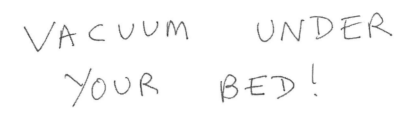

VACUUM UNDER YOUR BED!

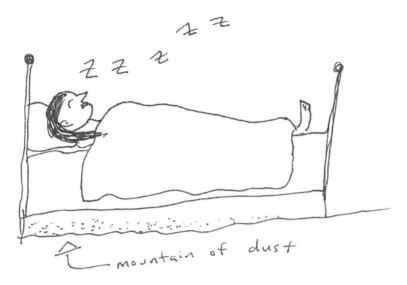

← mountain of dust

Now that we are mostly grown-ups around here, probably we're not too worried about monsters under the bed! 😈

But, if you had a strong enough magnifying glass... 😳

Unless you are a clean freak or the proud owner of a Roomba, there is probably a ton of dust under your bed! And dust is mostly made of dead skin. And dead skin is food for dust mites!

Dust mites are tiny arachnids - yes, relatives of spiders! And they poop and die, etc., too, and become part of the dust mess. It is this dust mite poop (and the powerful enzymes inside of it) that are the main culprits for dust allergies! I know, gross. Hey, I'm just the messenger. Anyway, excessive dust tends to trigger allergies, which can also disrupt your sleep!

If you lay down in bed and almost immediately start feeling stuffed up or itchy or feel like you're allergic to something, it just might be the dust and those dust mites around your bed! You may need to wash your bedding more often and/or clean up underneath that bed!

SLIGHT BEND IN ELBOW WHEN CARRYING GROCERIES!

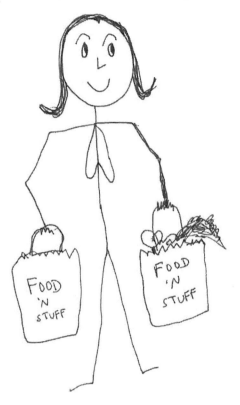

It's very tempting to just let your tired arms hang loose when you are carrying your groceries (and stuff), but... don't do it! Keep a slight bend in your elbows. This helps to engage your muscles, including your core, but most importantly, it protects the ligaments in your elbows! Ligaments are not really designed to stretch very far. Their job is to connect bones to other bones. If they become over-stretched, they don't always snap back! Think of pulling a can out of a 6-pack. The plastic ring stretches, but it doesn't snap back to shape! Unlike muscles, ligaments have almost no blood flow, which means that once injured, they heal very very slowly. Every so often, someone comes to me with elbow pain and then are surprised to discover that their elbow has come out of alignment! When we dig back to figure out what happened, it was often a heavy bag of groceries or a suitcase that was being carried with straight unengaged arms. And the older you get, the more vulnerable you are to this kind of injury. Also, there is no shame in using a little cart!

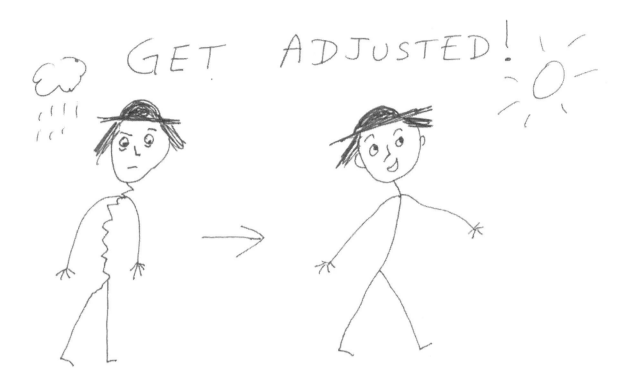

Am I a bad chiropractor for waiting until the 132nd Daily Nugget to mention getting adjusted? 😳 🐵

I guess I have a knack for forgetting to mention the obvious!

Anything with any kind of joint works better when the joints are in alignment!

There are 360 joints in the human body!

Chiropractors adjust more than just the spine.

Even a chiropractor like me - who is specialized and mostly doing NET these days - adjusts many different joints.

Today, I adjusted the following joints: several spines (of course), a ribcage, a shoulder, a jaw, an ankle, a skull (specifically, a sphenoid bone), a hip and a wrist!

Life is just better when you're well adjusted.

Whenever I would adjust my Gramma (during the year that I lived with her), she would open her eyes wide afterward and say, "Gosh! I thought I was just old!"

Chiropractic is an American healing art and is over 125 years old. Check it out!

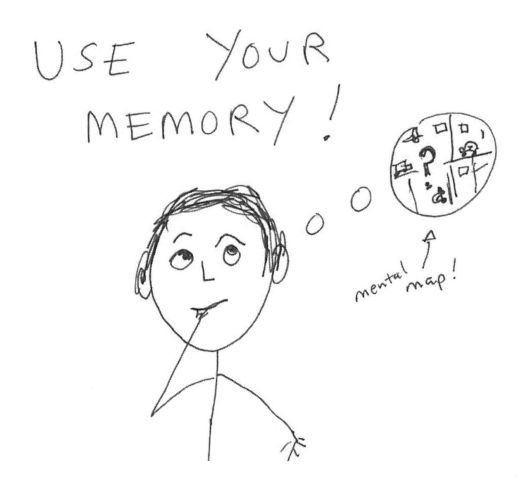

USE YOUR MEMORY!

mental map!

As we get older, our brainpower tends to slow down. It can still get the job done, but... it'll take longer.

So, it's helpful to think of your brain like a muscle. Use it or lose it!

It's nice to live in a time when we don't have to memorize so many things. Such as road maps! Remember those big fat map books we used to keep in the car?! (Actually, I liked those maps...)

GPS is indeed something of a godsend. But... it's also shrinking our brains.

Do you ever catch yourself turning on the GPS for a place that you already know how to get to? I know, sometimes you do it to check the traffic. Fair enough.

But other than that, turn it off if you don't need it!

If you **can** use your memory for a task, then use it!

Your older self will thank you!

LEFTOVERS ARE YOUR FRIENDS!

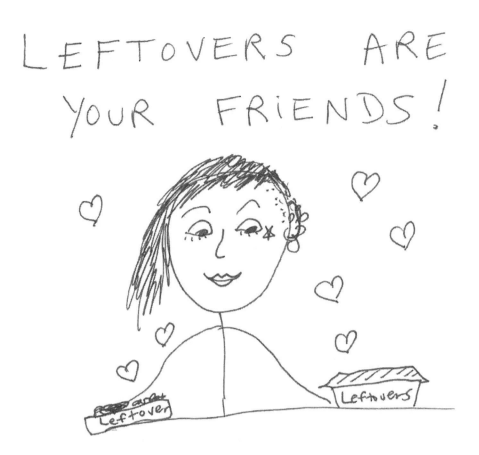

Does anyone love leftovers as much as that person in the picture? 🫨 (Yes: me!) Some people have a serious aversion to leftovers. I've even had to do intensive NET sessions with people who had unusually strong emotional reactions to the idea of eating leftovers! But appreciating and eating your leftovers saves you time, money, energy **and** is good for the planet. Did you know that Americans throw away about 30-40% of the total food we buy?! We are the most food-wasteful country in the world! When I was a kid, my dad would tell us, "Finish your food! There are kids starving in Africa!" I knew that whether I finished my food would not make a difference to a kid in Africa... but... turns out... I was wrong - in an unexpected way! The massive amount of food waste that we create mostly ends up in landfills. And guess what? It creates a shocking amount of those pesky greenhouse gases that contribute to climate change. And who does it hurt the most? The people who live in already hot places... like Africa! Work on developing the habit of treating leftovers as perfectly good and delicious food. It's a small habit that is healthy for you and the rest of the world. 😎 🌍

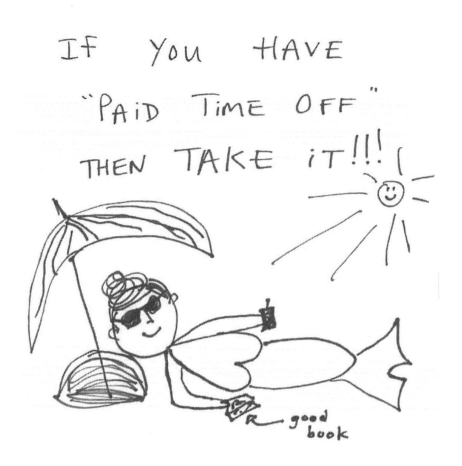

IF YOU HAVE "PAID TIME OFF" THEN TAKE IT!!!

R — good book

Apologies to all the gig workers, part-timers and self-employed people (like me!) who don't have any such thing as Paid Time Off. But the topic is still an important nugget to bring up because we're in America. And here in America, we seem to have a weird aversion to taking time off from work - even if it's **paid** time off! 😲 According to Forbes, Americans waste more than $200 billion a year (!) by failing to take their vacation time. Some of that can get rolled over into the next year, but many employers reset the clock on January 1, so about $65 billion of that is lost forever. Wowzers. It's true that work is important. But time away from work is also important - and it's important for your health! A big part of "happiness" is feeling like you're getting closer to a meaningful goal. And doesn't it always feel good to look at your calendar and see that you are getting closer and closer to a vacation or some time off that you've been really looking forward to? Unless you're saving that PTO for something reeeeally specific, you need to mark your calendar and just make it happen. You will never regret taking the time off. But you may well regret wasting it. Remember, one of the top 5 regrets of the dying is this: "I wish I didn't work so much."

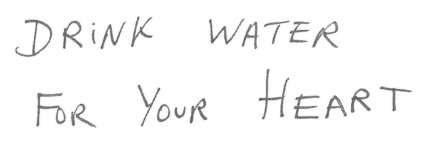

DRINK WATER FOR YOUR HEART

Another water nugget?

Water is so important!

Today it's all about the heart. ♥

If you drink a glass of water right before taking your bath or shower, it helps to lower your blood pressure! ♥

If you drink a glass of water before going to sleep, it helps to prevent a heart attack or stroke in the middle of the night. ♥

Interestingly, one of my mentors, the late Dr. Victor Frank, used to recommend a glass of water before bed to prevent morning low back pain. I say "interestingly" because in his healing system, a lot of low back pain turned out to be what he called "cardiac low back," which meant low back pain that was really being caused by stress on the heart! ♥

If you drink at least 5 glasses of water a day, you can lower your stroke risk by 53%! ♥

It sounds too good to be true, because water is ... well, it's "just" water!

But dehydrated bodies mean thicker blood which is harder to pump and more susceptible to forming clots. So, it's legit.

Love your heart ♥ drink more water!

THE 9 MAGIC WORDS FOR PEACE

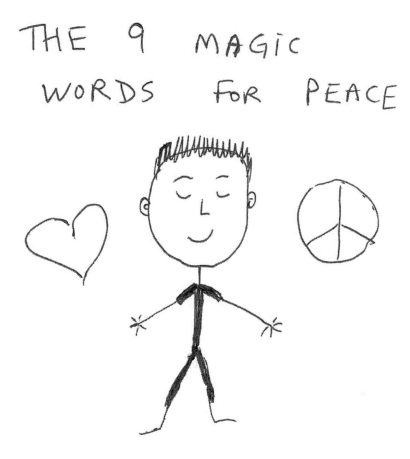

The other day, I was listening to an old podcast by a friend and fellow NET colleague (who suddenly passed away a few years ago), and it inspired today's nugget. The colleague was Dr. Michael Kudlas, and his podcast (Speaking of Health) lives forever online!

In this episode, towards the end, he says that if you're mad at a loved one, and you don't even want to talk to them, then you should take their picture, look at it, and repeat the 9 magic words: **I love you. God bless you. Peace, be still.**

And, he adds, if you can't say the 9 magic words, then try the 11 magic words:
I love you. God bless you. Peace, be still. You jerk.

I thought that maybe Michael made up those words, because he was just that kind of guy!

But turns out, it's a prayer from the Institute for Individual and World Peace (IIWP).

On their website, they recommend that you repeat the simple prayer for yourself.

Take a few deep breaths, put your hand on your heart, and say the words to yourself:
I love you. God bless you. Peace, be still.

And then say it separately out into the world.

When I was a grumpy tween and teen, I used to really hate those annoying hippies and their tie-dye shirts and their peace signs!

I used to run around crossing out the peace signs and replacing them with anarchy signs.

I still prefer black to tie-dye, but... now I say, give peace a chance!

STRETCH YOUR WRISTS!

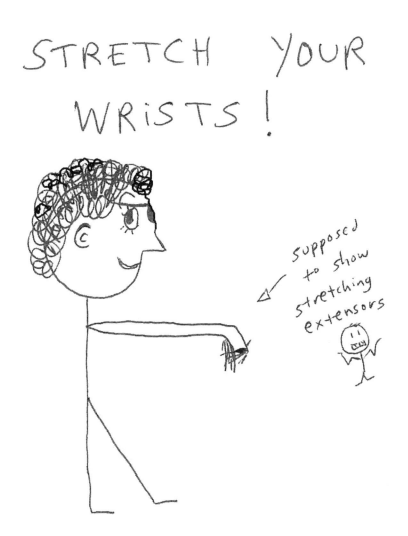

supposed to show stretching extensors

Everyone in Daily Nugget Land could use more wrist stretching!

Typing and tippy-tapping on little devices every day puts a lot of strain on the wrists.

Here are some basic wrist stretches:

Extensor Stretch: stand with your feet shoulder-width apart and, with your elbow extended, lift your arm so that it's parallel to the floor. Bend your wrist so that your palm and fingers are facing downward. Use your other hand to gently pull until you feel the stretch. Hold for about 30 seconds.

Flexor Stretch: stand with your feet shoulder-width apart and, with your elbow extended, lift your arm so that it's parallel to the floor. Bend your wrist so that your fingers are pointing upward. Use your other hand to gently pull the fingers back until you feel the stretch. Hold for about 30 seconds.

NO KNEES OVER THE TOES when...

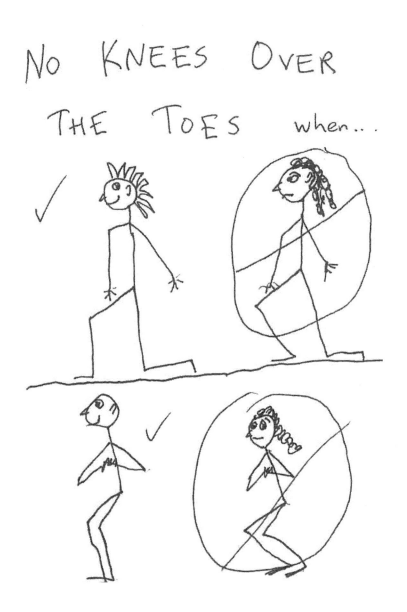

When you are doing exercises such as squats and lunges, don't let your knees go out further than the tips of your toes!

This can put too much stress on your knees and can make you more prone to injury.

And if you're not the kind of person who is doing squats or lunges anyway, this nugget still applies to your life (probably). Do you have stairs in your life? Same rule applies. When you are walking **up** the stairs, pay attention to where your bent knee is in relation to your toes. Is your knee moving way in front of your toes? If so, that's not good for your knees! (Don't think about this when you are going down the stairs, though, as it looks confusing. The biomechanics of coming down the stairs are not the same as in the squats and lunges!)

TURN OUT YOUR FEET AND KNEES WHEN WALKING ON STAIRS!

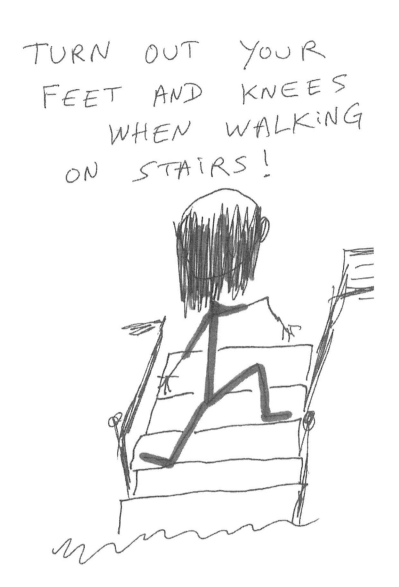

I know, it feels weird at first and it sounds weird, too, but... this is the way to do it if your knees are giving you trouble with stairs!

When going up or down the stairs, turn your feet outward (not pointing straight ahead) and turn your knee outward as well, so that it is pointing in the same direction as the foot. When activating your weight-bearing leg, the muscle that you want to pay attention to is actually your butt muscle (your glutes) - NOT your quads!

You will take pressure off your knees and have a nicer butt, too. 🍑

OLIVE OIL IN THE COFFEE...?

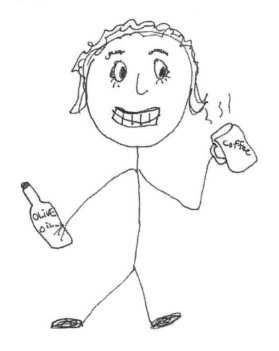

Is it April 1 already? 😵

No, this is for real! Still, I don't expect many of you to adopt it.

I know, the black coffee drinkers are just shaking their heads in disdain anyway since they don't add **ANYTHING** to their coffee...

And I know, the first, next and last question is: WHY?!?!

Well, **WHY** is because most people are a lot healthier when they eliminate dairy from their lives. Even if coffee creamer is the "only" dairy you use, it might be hurting you more than you think!

Years ago, I remember having this argument with a patient who was showing all the signs of dairy sensitivity, but he said it wasn't possible because the **ONLY** dairy he was using was a splash in his coffee. Well for the sake of science, he agreed to stop it for at least a week.

He came in the next week, stunned to report that he had lost more than an inch around his waist just from eliminating that daily splash of dairy!

Olive oil sounds vile, but... it's not as bad as you think! It cuts the bitter acidity of the coffee, and it's a healthy oil. Just don't look at it too hard.

That green oil slick is kind of disturbing to look at.

TAKE THE HOLMES - RAHE STRESS INVENTORY

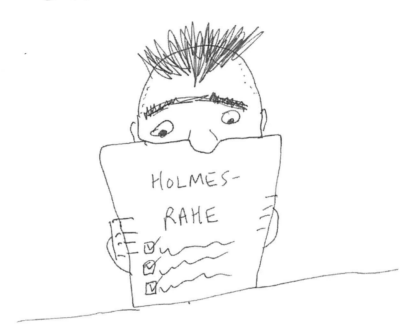

What is the Holmes-Rahe Stress Inventory?

(It sounds boring.)

It's a widely used measure of stress that can accurately predict your odds of experiencing a stress-related health breakdown in the next 2 years!

Why is this a helpful tool for you?

Because sometimes, you don't even notice just how stressed you are until it's too late!

Once in a while, take the Holmes-Rahe Stress Inventory to get a sense of where you're at, objectively.

You can download it for free at https://www.stress.org/holmes-rahe-stress-inventory

Sometimes, you can't do much about the stress.

Life is life! But sometimes, you can get NET, which helps a lot.

And when you can't get NET, don't forget about FAST!

TOWEL ROLL FOR YOUR NECK!

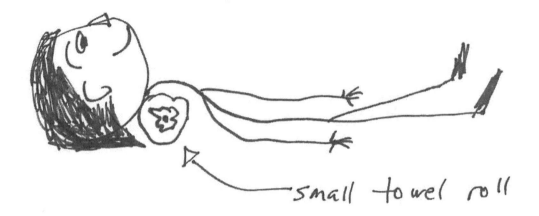

small towel roll

Apparently, my phone thinks that I am spending too much time with my neck in flexion.
(I have to grudgingly admit that it's right.)
It keeps showing me ads for the latest greatest neck cradling device.
It looks an awful lot like the former latest and greatest device...
which looks an awful lot like the **former** former latest and greatest...
because you know why??
Because the human neck is still designed the same as always, and we are still spending too much time in flexion, and the solution is still to spend more time with the neck curved in the direction that it was designed for!
But you really don't need to buy one of these special curved foam things to lay on.
You can still use what my old mentor, Dr. Kerby Landis, was recommending to his patients more than 50 years ago:
A simple towel rolled up and held in place with rubber bands.
It should be a large enough roll that you can feel a gentle stretch in your neck, but it shouldn't be so big that your head is moving back into forward flexion!
Save your money for something more fun! Just use your towel for your neck.

"HUNGRY?"
DRINK A GLASS OF WATER FIRST!

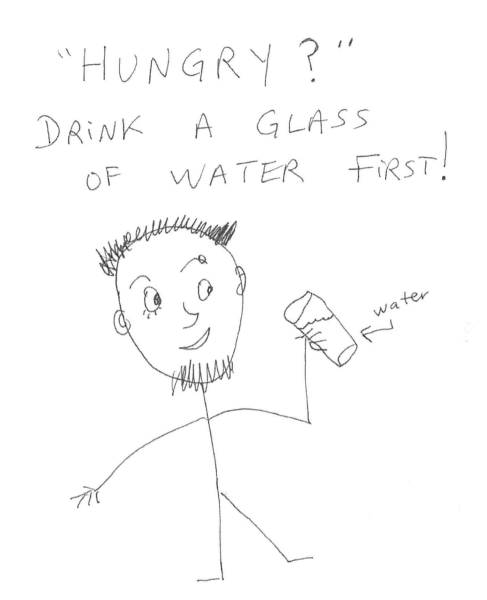

Oftentimes, when you think you are "hungry," your body is really thirsty!

It sounds crazy, but sometimes, the signals feel exactly the same.

So, next time you think you are "hungry," go drink a glass of water, and then wait a few minutes.

If you were really thirsty, then you won't feel hungry anymore!

If you were really hungry, well, then you'll still be hungry.

But you'll be surprised at how often your body was just asking for water.

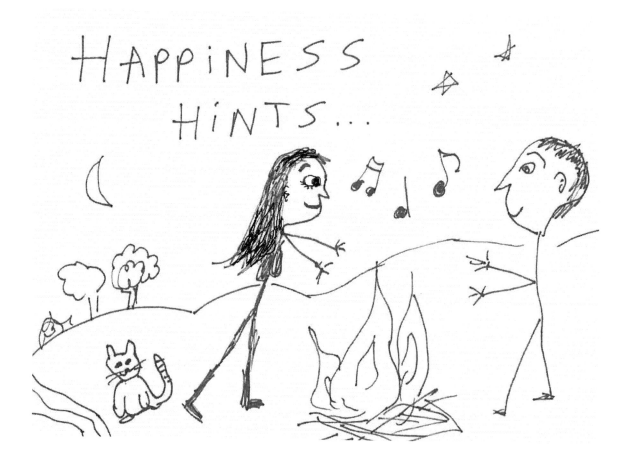

HAPPINESS HINTS...

Surprise!

I just read a great book. 😊

It's called *Spent: Sex, Evolution and Consumer Behavior*, by Geoffrey Miller.

It's basically an evolutionary psychology book about consumerism.

But I really wanted to share a self-inventory that Geoffrey adds at the end of the book. There are lots of components to "happiness," and this book doesn't cover them all, but there are many things that we have evolved to find deeply satisfying, and modern life has eliminated many of them!

So now, to benefit from that long evolution, we have to make a concerted effort.

Apologies in advance for this long "nugget." You don't even have to read the whole list to get the idea.

The idea is, you want to **honestly** write down the number of times in the last month that you have experienced each thing on the list. The goal is to reach at least 100 if you are feeling unhappy with your life. You will probably get the gist of it just by looking at the list!

Here it is:

154

* Rocked a newborn baby to sleep
* Made up a story and told it to a child
* Felt the sunrise warm your face
* Satisfied a genuine hunger by eating ripe fruit
* Satisfied a genuine thirst by drinking cool water
* Shown courage in protecting a child from danger
* Shown leadership and resourcefulness in an emergency
* Shared a meal with parents, siblings or other close relatives
* Gossiped with an old friend
* Made a new friend
* Made something beautiful and gave it to someone
* Repaired something that was broken
* Improved a skill through diligent practice
* Learned something new about a plant or animal that lives near you
* Changed your mind about something important on the basis of new evidence
* Followed good advice from someone older
* Taught a useful skill, charming art, or interesting fact to someone younger
* Petted a furry animal such as a dog, cat or monkey
* Worked with earth, clay, stone, wood, or fiber
* Comforted someone dying
* Walked over a hill and across a stream
* Identified a bird by its song
* Played a significant role in a local ritual, festival, drama or party
* Played a team sport
* Made a physical effort to achieve a collective goal with others
* Sustained silent eye contact with someone to show affection
* Shamed someone who was behaving badly, for the greater good
* Resolved a serious argument using humor, emotional self-control, and social empathy
* Sang, danced, or played instruments with a group of people
* Made a friend laugh out loud
* Reached a world-melting mutual orgasm with a sexual partner
* Experienced sublime beauty that made your hair stand on end
* Applied the Golden Rule by helping someone in need
* Warmed yourself by an open fire under the stars
* Experienced an oceanic sense of oneness with the cosmos that made you think,
  This is how church should feel.

SOAK YOUR FEET !

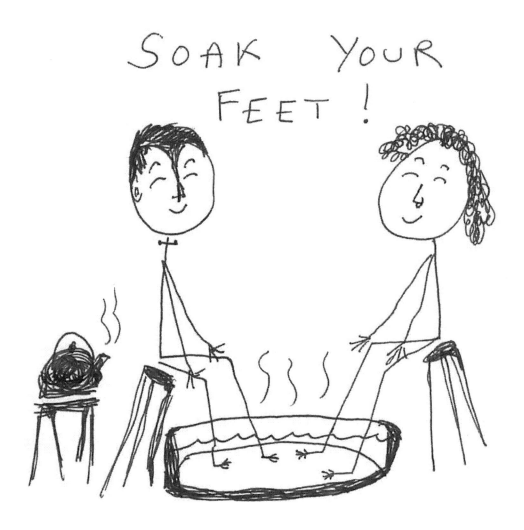

When was the last time you soaked your feet?

I used to do it a lot as a little kid, because I thought it was fancy!

(It annoyed my parents because it made a wet mess on the floor.)

But now that I'm older... much... much... older... it just **feels good!**

You can use a bathtub, a wash basin, or a foot tub.

You can make different types of foot bath depending on what you put in the water.

The simplest one is this:

Add about 1/2 cup of Epsom salts to your warm foot bath.

If you just do the Epsom salts, this will help to relax and soften the foot muscles!

You can take it up one notch by adding a few drops of a relaxing essential oil mixed with a carrier oil and adding it to the bath water.

A nice foot bath should last at least 15 minutes, but you could go as long as an hour. (If you plan to go long, keep some hot water nearby to add to your water to keep it warm.)

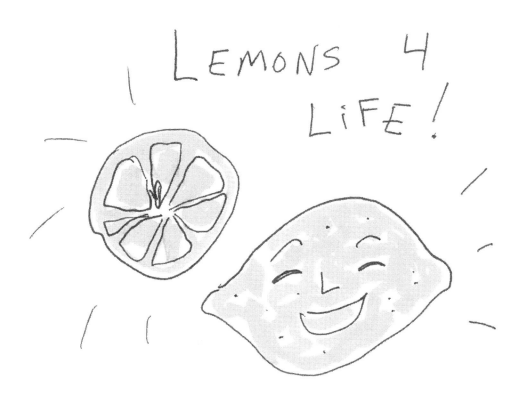

When life gives you lemons... ◌ ◌ ◌
use them!!!

Lemons really are very good for your health.

A simple practice is to start the day with a warm glass of lemon water.

Lemons are high in vitamin C and antioxidants and can help prime the stomach for digestion. They also have a net alkalizing effect on the body, which we need! The typical American diet and lifestyle leaves many people running too acidic, which them causes the body to pull calcium from bones and muscle to bring the pH back to neutral!

Also... lemon is not just a generic scent added to many cleaning products.

It **is** a really good cleaning product!

This is extra great for those of you lucky enough to have big lemon trees in your backyard and more lemons than you know what to do with!

GET A BIDET!

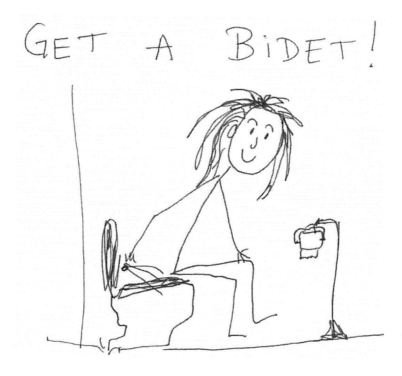

What does using a bidet have to do with your health?? Well, it might not be as big of a deal as getting enough vitamin D or getting your exercise! But any little thing that you can do to improve hygiene or make the world a better place is a good thing. Is it better hygiene than just toilet paper? YES. If you've ever had the unpleasant experience of picking up some dog poop and accidentally getting some on your hands (or changing a messy diaper) would you consider your hand "clean" if you just wiped it with some dry toilet paper? Ew. No. You wouldn't feel clean until you got to wash with some water! But does it make the world a better place? YES. Because (1) you will use a lot less toilet paper, which is better for the environment and will save you some money, too! And (2) most other people in the world use some kind of bidet. Americans are the biggest consumers of toilet paper. By using a bidet, you are connecting in a new way with people all around the world! They are simple to install, and simple ones are just around $35! You can even get little travel bidets for camping or traveling. I got my first bidet during The Great Toilet Paper Crisis of 2020, and I haven't looked back! And lastly... I haven't seen any research on this, but... I bet using a cold-water bidet is good for the vagus nerve, too... just sayin'...

FACE FORWARD FOR [some kinds of] IMPACT!

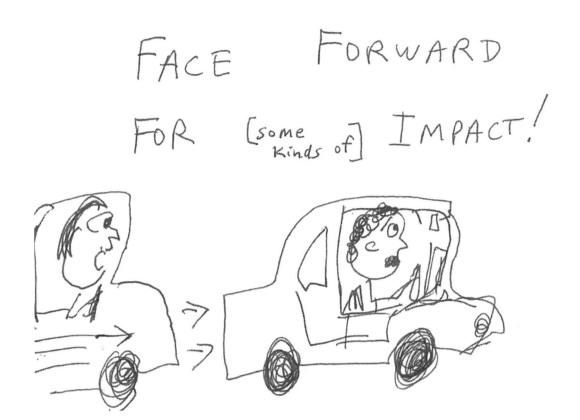

Of course, the best and healthiest thing is to **not** get into any impacts with cars, etc.!

But life is life. When you're about to get rear-ended, you rarely have much time to think about which direction your head is facing.

But if you do have a moment to choose... then choose to face straight ahead! Sit upright with your head against the headrest and as much of your back against the seat as possible.

This is the "best" position in terms of minimizing the injury to your neck, because your head will move in the direction that the joints face, and you will get some whiplash anyway.

But if your head is turned to either side while getting rear-ended, then your neck will whiplash in a direction that is basically "against the grain" of the planes of movement for the vertebrae in your neck, and you will have a much worse injury that will take longer to heal! This is part of why getting T-boned makes for a worse injury than getting rear-ended.

By the same principal, if you feel a sneeze coming on, try and keep your head facing forward.

If you don't have a hanky to sneeze into, then bring your elbow up to your face rather than twisting your neck too far down to your elbow. If you need to turn away from other people, then turn your whole body away so that your neck can be in a straight line and not twisted. Sneezing puts a lot of pressure on the discs! (This is why sneezing is so painful if you have a bulging or a ruptured disc, and it's why sometimes a big sneeze can *cause* a disc bulge!)

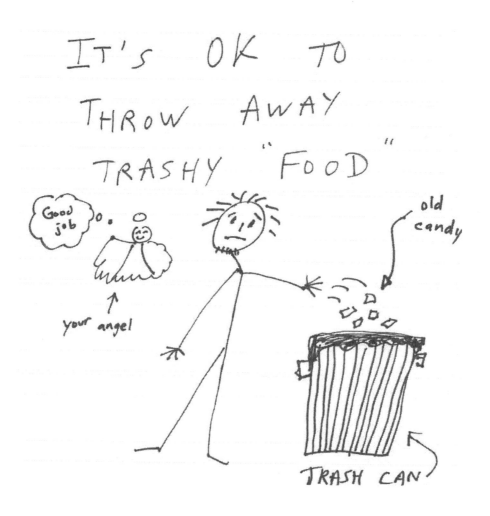

I dunno if this happens to anyone else, but... I often have a ton of leftover candy after Halloween and no matter what my "intentions" are or were, I usually end up eating a lot of it. The good stuff vanishes first, of course! And by the end, it's just a sad little bucket of plain Hershey's mini bars and lots of lemon and orange Starbursts! From childhood, I was always taught to never waste food. So, I would eventually eat every last lemon Starburst and waxy plain Hershey's chocolate! But finally... I was able to just pour the dish of sad candy into the trash. Yeah, yeah, I shouldn't have bought it in the first place if it's so bad. I know, I know! But, once it's done, if you are afflicted with the "don't ever waste food" voice, remember this. It's not **really** *food.* It gives you zero nutrition. (Or if it does, it's negated by the resources it's taking away!) It does nothing whatsoever nice for your dental work. It won't help you sleep better. It won't make you happy (for more than a few seconds?) If it vanished mysteriously, you wouldn't actually be "missing out" on *anything!*

So... it's OK to throw it away.

LET YOUR LIGHT SHINE ... EVEN IF IT'S JUST A LITTLE BLINKY LIGHT....!

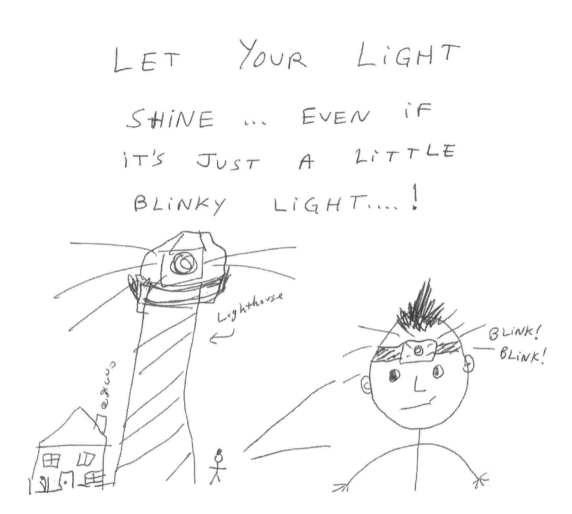

You hear a lot about the various shades of darkness overcoming the world these days... amiright? And you also probably hear about how you just gotta let your light shine! Maybe like a big powerful lighthouse in the darkness! Or at least a bright steady candle in the window? Honestly... some days... you're doing good to just get out of bed and bathe and show up at all! Yes? Well, good news! All kinds of light can be seen in the darkness. Even a tiny ass LED blinky light! So when you can't summon the power to shine like the sun, at least shine like a blinky light, shooting enough light into the world to help someone somewhere somehow, even just a little. You can even use it as a mental mantra when you're walking down the street and don't know what else to focus on:

I'm a blinky light in this world of darkness...

I'm a blinky light of love...

I'm a blinky light of The Light...

My blinky is eternal...

Amen.

161

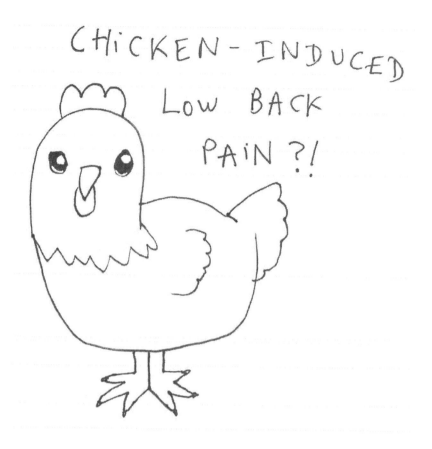

CHICKEN - INDUCED LOW BACK PAIN ?!

Chicken-induced low back pain? Come on now. Are we scraping the bottom of the nuggets barrel?? No, it's true! This particular type of low back pain tends to hit women, who are more sensitive to the intense hormone content of most commercially grown chickens in the United States! (For some reason, chicken also tends to adversely affect people with type B blood. I don't know that I totally buy the current reasoning behind it, but... it's a thing!) So, if you happen to eat a lot of chicken AND have a lot of mysterious low back pain, consider eliminating the chicken from your diet. Same with if you have type B blood and are currently eating a lot of chicken. Is "free-range," "hormone free, " etc. better? Yes, of course, it is! But I would eliminate chicken all together if you are trying to figure out whether it's affecting you. This is because what a label says and what the truth is can be... let's say... complicated in the U.S.

And yes, I learned to draw this chicken by watching a "how to draw a chicken" video on YouTube!

THE EPLEY MANEUVER FOR VERTIGO

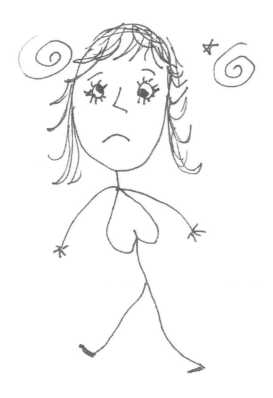

Most people experience vertigo (dizziness) at some point in their lives.
Sometimes you know what caused it - like if you ate an entire certain kind of brownie even though you were forewarned that it was no ordinary brownie and that you should only eat a little bit of it! - and sometimes, you have no idea what caused it. 😵
And for this reason, everyone should know about The Epley Maneuver.
One of the most common forms of vertigo (called benign paroxysmal positional vertigo or BPPV) is caused when a teeny tiny crystal inside of your ear dislodges and lands inside the little curly tube, causing you to feel dizzy, especially when you move in certain directions!
The Epley maneuver is a simple way of getting that crystal to roll out of the curly tube. If the dizziness feels a little better after doing the maneuver, then do it again! You may need to do it a few times to get full relief. If the Epley maneuver does not help at all, then you may need to get to a doctor to find out what's causing it! You don't want to mess around if it's an infection or something worse!

163

Here are the basics of how to do the home version of the Epley maneuver:
(You may find it helpful to watch a video of the home Epley maneuver first.)
Your healthcare provider can tell how often to do this procedure. They may ask you to do it 3 times a day until your symptoms have been gone for 24 hours. They will also tell if your right or left ear is causing your symptoms.

Follow these steps if the problem is with your right ear:
* Start by sitting on a bed.
* Turn your head 45 degrees to the right.
* Quickly lie back, keeping your head turned. Your shoulders should now be on the pillow, and your head should be reclined. Wait 30 seconds.
* Turn your head 90 degrees to the left, without raising it. Your head will now be looking 45 degrees to the left. Wait another 30 seconds.
* Turn your head and body another 90 degrees to the left, into the bed. Wait another 30 seconds.
* Sit up on the left side.

Follow these steps if the problem is with your left ear:
* Start by sitting on a bed.
* Turn your head 45 degrees to the left.
* Quickly lie back, keeping your head turned. Your shoulders should now be on the pillow, and your head should be reclined. Wait 30 seconds.
* Turn your head 90 degrees to the right, without raising it. Your head will now be looking 45 degrees to the right. Wait another 30 seconds.
* Turn your head and body another 90 degrees to the right, into the bed. Wait another 30 seconds.
* Sit up on the right side.

IF YOUR DENTIST SAYS TO WEAR A NIGHT GUARD.... DO IT!

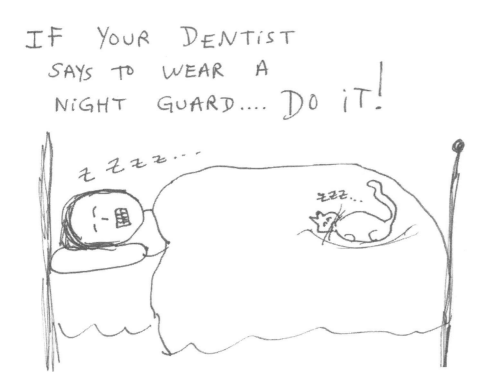

Having to wear a night guard or retainer when you go to bed is not one of the sexier things in life. But if your dentist says you need to do it, then DO IT!!! You may think it's only for cosmetic reasons -- to keep your teeth in alignment after expensive orthodontia or to keep them from wearing down into creepy little nubs - but there are plenty of other reasons to wear them! The obvious thing for the night guard is that you don't want to crack and eventually shatter your teeth from all that intense night grinding! Replacement teeth are expensive, and just leaving the spaces blank is not good for your future health. You need your teeth for chewing your food - obviously - and they are a part of the structural integrity of your head. One creepy fact that I did not know until adulthood is that everyone starts to lose bone density in their jaw starting around age 30! 💀 And that is why old people seem to all have crooked lower teeth even though they looked normal in their younger years! It's thanks to the bone loss. So, if your dentist recommends a retainer to keep those teeth in place, then wear that. And if you are losing bone density, don't just consider your calcium intake, but remember to keep your vitamin D levels up! And listen to your dentist!
(And remember that tooth grinding is almost always tied to *stress* and possible liver/gallbladder issues. Are you getting your NET?)

"I CAN'T DRINK WATER" = maybe COPPER toxicity

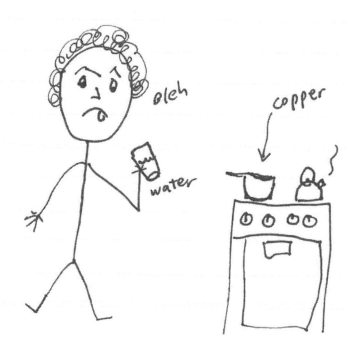

Here's a weird symptom you may have (though of course I hope you don't).

You "can't" drink water - you can only tolerate sips of it at a time.

If this is happening to you, and you have copper pipes, copper cookware and/or use copper-based algaecides in your pool or hot tub, then you might be experiencing copper toxicity!

In this case, eliminate the copper source - stop drinking water from those pipes, stop using that cookware, use a different algaecide - and add nutrition that can counter the effects. That means adding zinc, sulfur-bearing amino acids (like those found in eggs, onion and garlic), vitamin C, iron and pectin. Symptoms should be better within 3-4 weeks.

Water is so important! If there is any reason that you "can't" tolerate it, get it figured out! Copper water bottles are kind of trendy in certain health circles. While they **can** be used safely, they can also cause a lot of problems - **especially** if the water you put into them is even slightly acidic! (Note: San Francisco water is clean, but it is slightly acidic.)

TRAVEL SUPPLEMENTS — THE ESSENTIALS!

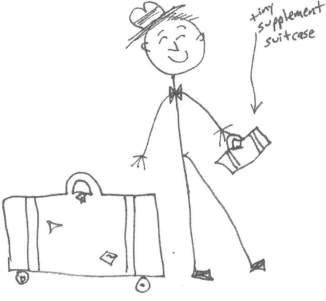

tiny supplement suitcase

Should you pack supplements when you travel? **YES!** Even if you are traveling within the country, travel food is just not as good as home food, so you will need some support. But if you're traveling internationally. then you **definitely** want to pack some supplements! Because even if their food is "clean," you will be exposed to foreign microbes that your body is just not used to handling. And if you're only there for a short visit, you won't have time to adapt. And you don't want to waste your vacation time feeling sick and running to the bathroom in a panic! OK... this is a long one.

#1 basic supplement to pack for domestic or foreign travel:

A good digestive enzyme. When it comes to foreign travel, you will want to bring one that has added hydrochloric acid (HCl or betaine HCl). The extra acid will help to break down foods and some critters that you are not accustomed to. Travel is stressful, too, and your body tends to lower stomach acid production under stress. Examples of good acid-enhancing digestive enzyme supplements are Hydro-zyme (Biotics Research) and Zypan (Standard Process).

#2: basic immune support supplement for domestic or foreign travel. Most of the people I know who caught COVID despite precautions at home caught it while traveling! There's no getting around it: traveling involves passing in close proximity to tons of strangers in a stressful and crowded environment. COVID or not, you don't want to get sick while traveling. Immune supplements could include antioxidants like vitamin D and vitamin C, or zinc, anti-virals like L-Lysine, and glandular extracts like spleen and thymus extracts. I am fan of blends, such as Bio-FCTS (Biotics Research) or Congaplex (Standard Process).

#3: additional **anti-microbial / anti-parasite support** for international travel. The #1 consistently effective product I have found for this purpose is TriGuard Plus (Oxygen Nutrition). It is a liquid, and you can take it directly, or put a dropper full into a glass of water. While traveling in a foreign country, drink 1-2 glasses of this TriGuard water a day, and even consider mixing some into the water that you use to rinse when brushing your teeth! We've used this even on group trips to India and China where everyone else on the trip got sick except for the people using the TriGuard Plus! This is not a supplement that you would use daily under normal circumstances, as it works to specifically kill things as opposed to building up things (like vitamin D, etc.) If you are traveling to a place where parasite risk is high, then bring some kind of oregano oil supplement (such as A.D.P. from Biotics Research) to take daily.

#4: a **fiber supplement** if you will not have access to enough fresh fruits and vegetables. No one wants to be constipated on vacation! Remember, though, if you take a fiber supplement, you need to take it with a bunch of water! Bottled water is best when traveling to foreign countries.

#5: Not everyone needs this, but, if you are prone to constipation and ensuing hemorrhoids, then **Collinsonia Root** is your friend. This is a great herb for blood vessel support. Standard Process has a very clean and potent formulation.

#6: ER 911, Allergy Remedy and **Day & Night Vitals.** These NET homeopathic remedies can be a lifesaver when traveling! The ER 911 helps with any stress (airport stress, turbulence stress, etc.) and the Allergy remedy helps if you are sensitive to the various chemicals, cleaners, pollens, etc. that are unfamiliar to your system. The Day & Night Vitals remedy was specifically designed to help with jet lag, and it can help you to acclimate to the new time zone and get back to normal when you come home! And that sums it up! You can add more and go crazy, but those are the basics. If you are traveling and planning to drink more alcohol and/or eat more rich foods than usual, then it's also smart to pack a liver support supplement, such as Livaplex (Standard Process).

For individualized specifics, you can always e-mail me or call/text the office (415-864-2975) for a video consultation.

Happy traveling!

FOR ANY TOUGH TASK, FIND AN ACCOUNTABILITY BUDDY!

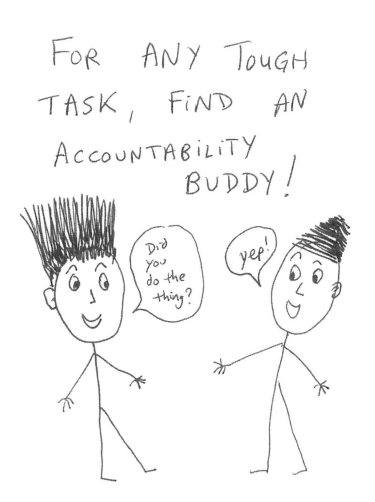

It's hard to do hard things! And sometimes, it's hard to do "easy" or "simple" things, too!
Why is it soooooo hard to do "simple" things that we know are "good for" us?!?!
It's because we are fighting deep and primitive automatic impulses.
So, to overcome the urges, we can use OTHER deep and primitive impulses to help us in the battle!
Such as: the deep and primitive impulse to gain approval from someone we like and respect.
Enter: the accountability buddy.
It can be someone who signs up for an exercise class with you and makes sure that you go every time (or else pay them a penalty fee).
It can be having lunch with someone who is also trying to follow the same kind of diet as you.
It can be sitting with someone on zoom or Facetime while you are just both sitting there working on a writing project without clicking over to distracting places!
Some of you have complimented me on my consistency with putting out the Daily Nugget.
Well, guess what?
I have a bunch of accountability buddies.

YOU!

Once upon a time, I just had the idea for daily health nuggets.

Then I procrastinated until one day I mentioned it on my blog and created a sign-up form.

I didn't think that anyone would read it or notice, much less sign up for it!

And I figured that would buy me some time to create the nuggets.

But then someone signed up! 😵 (Hi, Barbara!)

And I had to scramble and make a nugget to send out!

And then someone else signed up! (Hi, JC!)

And then TWO people were counting on me for these daily nuggets!

So, even if I don't feel like it, I always have to stay ahead of the curve - ahead of Barbara and JC! - to keep up the appearance of smooth sailing. 😄

And now I have all of you, and here we are, on nugget #158!

Find an accountability buddy, and step by step, you will get your thing done!

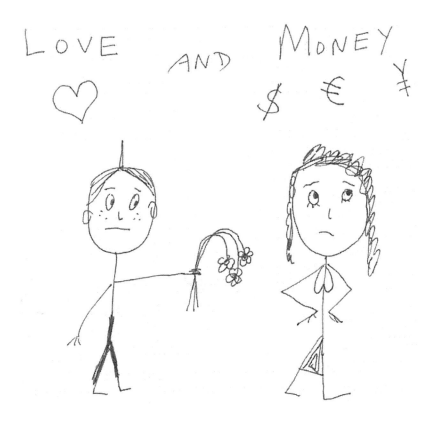

Stress is a huge underlying cause of sickness and dis-ease, right? And what's a huge cause of stress? LOVE and MONEY!!! In NET, we say, "There's two things in life, love and money..." But isn't it weird how sometimes we think that we are "just not good at" love or money...and yet... we didn't bother to learn very much about them except through trial and error??? For some reason, it doesn't occur to us that maybe we should study and practice those things if we want to be good at them. Maybe we shouldn't count on magical thinking to save the day in these areas that are so important to a healthy life. 🤓 I like books as a starting point. So here are a couple of book recommendations for studying LOVE: *The Art of Loving*, by Erich Fromm and *Love Unf*cked*, by Gary John Bishop. And since we are big Enneagram fans around here, here is a great money book written by an accountant who noticed that different Enneagram types tend to have different money problems! Plus, this book tackles money AND love! Money: *From Fear to Love: Using the Enneagram to Create Wealth, Prosperity, and Love*, by Margaret H. Smith, PhD. and here's a great MONEY book: *I Will Teach You to Be Rich, Second Edition: No Guilt. No Excuses. No BS. Just a 6-Week Program That Works*, by Ramit Sethi

Love and Money will always be challenging to one degree or another but isn't it nice to have new and different challenges in those areas, and not the same old same old?!

171

WRITE DOWN YOUR GOALS!

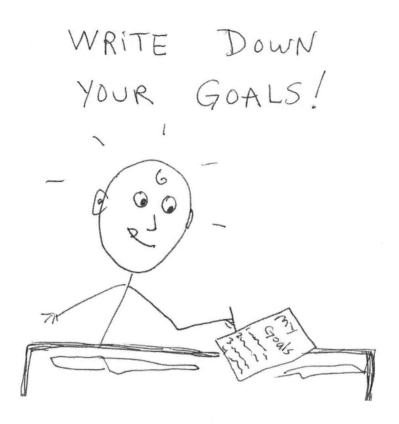

Write down your health goals? Sure! Write down all your goals! I know, I know, it's such a pain to keep track of **one more thing**. But you know what's weird about this whole goal-writing thing?? There are studies that show that writing down your goals makes a difference even if you never look at it again! Writing it down helps to get it into your brain.

And then your brain does the rest. Obviously, if you are serious about reaching a goal, you have to do more than just write it down to make it happen! But writing them down helps... a lot! Once a year - usually January 1 because why not - I like to write a list of 100 things I'd like to do that year. I've never achieved **all** the things in a year, but even when I forget about a list and return to it the next year, guess what? I usually achieve at least half of the list!

And you know what else is weird? In school, if you get 50% on a test, that's a big fat F! But on your 100 goals list, if you achieve 50 goals, it's like, "Holy shit, I achieved 50 goals this year! Yay me!" 😊 🙆 🎉 But to reach a lot of goals, make a long list. And don't be afraid to add "easy" things that you'd like to achieve, but just never have. For example, "Walk all the way across the Golden Gate Bridge." or "Learn to play one new sport, like pickleball." or "Go bowling with my friends." You get the idea! And yes, it's OK to put your list onto a Google spreadsheet or something. It doesn't have to be paper.

L - LYSINE
The Unsung Hero of Anti-virals!

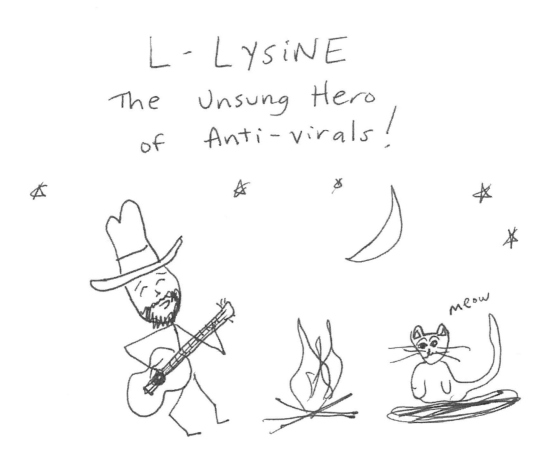

If this were Family Feud, and the question was, "name a supplement you take when you're sick," then you would slap your hand on the buzzer and yell, "VITAMIN C!!!"

And, probably, it would the #1 answer!

Everyone thinks about vitamin C.

But you know what might not even be on the board but should be? (Even more than vitamin C, in my opinion!)

L-LYSINE.

L-lysine is an essential amino acid (meaning that your body cannot synthesize it and needs to take it in) which plays a big role in immune health, among other things! It is widely used to fight common viral infections, such as herpes. (Lip balms, etc. for cold sore usually contain L-Lysine to speed healing).

I think this is the part where I'm supposed to say, "As far as dosing is concerned, speak to your doctor!"

Ehem.

But something else that people should really know is that if you are fighting something that can benefit from L-Lysine, then you will want to **avoid foods that are high in arginine**, which is like the body's counterbalance to lysine. The body needs both, but in certain ratios!

So, foods to AVOID (high arginine foods) include things like chocolate, nuts, and dairy. (I once had a friend who was struggling to get rid of a cold sore - and her stress-eating food of choice was chocolate peanut butter cups! No wonder she couldn't get rid of them!)

Foods that are high in lysine include eggs, meat, fish, spirulina, and tofu. But if you are trying to get a therapeutic dose, then supplements are the way to go.

I don't carry many supplements in stock anymore, but I always carry a good quality L-Lysine. My favorite brand for this particular product is DeeCee Labs. It has an added boost due the glandular components it contains, so - warning - it is not vegetarian friendly!

And the cowboy in today's drawing is singing an ode to L-Lysine. And that cat is listening because they make L-Lysine treats for cats! (Cats are susceptible to a type of herpes virus that shows up as cloudy eyes. My cat had it, and we would give him some L-Lysine treats and his eyes would clear up within a day or so. Worked way better - and way more economically - than the prescribed kitty anti-viral eye drops!)

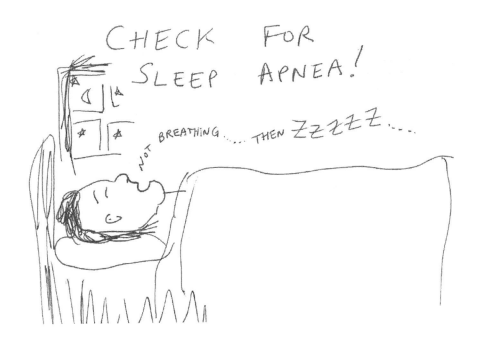

Sleep apnea is no joke. It's the name of the condition where people stop breathing for a few moments (or longer) while they are asleep. If you have it, you probably don't know about it! After all, it happens while you're asleep. If you are a snorer, then you are more likely to have it than a non-snorer. If you sleep alone, you might not even know if or how bad you snore! But if you snore, or feel tired and sluggish when you wake up, or have brain fog, and **certainly** if you have a partner who has noticed that you sometimes stop breathing while you sleep, then pleeeeease go get checked for sleep apnea! These days, you don't even have to go into a weird lab overnight. They can test for it by sending you home with a small device to wear while you sleep! Aside from feeling like crap while you're awake, what's so bad about sleep apnea? Well, for one thing, it can kill you! As you know, I'm a pretty "death positive" person. We all have to go sometime somehow, so that can't be helped. But! I really hate it when good people die prematurely of **avoidable things**! One of the most awesome and creative people I ever knew, my old neighbor Lisa Snare, died suddenly one night from sleep apnea. She went to sleep, and she didn't wake up. And another person I know had a stroke in the middle of the night thanks to sleep apnea! Anyway... don't put it off and don't be afraid of the treatments (such as CPAP machines, etc.). Just take it one step at a time. Breathing and sleep are two of **the most important components of life**.

So, check yourself out and/or keep pestering that stubborn snoring partner of yours!

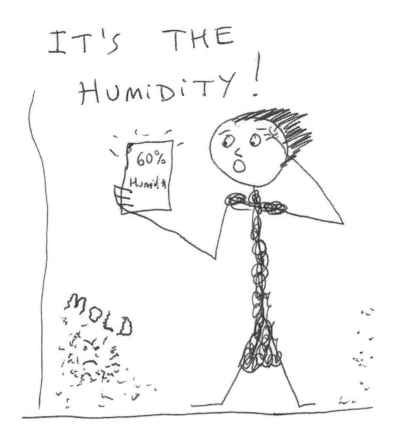

Humidity matters! Maybe you are lucky enough to live in a place where it's an even 40-50% humidity all the time, but, if you're not, then you need to pay attention! One of the most awful things in the world of health challenges is **mold**! Mold can be relatively benign like that green bread mold. Or it can be that nasty black mold that gets into your house and requires professional cleanup! And if you've ever had a mold infection inside of your body, then you know what a nightmare it can be to get rid of it! As with many nasties, prevention is best. What's one way to prevent mold in your home? Keep the humidity in the right zone! The ideal humidity zone for health is between 30-50%. Mold can grow starting at around 55%. San Francisco (where I spend most of my time) can be a pretty damp city, especially in the foggy season! I once lived in an apartment where the shadier north-facing room would sometimes hit 65-75% humidity! Ew. And yes, it was prone to growing mold on the cold wall that was made of cinder block behind the paint. I got a good dehumidifier and never had a mold problem in that room again! How do you know what the humidity is in your home? You get a little humidity monitor for about 10 bucks! And on the rare occasion when your home is too **dry** (maybe in those cold states where you have to run the heater all winter?) then it helps to have a humidifier, especially near your bed, so that you can sleep comfortably.

176

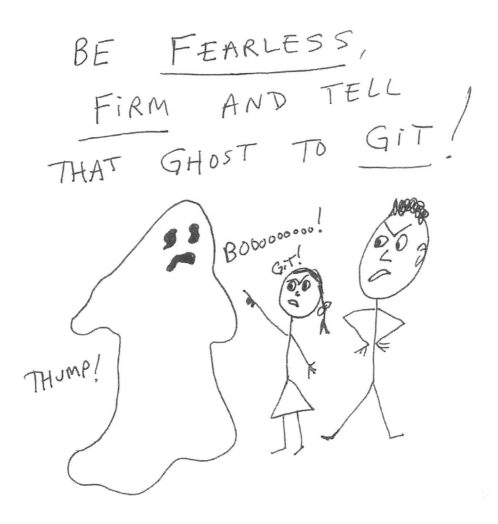

OK... so, why is this ghost fighting advice in the Daily Nugget??? It's mainly because **sleep** is such an important part of health, and... sometimes... for some people... in some old houses... in some old cities... ghosts [and stuff] can really mess with a peaceful night's sleep! Now, if you're hearing voices and stuff like that, make sure to get a mental health evaluation first. Schizophrenia is a thing. But if it **is** something like a ghost, then it may or may not help to burn sage (with the windows open) and use assorted prayers, trinkets, etc., but... the bottom line is a firm, fearless, direct order for the thing to get out! Git! Sometimes even a big ol' fashioned GTFO! And if it's just too scary for you, then you need to find someone to come in who **can** be firm, fearless, and direct. Remember, those things don't belong in our usual mundane day-to-day time and space. Even if they used to be people like us. (I guess this topic popped into mind because I've been listening to the **Spooked!** podcast lately. It's so good!)

EAT THINGS THAT ROT, BUT ... EAT THEM BEFORE THEY DO!

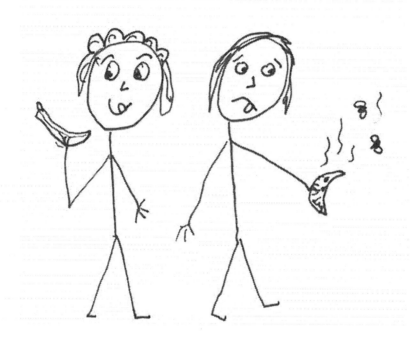

Here is one of the simplest health nuggets of all time!
Eat foods that rot but eat them before they do!
Pretty sure I read this in Michael Pollan's book, *Food Rules*.
I'm a hearty endorser of Michael Pollan's books in general!
And that really is it for today.
Simple! 😊 🧑

EXFOLIATE YOUR HINEY

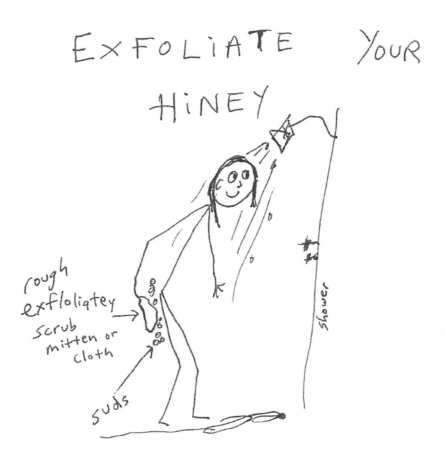

rough exfloliatey scrub mitten or cloth

suds

shower

Did you know that "hiney" is NOT a valid Scrabble word??? Even though everyone knows that it means butt??? Anyway... I wasn't sure what word to use because I don't exactly just mean butt for this one. I mean the whole part of your backside (including upper legs) that sits flat in a chair for hours and hours every day. Fortunately, not all of you do spend hours and hours sitting in one position! But some of you do. And if you're hairy (hello, fellas) you may run into this annoying and potentially dangerous (!) problem. If you have hairy legs and/or buttocks AND you sit for hours and hours a day, then you are vulnerable to ingrown hairs or blocked hair follicles, which can become infected, and potentially become large cysts or abscesses! Large cysts can be just painful and annoying and embarrassing, but if they progress to abscesses, then they can even lead to sepsis and become lethal! You think I am being dramatic? Dude. I just watched a documentary in which a guy **died** from sepsis from a butt abscess that he never got checked or treated (probably because it was too embarrassing)! (The documentary was **not** about the butt abscess, but I was just like... OMG, what a tragically ridiculous way to die!) I also have patients (so far, all men) who have had to take antibiotics and/or get the things drained by medical professionals because they waited too long - again, because it's embarrassing. This problem is almost always preventable with regular exfoliating. You can either do this with good regular scrubbing with a rough cloth, loofah, etc. or with a chemical exfoliant (which usually contains a mild acid).

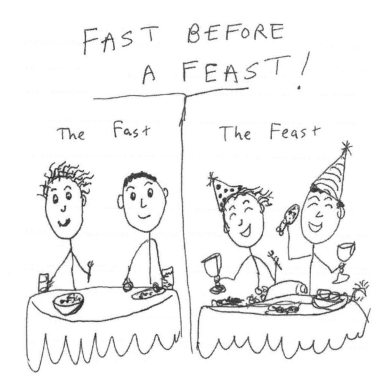

FAST BEFORE A FEAST!

The Fast | The Feast

Back in my Russian Orthodox days (yes, I officially converted to Russian Orthodoxy in my early 20s) I did a lot of fasting - and feasting! The Orthodox really know how to **FEAST!** (Any town with a big Greek Orthodox church can also attest to this.) But there was never a feast without a fast, and the bigger the feast, the bigger and longer the fast! Psychologically and emotionally, this made the occasion of the feast even more intense and wonderful! But also, it made for a culturally built-in check against going too crazy on rich foods for extended periods of time. It also matched a more "natural" way of eating, if you consider human history. For most of our history, day-to-day eating was simple, probably mostly vegetarian, and then once in a while, when you got lucky, you got to feast! It's only recently that humans have been able to feast at will -- and that is still not true in many countries or socioeconomic groups! So next time you have a big feast coming up - holidays, birthday, wedding, etc. - consider making an effort to eat light and drink only water in the days leading up to the feast. It's not about vanity or losing weight or whatever. Give it a try and see how you feel. How do you feel emotionally during the fast? How do you feel during the feast? How was it different from the usual? How did your body (and brain) feel after the feast? NOTE: For this context, **I don't** mean a severe fast like a water fast or a juice fast! It's a terrible idea to go to a feast right after **that** kind of fast! I mean just eating very simple and very light.

LINGERING COUGH?
RUB CHAPMAN'S REFLEXES!

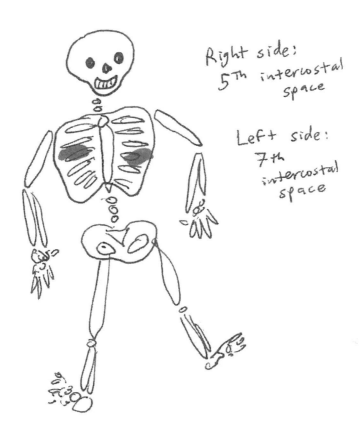

Right side:
5Th intercostal space

Left side:
7th intercostal space

OK...first of all, this image is not anatomically accurate (I know!) and also... the skeleton's right foot did not get blown up by a tiny landmine. I just got anxious and sloppy at the end of the sketching! So, what are Chapman's reflexes? Dr. Frank Chapman was an osteopath in the 1920s who discovered a system of neurolymphatic (some people say somatovisceral) reflexes in the body that could be used to help speed the healing process. For example, the points we're talking about today (the thymus and the spleen) are used for improving immune responses. Ever get one of those lingering coughs that is hard to shake even after you've recovered from a cold or other pesky illness?

You can often speed that cough along its way by massaging the Chapman's reflex points for the thymus gland and the spleen.

The reflex point for the thymus is located on the right side of the chest, in between the 5th intercostal space. That means you start up at your collarbone and feel around for the first rib

181

you can feel, and then count the spaces in between the ribs until you get down to the 5th one. If your body wants/needs this point stimulated, there's a good chance that it will be sore once you find it! That's usually your big clue that you're on the right spot!

The Chapman's reflex point for the spleen us on the left side of the body, in the 7th intercostal space. So, yes, counting down from the top, find the 7th space. Again, this point will probably be sore if you need to massage it.

How long do you massage it? For about a minute.

Usually, Chapman's reflexes are rubbed for about 15-20 seconds, however, for this lingering cough, they usually need to be massaged for longer! Do this a few times a day, and you will notice that the points will become less tender as the cough gets better and better.

So, upon further research, the thymus point mentioned here does not appear to be one of Chapman's originals! But this is what I learned from the late great Dr. Wally Schmidt, who trained under the late great Dr. George Goodheart. And they work in practice! So... so there.

CHIA GEL!

for hydration,
fiber, protein and more!

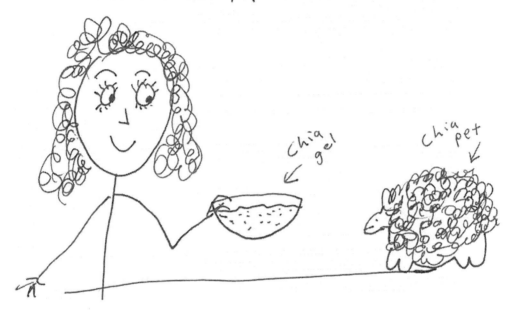

(Is anyone else here old enough to hear the Chia Pet commercial song in your head when you read the subject line today?) Well, today, we're talking about chia gel.

Those of you who just can't handle slimy / gel textures in your food, well, I guess you're off the hook for today's nugget. But if you can handle it, then you can get a lot of benefit from chia gel! Chia seeds can absorb almost 10 times their weight in water!

To make chia gel, you add about 9 parts water to 1 part chia seeds and wait about 5 minutes for the magic to happen!

Now... why would you want to do this?

Well, for one thing, ingesting a gel like this helps to support hydration, because the body absorbs the water more slowly. (This is why adding chia seeds to your smoothie is a good idea when it comes to improving your hydration!)

You can mix the chia gel with just about any beverage to add some flavor, or even just add some lemon and a dash of sweetener for a little snack.

Chia seeds are also an excellent source of protein, fiber, omega-3 fatty acids and more!

TAKE ADVANTAGE OF HEALTH TECH. !

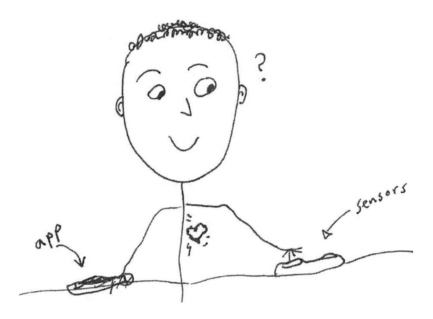

Most of the people reading this e-mail are already using some kind of health tech, such as a smartwatch.

Are you getting the most out of it?

Are you only looking at the numbers before and after working out?

Do you look at your health info (heart rate, heart rate variability, etc.) before and after stressful events? What surprising patterns do you see?

It was a home EKG monitor (KardiaMobile) that first detected the atrial fibrillation that I wrote about in my book, *The Issues are in the Tissues*. Without it, who knows how long it would have taken me to drag myself to the ER rather than try and sleep it off or something?! Prevention and early detection are key with so many things - especially heart stuff! - so take advantage of living in the age of easy techno-self-health-monitoring!

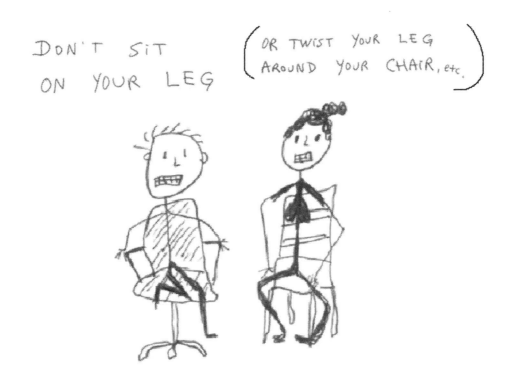

DON'T SIT ON YOUR LEG (OR TWIST YOUR LEG AROUND YOUR CHAIR, etc.)

(Who knew that it would be so hard to draw people sitting badly in chairs?!)
Some of you have some very strange ways of sitting in chairs. I know that this probably begins because you have to spend so much time in the chair, and it gets really boring! But time spent with your legs in exotic positions - like bent underneath your butt on an office chair or twisted around the legs of a chair - can really do a number on your knees! This is especially true if you have any history of injury to your knees. Sometimes it feels "OK" to sit in these weird positions, but any prolonged time spent in an unnatural position is putting strain on ligaments, and over time, those ligaments won't snap back to their old shape. Even just sitting cross-legged for a long period of time can put undue strain on the knee and can cause pain or injury once you do stand up! This is an extreme case, but... I have a friend who once managed to separate and injure his pubic symphysis (that tiny joint right at the center of the pubic bone) just by attempting to cross his legs while sitting in an awkwardly high chair! If you have chronic trouble with your knees or hips but are not sure "why," take a close look at what you're sitting or standing in/on for most of the day and what your body position is like during that time! It's best **not** to sit too much in the first place, but if you must, be kind to your knees!

185

SHOP FOR SHOES AT THE END OF THE DAY!

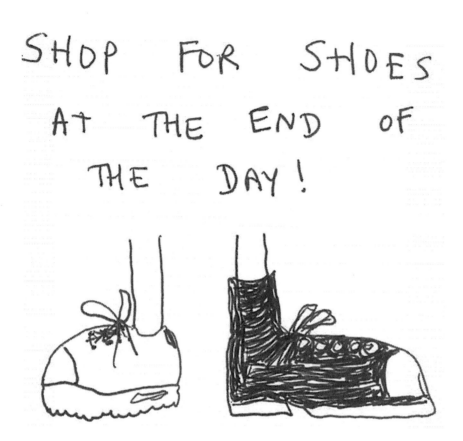

Why does it matter what time of day you shop for shoes?!

Well-fitting shoes are important to the health of your entire frame!

One of the mistakes that many people make when buying shoes is that they buy shoes that are too tight. Tight shoes worn for too long can contribute to joint deformations and injuries. And, since the feet tend to expand slightly over the course of the day, you will find the best fitting shoes if you try them on late in the day, with the socks that you are most likely to wear most often in those shoes.

Also, many people have one foot that is slightly larger or smaller than the other one! If you are one of these people, and you can only afford to buy one pair of shoes, then choose shoes that are a better fit for the bigger foot!

IF YOU HAVE A
SHOULDER INJURY,
KEEP YOUR ARMS & HANDS
IN FRONT OF YOU!

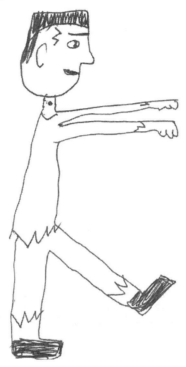

No, you DON'T have to go full Frankenstein's monster, but... that's just the image that popped into my mind. If you are healing from a shoulder injury, your "window of activity" is basically right in front of you. You can do lightweight activities such as typing on a keyboard or chopping vegetables. Even though it's good to exercise and stretch, it's usually NOT a good idea to stretch injured areas - especially if the injury involves ligaments! Here are some "don'ts" for shoulder injuries: **DON'T** reach into the backseat of the car! **DON'T** reach behind you in general! **NO** push-ups or bench presses! **NO** yoga! **NO** Pilates or rowing machine! **NO** butterfly exercises. **DON'T** sleep on your stomach or your back with your arms above your head! **DON'T** lean on your elbows while at your desk, while lying in bed, on the couch or in the car! Sometimes, if you are healing from a shoulder injury, you might even need to sleep on your side with a thin pillow under your waist and 2 pillows under your head and neck to give more space for the shoulder! (If your shoulder has been injured for a long time and is just not healing, you may consider looking internally and asking yourself, could it be my **liver**? Sugar handling issue? Food sensitivity? These are common hidden causes of chronic shoulder problems!)

PREPARE TO DIE!

(for a better LiFE ☺)

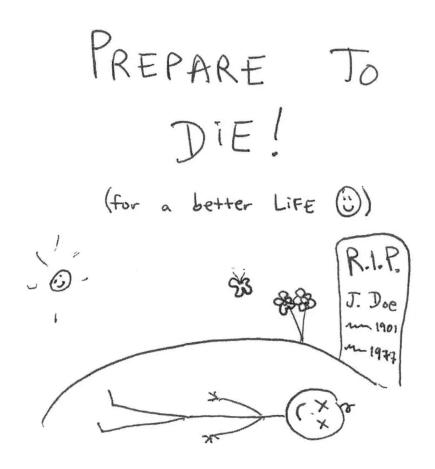

Unpopular opinion (or...actually, it's a fact): most of us are not going to make it to 90, no matter how well we take care of ourselves!

I mean, strictly speaking, most of us won't even make it to 80. That falls under the category of "who cares" when you're 16 or 20. But the older you get... as you cross the 50 mark and beyond... it starts to feel a little weird. A lot of 50-ish people I know (myself included) still call themselves "middle-aged" - even though only about 1.5% of people make it to 100!

Death is a part of life. It's an important part of life!

And, paradoxically, the healthier your relationship with death, the healthier your relationship with life can be. If you can prepare for your own death, not only will it help to enrich your own life, but it will also be a big mercy and a blessing to those you leave behind.

What do I mean by "prepare to die?"

That's a whole lot more than a single daily nugget can impart!

I recommend this excellent book: *A Beginner's Guide to the End: Practical Advice for Living Life and Facing Death,* by Dr. BJ Miller and Shoshana Berger.

I recommend it for everyone who will die one day. (hint: that's you, too!)

It sounds depressing, but it's not. Trust me. Would I lie to you? (No!)

HAD OPEN-CHEST SURGERY? GET YOUR RIBCAGE CHECKED! ←by a good chiropractor!

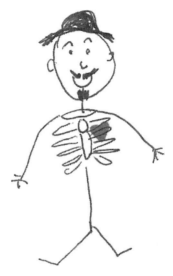

One of my favorite people in the world (who doesn't receive the Daily Nugget because he doesn't want to hear from me **every dang day**) told me that the way he found chiropractic in the first place was after his open-heart surgery! The surgery went well and all, but... when they closed him up, they didn't exactly line the ribs back up perfectly, so while he slept, his ribs made creepy noises that upset his wife! He told his surgeon about it, and she referred him to a chiropractor, who adjusted the ribs back into place, and the wife could sleep in peace! The creepy noise thing, as bad as it sounds, was fairly innocuous, considering all the other things that can happen when the rib cage subluxates after an open-chest surgery! Things like what?? Things like headaches, neck rigidity and pain, loss of range of motion, neurological entrapment of the brachial plexus, Thoracic Outlet Syndrome, symptoms of panic attacks and anxiety, pain while breathing, vertigo, difficulty swallowing, throbbing behind the eye, post nasal drip. All from a rib cage being out of alignment?! Yep, because soooo many muscles attach to the rib cage and it's also an area that is very rich with nerves! So.... I hope you never need open-chest surgery, but if you or a loved one ever does, once you're healed enough to handle gentle adjustments, see your chiropractor.

EASY DOES IT ON THE KOMBUCHA!

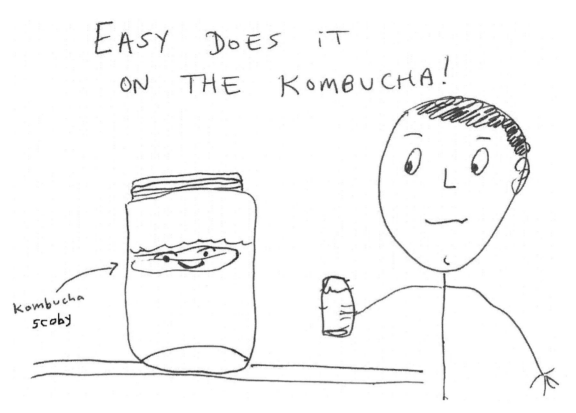

kombucha scoby

I'm a fan of fermented foods. They're good for you, and it's nice to have a variety!

But I'm giving this warning about kombucha because I often see people get into trouble with it. The trouble with kombucha is that it is very high in sugar!

Proponents say that no, it doesn't have much sugar, because the kombucha thing is eating it. It's true that the kombucha critter is eating the sugar.

But it's also true that there is plenty of sugar in that beverage that the kombucha is **not** eating.

So, when people go crazy with kombucha - consuming it daily, sometimes multiple times a day (especially if they're growing it at home), they can develop a lot of classic sugar problems. Like what?

Like hypoglycemia, fatigue, skin conditions, susceptibility to yeast or fungal infections, brain fog, interrupted sleep, headaches, etc.

So, if you're a fan of kombucha, it's OK to enjoy it every so often!

But treat it like a sugary drink and be mindful.

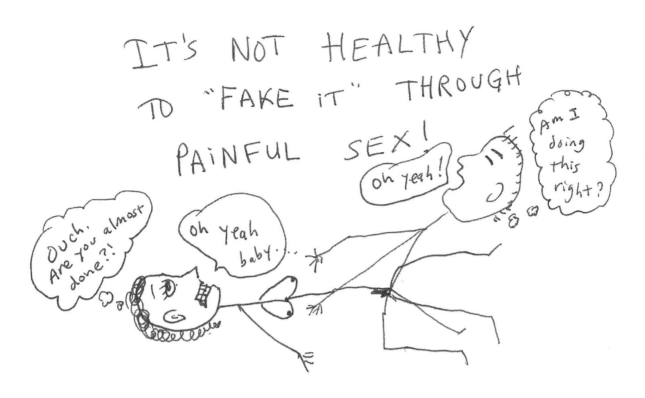

The only time that sex should be painful is if you **want** it to be painful! (And even then, it should only be the nice safe consensual kind of painful!)

For some reason, most people - especially women - make the strange assumption that there must be something "wrong" **with them** if sex is painful! And they often don't speak up about it. This gets even worse with age, as menopause nears, and reduced estrogen leads to vaginal atrophy. (That is just as unsexy as it sounds.)

Male partners of aging women don't help matters much, thanks to (1) knowing nothing about how women's bodies work and (2) having weird ideas about what it means to "be a man."

I sometimes have older male patients confide in me that they feel really bad - and unmanly - if they are unable to excite their partner enough to be able to have sex without "needing" lube. That is just ridiculous. Just because porn never shows the lube bottles doesn't mean that it's not being used copiously! Everybody should have a **good** lube at home! (And travel sizes for vacation!)

Anyway... there are various reasons why sex might be painful, especially following childbirth, surgery, or general aging.

If the pain is just from the atrophy of aging, there's some good news! It's an easily treatable condition thanks to estrogen suppositories and topical hormone creams. A good gynecologist will know all about it. (And yet, they often will not mention it unless you ask about it first!)

If the pain is from childbirth or surgery, then scar tissue may be to blame, in which case you will want to work with a scar tissue remediation specialist or other trained bodyworker. This sounds painful, but it's not!

If the pain is from a terrible partner, then you need to have an honest (if painful) conversation with the partner and sort it out. (Or get rid of the partner!)

Sometimes the pain is due to other injuries – old back injuries, leg injuries, etc. – and maybe you will need strategic pillow configurations to make it comfortable. Don't be afraid to speak up and arrange those pillows!

In any case, no matter what your plumbing is like down there, if sex is painful, then speak up and get some help!

You don't get anything great from pretending that it's OK.

It's like they say.... play stupid games, win stupid prizes!

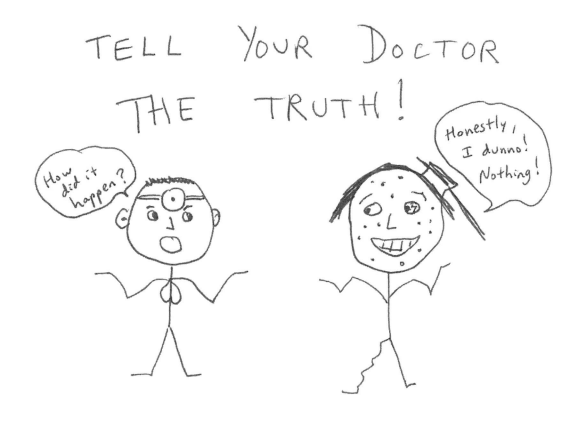

OK, this one seems pretty obvious, but I will say it anyway.
YOUR DOCTOR WILL BE ABLE TO HELP YOU MORE IF YOU TELL THEM THE TRUTH.
I get it, we've all lied - or at least withheld information - from medical professionals.
(We all have, right...? It's not just me?)
We might do it out of shame, or guilt...
..or maybe we feel like it's just none of their damn business!
Nevertheless, when a doctor is trying to figure out a plan of action, they need the right diagnosis, which means they need a proper - and truthful! - history.
Fair enough, doctors are only human, and you don't always feel good about telling any human about your private health stuff.
But if you feel like you can't even tell the truth to your own doctor, then, guess what? You probably need a new doctor.
I like to think that I am pretty open-minded and that my clients are comfortable with me, but then I later find out that they withheld info from me because they thought that I would judge them or laugh or ??? whatever else!
Inevitably, once the truth comes out, everyone feels better, and then we can get on to the business of **healing!**
Here is an example of a client who gave me false information about a "problem," which

193

resulted in me giving them a pretty useless "solution."

This person came in regularly for chiropractic adjustments for back pain. That was all well and good, and then one day, he mentioned that he was getting bitten by a bug at night, and did I have any suggestions.

Well, naturally, we ruled out bedbugs first. Next, he mentioned that he sometimes saw spiders in the room. So, I made suggestions about making sure that the bedroom and sheets were clean so that there wasn't any food for bugs. I also recommended a good natural insect-repellent oil and some natural antihistamine supplements.

I didn't hear anything about the mysterious bug bites for a while.

And then, recently, the client 'fessed up.

It wasn't bug bites.

He was waking up in the morning with long mysterious 3-pronged scratches down his back! Oh and also cold sensations of something brushing against his legs at night, and a strong smell at one specific spot in his bedroom (in the air in the middle of the room) sometimes.

All of this weird crap started when he moved into a new apartment, and it stopped after he moved into a different apartment.

Umm... dude... I can't believe I spent all that time troubleshooting for bug bites when what you needed was a dang exorcism!

Not sure whether or not I could have helped him with that, but... I'm just saying... even if it sounds weird or embarrassing or crazy... please tell your doctor the truth if you really want the best shot at the right solution!

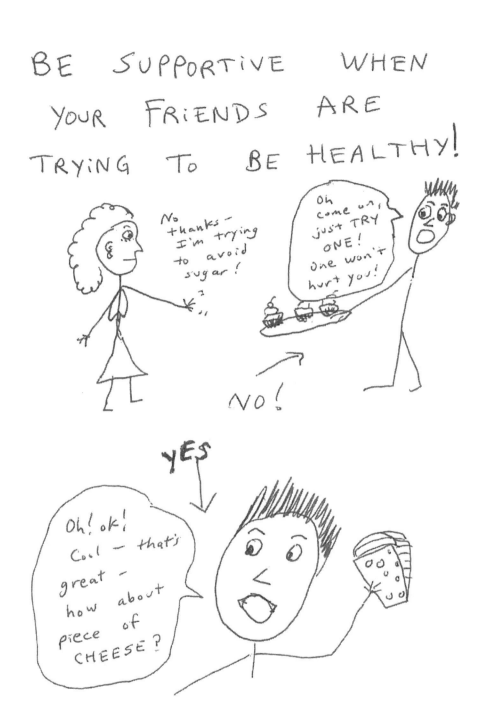

Now, I'm sure that everyone reading this has only ever been on the "trying to be healthy" side of the equation... and would never dream of thwarting anyone else's attempts to better their health! 😵

(Oh it's OK, you can breathe. We're all human here!) 😃

Seriously, though.

It's a real problem when well-meaning friends, family, coworkers, etc. pressure people to "have just a little" or "cheat" a little on this or that new healthy resolution!

The problem is not that the thing in question is so terrible.

It's true that "just one piece" or "just one drink" or "just one day without a workout" will not "hurt" you!

The **PROBLEM** is that there are **SO MANY** temptations and distractions that if a person can hold it together and do good on their health resolutions, then they should be lovingly supported in that endeavor!

Maybe **YOU** are the kind of person who can eat, drink, behave, whatever "a little" this that or the other without consequence, but you never know what someone else is going through or dealing with!

Even if you don't get it, just be supportive of your friend and pivot.

The pivot can be awkward.

Like our friend up there who offers "piece of cheese." 👻

It's OK! It's all part of the journey.

BTW - I thought of today's nugget because I just received yet another e-mail from someone who's enrolled in my *21-Day Sugar Challenge* who keeps running into well-meaning co-workers who try to hand her donuts in the morning! She is doing a great job resisting, but, wowzers. I don't think they realize how much more kind and helpful they would be if they just... didn't!

USE A STICK !

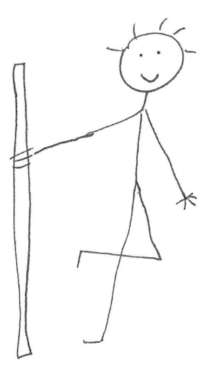

For what? For exercise!

Many years ago, Dr. Arthur Faygenholtz developed an innovative mix of stick-assisted yoga and tai chi while working with Paralympic athletes. He soon realized that this "Stick Yoga" was a great form of exercise for *all* people!

A few years back, I was leading Stick Yoga classes a few times a week. You can see my legendary video on YouTube ("Basic Long Stick Stretching Routine"):

https://youtu.be/xLbSQKywvG4

You don't have to do a full routine in order to make use of a long stick. Whether it's age or injury, there comes a time for most people when it's no longer safe or practical to do the same kinds of exercises that seemed so easy when we were younger. Most people just give up! "Oh well... I guess I'm just old now." or "I can't - I have a bad [foot, shoulder, knee, etc.]" The key to maintaining mobility over time is.... [get your pens out here!] ....REMAINING MOBILE.

In other words KEEP MOVING.

If you need to modify, **modify**.

I recently went to my first yoga class in about... oh.... uh... 20 years... and was shocked and dismayed to see that the mild neuropathy in my feet made it nearly impossible to sustain some very basic poses!

[cue sad trombone]

The cheerful voice of The Quitter in my head rang out, "Welp! I guess we won't be coming back to THIS class again!"

And then I remembered Dr. Faygenholtz and the STICK!

The Adult in my head went to the teacher after class and asked if I could bring a stick next time to help with balance, and he said YES.

So, I'll be back,

I tried the poses with the stick, and I can do them all! 😎

It's a good tool for your health arsenal!

It takes up very little space, and you can even make one yourself.

PINE NEEDLE TEA FOR LOTSA VITAMIN C !

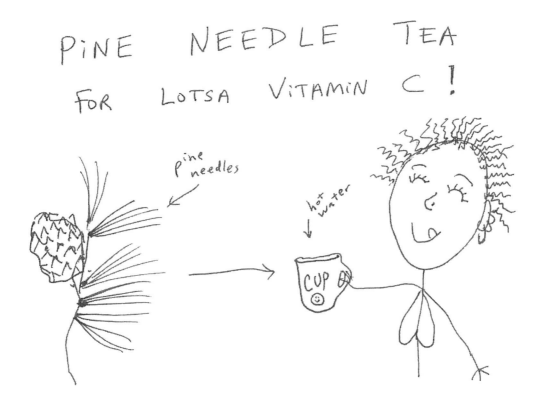

Did you know that a cup of pine needle tea has more vitamin C than a glass of orange juice?? It's true! What kind of pine needles are we talking about here, like, Christmas tree pine needles??? Probably yes! (Although, I've never bought a live Christmas tree in my life, so don't quote me on that!) The only pine species that you should *AVOID* for making tea are yew, Norfolk pine and some cypress. But your standard common pine trees out there? All excellent sources of vitamin C! For the tea, you will harvest the needles. Younger, more tender needles are preferable to older darker ones, and fresh is better than dried. (If dried, they should be recently dried and still have that nice evergreen smell to them!) Cut them up into about the amount you might use if it were tea and steep them in hot water.

When I first heard about pine needle tea (from my mom, shortly after she graduated from acupuncture school), I thought she was either making it up or had been duped into believing some (sub)urban myth! But no, it's legit, and apparently ALL the nature nerds have known about it forever. When I made it, it left some sticky mess on my cup, which is probably why it's not commercially produced. I'm sure dealing with pine sticky would not be profitable at scale.

But it made me feel very rugged and I do like the flavor of pine! 😎

Oh.. and ONE BIG **CAUTION** with pine needle tea!

DON'T DRINK IT IF YOU ARE PREGNANT, AS SOME FORMS OF PINE NEEDLE TEA CAN CAUSE ABORTION!!!

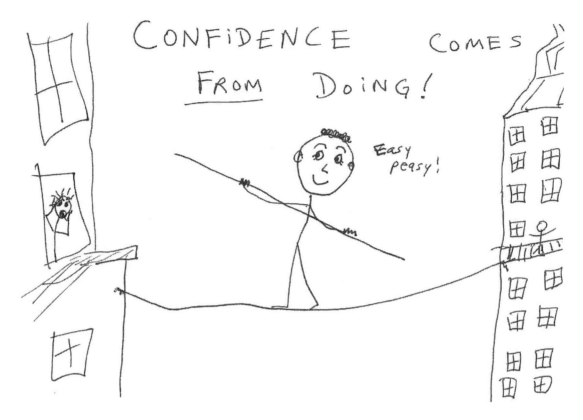

A lot of times, we avoid trying new things - including new healthy things! - because we are afraid and we lack the confidence.

"I think I'm going to work on building my confidence first... and **then** I'll go try that thing!"

And as much as I do love working with NET clients who are working on clearing their NEC's (basically, their "blocks") to certain goals, etc., I have to say that eventually... there's nothing left to "clear" until you just suck it up and take the **action!**

Confidence comes from familiarity with a thing, It's comes from that feeling of, "Oh, I've done this before... **lots of times.**"

It doesn't work the other way around!

"Instant confidence" sometimes appears in the form of a little bottle, powder, or pill, but... I don't recommend going that route, or your body will be needing a lot more than a few daily nuggets!

Good news for the introverts, though!

Introverts are already good at feeling uncomfortable, because they have to be uncomfortable so often just through the course of life!

Accept that it's going to be uncomfortable when you start doing the thing that you seek confidence with.

Know that each time, it will suck a little less, and someday... it might even be fun!

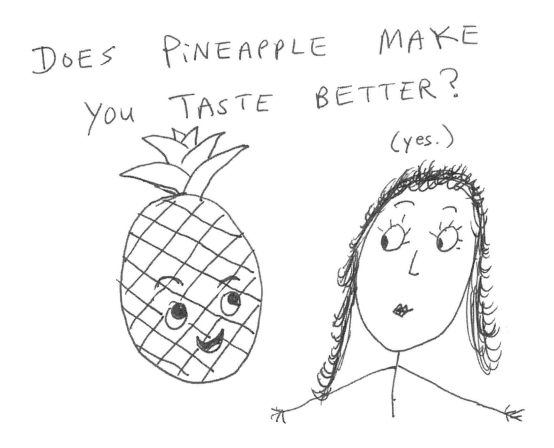

DOES PINEAPPLE MAKE YOU TASTE BETTER?

(yes.)

Pineapple is a pretty healthy food.

It's got tons of nutrients, antioxidants and contains the enzyme bromelain, which aids in digestion and also has anti-inflammatory properties. (If you've purchased the Bromelain Plus CLA supplement from the office, you may recall the instructions for use: take it with food to help with digestion and take it on an empty stomach to help with inflammation!) But the real question is... is there any truth to that rumor that eating pineapple makes you taste better? Not to cannibals, but, you know... for sexy time? The answer is, **yes.** The jury is out as to whether it's because of anything super special about pineapple, or whether it's because of its blend of anti-inflammatory properties, influence on pH, or ??? but it does seem to have a positive effect. <---based on my extensive research and interviews with both queer and straight experts! It's not that crazy, if you think about it. It's like how asparagus makes pee smell so pungent, or eating meat makes your sweat smell kind of meaty. One of the downsides of pineapple is that the high sugar content can be problematic for diabetics or people looking to reduce their sugar intake. For these people - and for anyone! - the perfect alternative is pineapple tea. So, whether or not you are anticipating getting any action, it never hurts to toss some pineapple into your smoothie or make some nice pineapple tea for your own enjoyment!

201

USE A DIGITAL MEAT THERMOMETER!

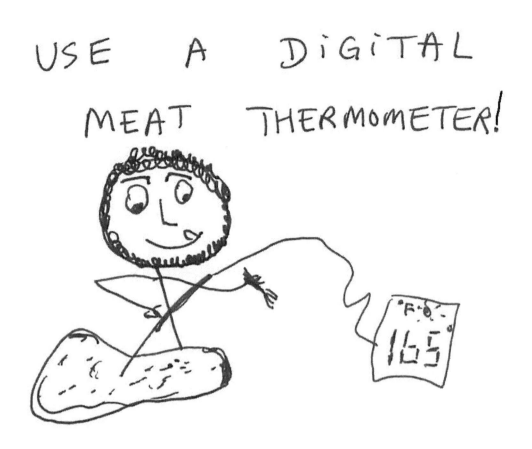

OK, this picture is not drawn to scale.

Unless the guy in the picture is a small domovoi (Russian house spirit)..? Anyway, I thought that these days, everyone uses a digital meat thermometer when cooking meat. But I found out that one of my friends just kind of eyeballs it! And guess what? The Thanksgiving turkey was under-cooked, and everyone (EVERYONE!) got diarrhea! I know, I know, never woulda happened if they'd just gone vegetarian. So, if you cook meat, **use a digital thermometer!** They are inexpensive, and they may save you from some nasty parasites or bacteria! Here are the basic safe temperatures for eggs and meat:

Eggs and all ground meats must be cooked to 160°F.

Poultry and fowl should be cooked to 165°F.

Fresh meat steaks, chops and roasts should be cooked to 145°F

Bon appetit!

(And no, I do not check the temperature on my eggs. I live crazy like that! But I draw the line with the meat.)

p.s. 150 degree juicy turkey kind-of-controversy update! It turns out that you can kill salmonella at 150 and have a juicy and safe turkey IF you sustain the 150 for at least 3.8 minutes.

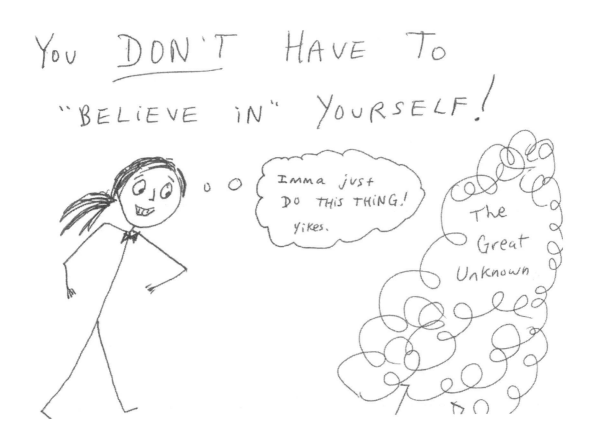

Well-meaning "motivational" resources tell us that we need to "believe!"

Specifically, BELIEVE IN YOURSELF! ✦

Stuff like that. The problem is... a lot of the time... we are not feelin' the believin'!

So, we procrastinate. And stuff. But guess what? To make meaningful changes in your life (including your health) you **don't** need to "believe in yourself" or "feel motivated" or any of that! You just need to **do something!** (Usually something specific.) Do you "believe in yourself" when you go to the bathroom and then clean up afterward? Do you "believe in yourself" when you do your laundry or pay your bills? Probably not! You just do those things because those things have to be done, regardless of how you are "feeling." Feelings matter, of course! BUT... only ACTION gets things done. Next time you are wanting to try or **do** something, but your brain gives you a lame excuse about lacking confidence or not "believing" in yourself, just suck it up and take an action step anyway! The human condition is ridiculous, but we're human, so we're stuck with it! Now go **do** something good for your health! ✦

SOMETIMES..... LEAVE THE PASTE ON YOUR TEETH!

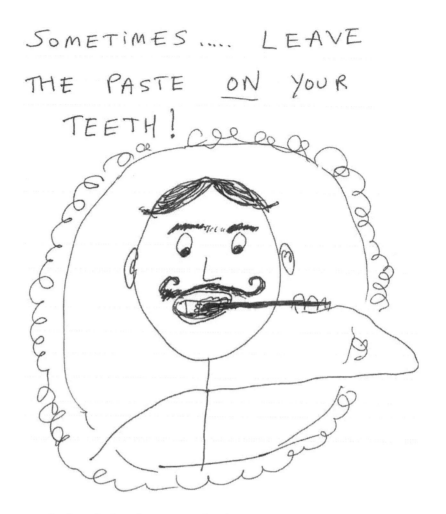

You put the toothpaste on the brush, brush your teeth, rinse, and that's that.
Right? Well, did you know that sometimes it's good to leave the paste on your teeth for a few minutes?? This is true mainly in 2 instances. (1) For people with very sensitive teeth, it can be helpful to take a sensitive-tooth toothpaste (such as Sensodyne) and just put it on the sensitive teeth and let it sit there for a couple of minutes before brushing. This can help to plug the tiny holes in the teeth and reduce sensitivity even more over time.
(2) There is a type of paste called "remineralizing pastes" which help to replace lost minerals (such as calcium) for people who have weak teeth. An excellent brand of remineralizing paste is **MI Paste**. This kind of paste goes on your teeth, and you just leave it there for a few minutes and then rise. You don't use it for daily cleaning; there are no abrasives in it. But it really does work to strengthen teeth. My old dental hygienist said that she used to get a lot of cavities due to weak teeth, but she never did anymore after using the **MI Paste** regularly! Dental care is expensive! (Plus, we're not sharks! We can't regrow teeth!) It's always worth going the extra mile to keep your teeth strong and healthy!

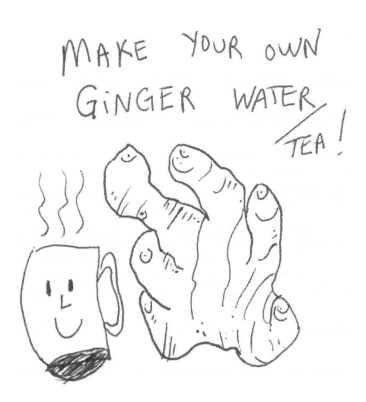

MAKE YOUR OWN GINGER WATER/TEA!

OK, that gigantic ginger root is not drawn to proper scale against that smiling beverage mug, so... sorry about that! (I was drawing it from a YouTube video for beginners.)

Anyhoo...

I can't believe it's taken me this long to make a ginger water nugget! Thanks to Virginia and Kat for the reminder!

Ginger water or ginger tea is one of the easiest and healthiest beverages you can whip up for yourself. The anti-inflammatory and antioxidant properties of ginger are well-known, and it can also help with immune function and sugar handing issues.

The best way to make it is to use a grater to grate some fresh ginger into a cup and just add water. If you want to make bigger batches at a time, you can add about 2 teaspoons to about 4 cups of hot water, let it steep for about 10 minutes, and then strain out the ginger and drink the water (hot or cold).

Don't go overboard - too much ginger can give you an upset stomach or gas!

Ginger can be such a pain to grate. But I learned the hack for this! Peel the outside ahead of time and freeze it! Then, when it's time to grate the ginger, just grate off of the frozen piece. The frozen ginger grates like a charm!

IODINE FOR SKIN FUNGUS

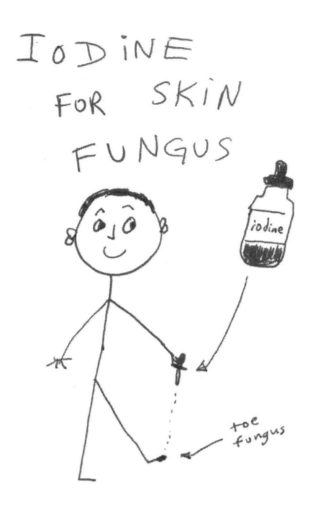

Thank you to **Dr. Jae Reed** for pointing out this very handy nugget: iodine is a great anti-fungal! It has strong antimicrobial properties, and so of course it makes sense that it would be a good anti-fungal! Why else would they swab a bunch of iodine all over people's skin right before surgery?! Just a single drop of liquid iodine can kick off the healing for a toenail that has become infected with a fungus. If you don't love the idea of iodine-stained toenails, though, fear not! There is such a thing as "white iodine," which is regular iodine that has been decolorized. Medical grade liquid iodine (which you can buy over-the-counter at any drugstore) can be safely used topically. Don't drink it!

There are safe iodine supplements, but they are made from a different form of iodine. But taking iodine as a supplement will not necessarily help with internal fungal or yeast infections. This nugget is all about topical fungal infections of the skin and nails!

To keep it simple, apply a drop of liquid iodine to the affected area twice a day until gone. For skin, this usually takes less than 2 weeks. For toenails, it can take longer, but you should still be able to see the results in action early in the process!

APPLE CIDER VINEGAR IN SALT GARGLE

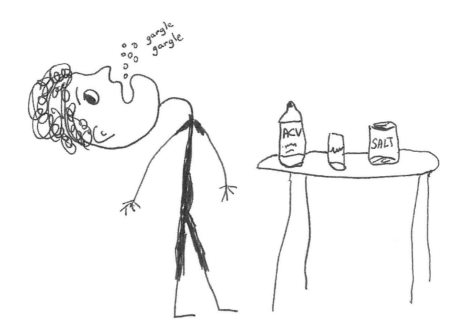

Everyone knows that a salt water gargle can help with an itchy or scratchy throat, right?
The salt water helps to wash away mucus and reduce inflammation.

But some people really hate to do it because of the taste!

Now, I know that it doesn't sound like adding apple cider vinegar to the mix would improve the taste, but I have it on good authority that it does!

If you are an exacting kind of person, here is the basic recipe:

Mix 1 teaspoon of apple cider vinegar with ½ teaspoon of salt and 8 ounces of warm water.

Mix, gargle, and feel better.

How long do you have to gargle? 15-30 seconds is plenty of time. Some people recommend two sounds to make sure you get as much of the mucus out as possible.

TEA BAGS ON THE EYES

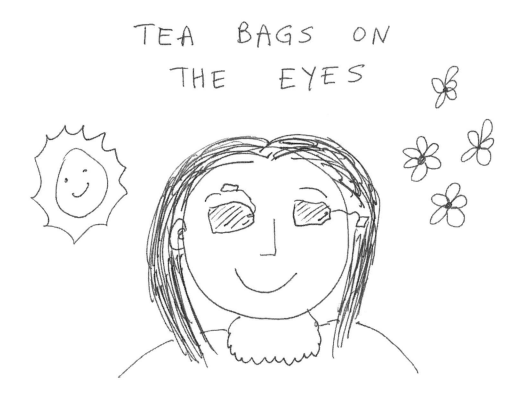

This is an oldie but a goodie.

Lay down with warm (not hot!!!) or cold tea bags on your eyes to help soothe puffy, irritated, or tired eyes.

You just steep the tea in hot water as if you're going to drink it, and then take the teabags out of the water, gently squeeze out the water, and then when it's cool enough to be safe (or some people like to put it in the fridge so they can have a cold teabag on their eye) and then lay down and just put on your closed eye and relax for around 15-30 minutes.

It's true that the tannins and antioxidants in tea really do have anti-inflammatory and healing properties.

But you know what else is good about this one?

You can't be looking at a screen while you have teabags over your eyes!

So just relax and enjoy.

(Maybe listen to a good audio book.)

If you want to get all complicated about it, yeah, yeah, certain herbals and all are slightly better for this or that, but let's keep it simple! Just use standard black, green, or white tea.

IT BURNS!

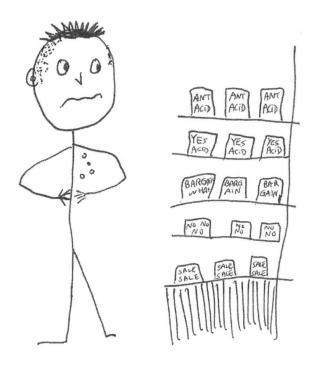

When is too much acid too little acid? Specifically, we are talking about "heartburn" or acid reflux. When people have this problem, they think that they have "too much acid." Their doctors usually assume this, too, and the solution is a prescription for antacids! While some people really DO have excessive stomach acid, the fact is that most people have **too little** stomach acid! Why would "too little stomach acid" cause a burning sensation?! Because the body works extra hard to splash that little bit of acid all around to get the job done! Some of it splashes up and irritates the esophagus. And why would so many people be making too little stomach acid?! The main reason is **stress**. The body naturally makes less stomach acid when it's under stress. This is because blood and resources are focused on the skeletal muscles (so you can fight or run away) when stress is high! The other reason is old age. We make less stomach acid as we age. This is why a lot of old people don't eat meat anymore. It becomes harder to digest! How can you tell if your heartburn is from too much or too little acid? One sign that you are probably low on stomach acid is if it's tender or painful when you press into the area just below your xiphoid process (the little bump at the bottom center your rib cage). If that spot is tender, then you may need to use some form of a "betaine HCl" supplement. Fixing a low acid problem in the stomach is often the first step in balancing out many health conditions!

IF ALIENS/UFO's/DEMONS
KEEP PROBING YOUR BUTT...
THEN YOU NEED MORE
WATER AND FIBER!

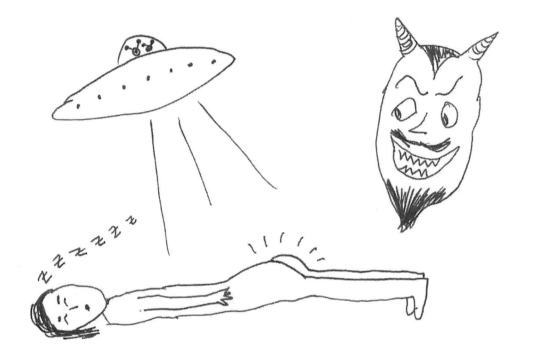

I always used to just laugh off the alien butt probe stories. I mean, come on. Why would advanced civilizations come here just to abduct people in their sleep and probe their butts at night?! But it's such a common story (as far as weird stories go) and it seems reminiscent of older tales (pre-UFO and aliens I guess?) of nighttime butt attacks from demons or other unseen entities! And like the aliens... why would demons be so interested in human butts??? These were just random flitting thoughts of mine until I met my first credible (?) person who swore that he was sometimes attacked in the butt at night by demons.

It wasn't every night, but it was occasional, and the attacks lasted about 15-20 minutes, causing quite a lot of pain and discomfort right exactly at his butthole! And then it was over, and he could go back to sleep. I never did ask him what made him think that these were demonic attacks. I was pretty young and I just wanted to play it cool. Like, "Yeah, yeah, demonic butt attacks, I know allll about that. Sure." But then, over the years, once in a while, people would confide in me that they would sometimes get this terrible pain right there in the middle of their butt! It happened in the middle of the night, and it scared them, but it would pass after maybe 15-20 minutes. Did I know what it could be? Were they cursed? **could** it be remnants of an alien butt probe? I didn't know... but I do know this:

If there's a **non**-supernatural explanation for something, then chances are, the answer is **not supernatural!**

It took me many years to figure it out (because not very many people speak up if they have this problem!) but I think I finally got it, thanks to an unusually good sport of a client who we'll just call B.

B noticed that on the days after she had the pain at night, she would pass an unusually hard poop. She asked if this could have anything to do with it, and if yes, WHY?

And finally, it made sense!

My theory is this: nerves to the butthole (and the area right around it) emerge from the little holes in the sacrum, at the base of the spine. On that side of the sacrum (the inside), that is also where viscera like the intestines can be found. My theory is that if someone has eaten a bunch of something very dry and low fiber, without enough water, then they will have an extremely hard poop which can press against those nerves coming out of the sacrum as the poop is making its way down the large intestine! This activity (moving the poop along) usually happens during the night. Which is why most people poop in the morning.

B, the good sport, was willing to test out this theory of mine. She said that the theory did make sense, because on the day before the "attack," she barely had any water, but she did eat a large amount of dry food (a tube of Pringles) in one sitting. So she intentionally did the bad thing - very little water plus a lot of dry food - and sure enough, right on cue in the middle of the night, the butt attack! A few days later (after giving her body a rest by eating healthy foods and drinking plenty of water) she drank tons of water all day and then ate the same dry food that provoked the attack earlier. No attack. Further observations in her case seemed to confirm that this unwelcome nighttime attack only happened if she had eaten a bunch of dry food and very little water during the day.

Mystery solved??

I guess you'll know if you see me as a guest on The "History" Channel! 😐 👽

But anyway... You can never get too many reminders about drinking enough **water** 💧 and getting enough **fiber** 🌿 in your diet!

Your butt - indeed your whole body - thanks you!

YOU CAN'T ALWAYS HEAL "NATURALLY"

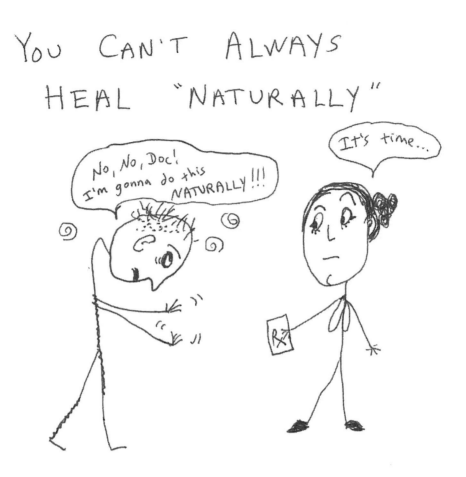

Oh boy, am I gonna get an earful on this one...

Look. I've been a chiropractor for more than 25 years.

I'm a big proponent of "natural healing," and I do believe that pharmaceuticals and all that tend to get overused and misused in the USA.

Dangerously so!

AND/BUT STILL...

I'm sorry to say but I have to say... *you can't always heal "naturally."*

WHY NOT?

Well I'm gonna tell you why not!

Why not is because we no longer live in a "natural" world.

We've reached a point of no return, where the stresses and strains on our bodies are beyond anything that Nature and evolution could have prepared us for. It's too much. Everything is weird, from the food we eat to the things we drink to the hours we work to the number of people we try to be "friends" with to the electromagnetic environment to the information in the DNA we pass to our children to the [fill in the blank]...

I'm not trying to freak you out or depress you. It's just the way it is!

You can't expect to be able to handle all modern health challenges with purely "natural" remedies. Because the problems are coming from living under very unnatural circumstances.

I can get and admire the impetus behind wanting to live a more natural life.

We SHOULD live a more natural life!

But we should also be honest and realistic about the life we're really living.

The main purpose of this Nugget is to help relieve any guilt that some of your may be experiencing over wanting to live a "holistic life" but still relying on certain "artificial' medications, treatments, etc. for some kind of health problem. (This is especially prevalent in people with mental illness who feel like they "should" get off of their medication even though they do feel better when they are on it!)

Always go for the simple and natural way first.

You will often be pleasantly surprised!

But there is NO SHAME in going the "unnatural" way when that's what it's going to take.

This is the world we're living in right now.

Take a deep breath.

It's fine.

(even though it's not fine. you know what I mean?)

USE EWG'S DATABASE TO CHECK PRODUCT TOXICITY

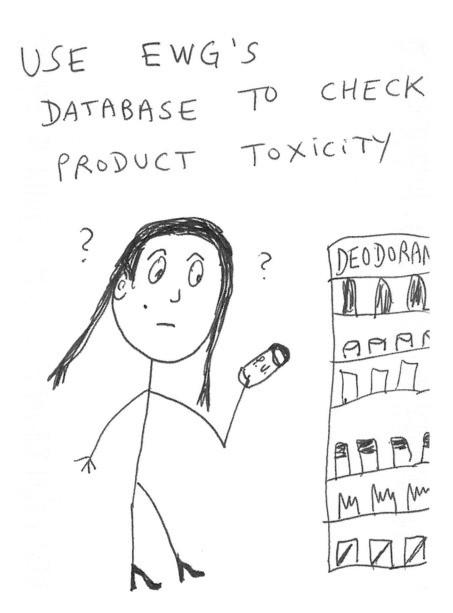

If it has the word "database" in it, can it really be simple enough for a Daily Nugget??

For today, sure!

Toxicity is a complicated topic. When we pick up personal care products (like deodorant) and look at the ingredient list, our brains tend to go blank.

That stuff can't be good. Is it good? Is it bad?

Just how bad are we talking??

Fortunately, there are nerds who have studied the data, and now we can get a general idea of how good or bad a product is (in terms of toxicity) thanks to some simple tools.

EWG (Environmental Working Group) is a 501(c)3 nonprofit that is committed to informing people so that they can make healthy and informed choices when it comes to environmental toxicity.

Their website has a huge database of commercial products.

You can search for a specific product here:

https://www.ewg.org/skindeep/search/

The lower the score, the cleaner and safer the product.

(For example, my hippie brand that I like for deodorant - Soapwalla - scores at a 1, which is as clean as it gets! Whereas the Axe family of products scores as moderately toxic, mostly at 6. The worst score would be 10.)

If your product is not on the list, you can cut and paste the ingredient list (from the manufacturer website, store website, etc.) into EWG's custom report generator here:

https://www.ewg.org/skindeep/build_your_own_report/

An even easier way to jump right to your results is to Google "[product and brand] EWG" within quotes and it will take you right to the results page!

"But how am I going to remember all that when I'm at the store?"

EWG has an app! It's called The Healthy Living App.

Using the app, you can scan barcodes right there at the store and see the toxicity score.

We can't escape all the toxicity in the environment, but every bit helps - especially when it comes to products that end up on your skin!

(Thanks, Kat, for the tip!)

USE MUSIC TO HELP WITH TOUGH TASKS!

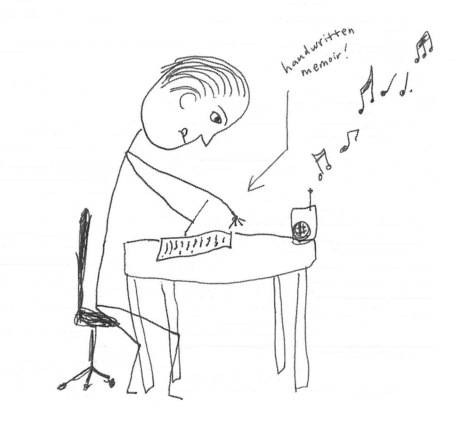

handwritten memoir!

When there's a tedious task that you want to do for your own well-being (like exercising or writing your book), sometimes it can really help to use some of your hidden brain powers! One of those hidden powers is the brain's tendency to pair things together.

Scents and sounds can be used to "program" the brain into leaning towards certain activities and behaviors. Yes, in a way, you are training yourself as if you are your own dog!

The writers among you may already know this trick, but others may be surprised to know that a common tool used by writers is to have a specific piece of "writing music" that they **only** listen to while writing! This helps to cue the brain into thinking "it's time to write!" and it helps to support the activity. For something like writing, it's best if the music is just instrumental, with no discernible vocals. (In case you're wondering, my "writing music" is a collection of German military marching band music. Sometimes bagpipes. It's from my dad's collection. Long story!) Same with exercise. Some people have very specific music that cues their brain to know that it's time to do very specific types of exercise!

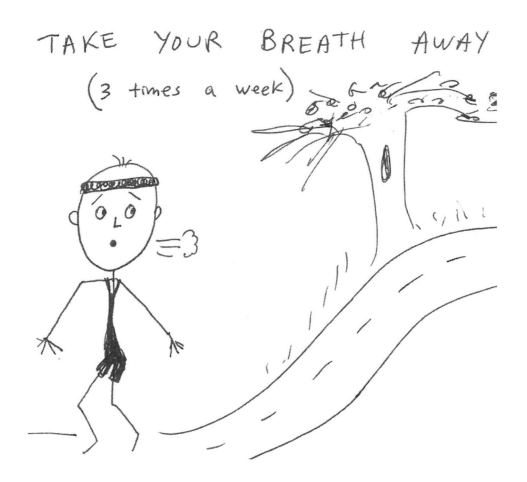

TAKE YOUR BREATH AWAY
(3 times a week)

One of the basic "general health and longevity" tips out there is that you should do **something** at least 3 times a week that causes you to lose your breath.

Not lose your breath for so long that you pass out!

Or to any ridiculous or dangerous extent.

Just, you know, that you exerted enough effort at something that it was a real challenge!

So, this can be a sprint, or a quick and intense dance, or riding your bike up a big hill or going up a ton of stairs or... you get the idea!

I guess one of the "nice" things about being "out of shape" is that it doesn't take as much effort to hit that "took my breath away" point 😆

It gets harder the fitter you get, but you also don't mind because you're more fit.

SALT CRAVINGS
OFTEN = ADRENAL FATIGUE
(a.k.a. STRESS!)

I think that most people like salty things. It's one of those things we've evolved to enjoy. Sweet, salty, fatty, crunchy... But if you **crave** salty things, like, can't get enough!!! then... you probably have adrenal fatigue - also known as **chronic stress**. What's "chronic" anyway? According to the U.S. National Center for Health Statistics, something is chronic if you've had it for more than 3 months. Any chance you may have been under stress for more than 3 months? If you have chronic stress and the inevitable adrenal issues that come with it, then there are lots of things you can do. Supplements, mindfulness, meditation, **NET**...

But one of the simplest "supplements" you can use is our good old friend, raw sea salt! Yep, just put some in a little baggie and take a few pinches throughout the day with some water. At first, the salt will taste **great**, and you will enjoy it and maybe use it a lot. But as your electrolytes and minerals come back into balance, you will not crave it so much, and it won't taste as exciting, and you won't use it as much. But if the stress stays intense, then the raw salt supplement will help. It's also helpful to take some raw sea salt after a hard sweaty workout. It helps to replace electrolytes and will also help to minimize muscle fatigue!

THE RIGHT PILLOW
is A TREASURE!

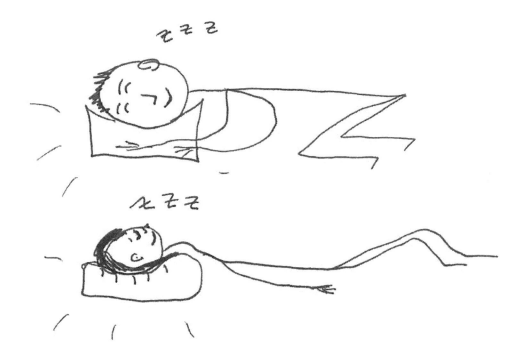

A good pillow is such a basic and important part of having a happy neck that you would think there would have been a nugget about it ages ago!

And of course I have thought about it. A lot!

The problem is... there are sooo many kinds of pillows out there and so many kinds of bodies... that there's no such thing as **the** best pillow.

There's only the best pillow for you at a given time.

At a given time??

Yeah, sorry... even for the same person, the ideal pillow can change and vary over time depending on what your neck needs!

For example, after being in a car accident or similarly injured, you may need a taller pillow than usual to help decrease the inflammation and swelling around your neck and head!

A person recently told me that they've have great success using a U-shaped pillow to help them quit stomach sleeping.

219

Some people feel that they need a more firm pillow with a little curve to it when they feel more tension in their neck.

People usually need a flatter pillow in a really soft bed and a somewhat taller pillow on a really firm bed depending on how far their shoulder does or doesn't sink into the mattress. You get the idea.

But **in general**, the guideline is that when you're in your sleeping position, your neck should be pretty neutral and in line with your spine.

So if you're on your side, your head should not tilt up or down in relation to your spine.

And if you're sleeping on your back, then your pillow should support the curve in your neck. Many people do well with a pillow that provides some gentle traction to the neck.

Personally, I am a fan of "butterfly" style pillows. They give great support when side or back sleeping.

The bottom line is, if your neck feels achy, stiff, or sore first thing in the morning, but then it mostly resolves as you get to moving around, then chances are, you're using the wrong pillow.

I know, it's a hassle to try different ones, but you just have to. 😑 🐵

OPTIMAL EXERCISES CHANGE WITH AGE!

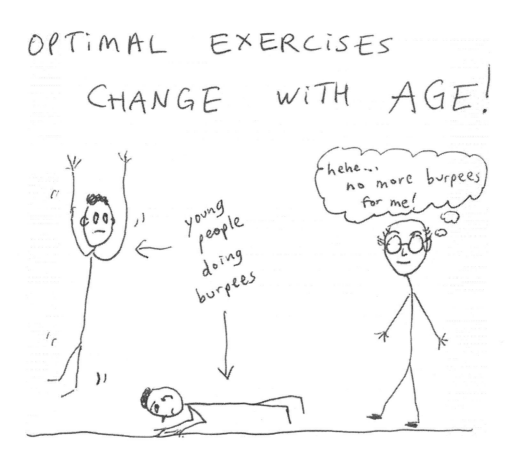

As we get older, there is a tendency to focus on what we "used to be able to do" and less on what's best for the body we have right now. The truth is, our bodies have different needs - of all sorts! - at different stages of life!

The things that are great for one age group might be terrible for another one!

Take cardio exercises, for example.

When you're in your 20s, if you wanted to lose some weight, you might take up running and just burn it off! But if you're in your 60s, then that would be a terrible idea. Cardio is not nearly as effective for fat-burning in your 60s, plus you're more likely to hurt yourself. So for a 60 year-old looking to lose weight, the way to go is strength-training and a focus on building muscle mass in combination with diet.

For young people, one of the most efficient full-body exercises ever is the dreaded burpee!

A burpee is a jump, squat, plank, and push-up all in one short brutal exercise.

It's a powerful tool.

For people of a certain age.

It's a terrible exercise for older people, because of all the ways it can aggravate old injuries and cause new ones!

Sure, there are always exceptions to the rule, so don't send me YouTube videos of old people doing burpees! It's not a good idea for **most** old people! (including me, and I'm just a baby old person!)

So, if not a burpee, then what is the best strength-training exercise for, say, women over 60? It's the leg press!

Leg presses target the largest muscle groups, help to stabilize the low back, and perhaps best of all, prevents - and can even reverse! - bone loss! It is a great bone-strengthening exercise that also helps to prevent fractures.

Older people also benefit from fewer days a week of intense strength training than younger people. (For example, 1 or 2 days a week of strength training is enough for most women over 60.)

(By the way, if there's a sport you **love** to do - and it brings you great joy - then find a way to keep doing it or stay involved with it in some capacity your whole life!)

And finally... less intense exercise as we age doesn't mean to stop moving around! We all benefit from plenty of movement at all ages.

So, keep moving, with passion and purpose!

(but you can eventually say goodbye to burpees!)

WORK ON PRESUMPTION OF GOODNESS

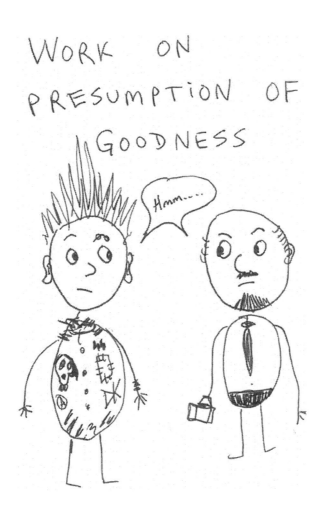

Why is it so easy to presume that people are basically up to no good? (Especially "**those people**?" As in... **those people** who are most different from us!) Well, as with most of our annoying traits, it's because we evolved that way! Think about it. Throughout most of history - and certainly during the time we call "pre-history" - which would have been the safer bet? Option A: assume that strangers equal danger and prepare to hide, fight, kill or be killed! -or- Option B: assume that strangers are just friends you haven't met yet and go say hello! It's safe to say that we are mostly descended from people who chose option A. Fortunately for us - people who have access to the Daily Nugget - the **vast** majority of the people we encounter on a day-to-day basis are basically "good people." Even the saltiest of characters we encounter during an average day are unlikely to kill or even really harm us. But the presumption of malice, which we project onto all sorts of people, causes tons of anxiety and stress that doesn't need to exist at all. Sure, some people really **are** up to no good! But mostly it's none of our business. See if you can tell a difference in your quality of health and life if you consciously work on presuming goodness instead of badness. For one week, try and project positive or good assumptions onto strangers, and see how you feel!

SEE THE WORLD THROUGH ROSE
(or purple or blue or green or yellow or ...)
TINTED GLASSES?

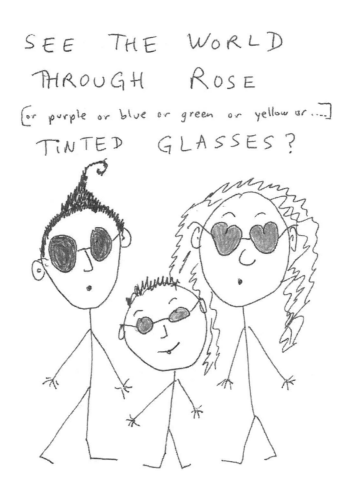

I never really understood that saying, "to see the world through rose tinted glasses" until the day when someone actually handed me a real pair of rose tinted glasses! I put them on, and... wow! The world really did look different! It had a different feeling. Somehow, it felt "better." (Although I wouldn't have wanted to wear them **all** the time - it also felt kind of disorienting.) Beyond just the preference that some people have for these rose-tinted glasses, there really is such a thing as "color therapy." This is where people wear glasses with specific color tints for about 30-60 minutes a day for specific health reasons. At first, this sounds like sooooo much baloney. Really? Color tinted glasses for health? Oh-kay. But... there is lots of research to support that different colors really DO evoke different states of mind and different feelings! This fact is used **all the time** when it comes to advertising and marketing. And you know it's intuitively true. Why don't people paint nurseries in bright crimson red? Why doesn't the bride ever wear brown? Why aren't firetrucks painted grey? So why not add some color therapy into the mix if you are looking for extra ways to support a solution? (My dentist hands out colored glasses as soon as the patient sits down for a procedure!)

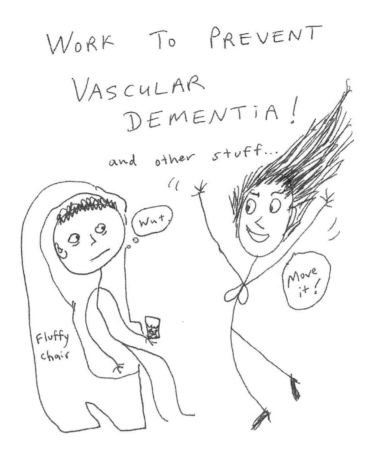

"Vascular dementia" is a term I only recently ever even heard of! 😵 My personal experience with dementia has been with Alzheimer's Disease, which my great-grandma had. And so, naturally, I've been worried for years about developing Alzheimer's! I worried about creepy plaque growing on my brain, and possible aluminum toxicity and all that jazz! But really... I should have been more worried about **this** thing: vascular dementia. Vascular dementia is a type of dementia that develops due to a deterioration of the blood vessels that feed the brain! And so, the brain deteriorates because it's just not getting all the oxygen and nourishment that it needs! It's obvious when you say it, but... I just never thought about it!

*Of course, wimpy circulation would affect the **brain!*** 👤 (And this is probably why, when I do high-intensity upper body aerobic workouts, it feels like a pencil sharpener for my brain! I really do feel "smarter" during and right after those workouts!) There was even a recent article on CNN that highlighted a study showing that (surprise!) "vigorous activity" (even for short amounts of time) seems to have the most protective effects on brain health. So, make sure you get a few minutes of "vigorous activity" in more days than not! Even if it's just running around waving your arms vigorously and yelling, "OMG WHAT AM I GOING TO DO???"

BODY SCAN MEDITATION FOR STRESS RELIEF

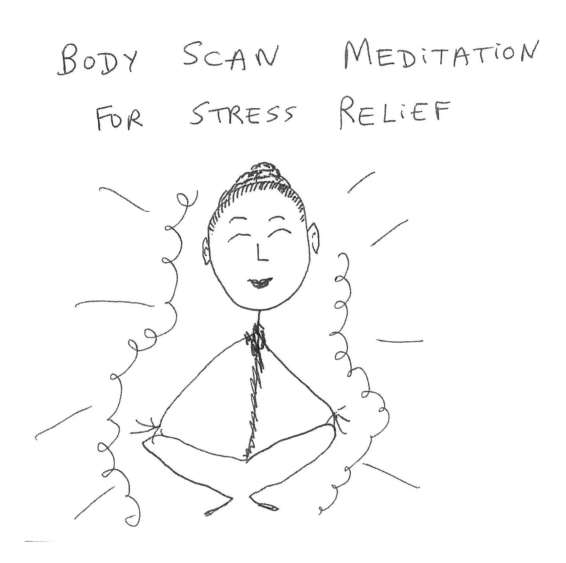

A "body scan" meditation is a simple meditation technique that helps you to get in touch with what is going on in the present moment with your body. It's a basic part of what is known in the healthcare profession as **MBSR**, or Mindfulness Based Stress Reduction. Body scan meditations generally involve sitting still or lying down, breathing slowly and deeply, and focusing on specific parts of the body (usually from head to toe) and simply paying attention to what's happening. Once you've gotten the hang of it. You can easily do a body scan yourself! But in the beginning, it can be really helpful to listen to guided meditations that walk you through the process. In this crazy world, you can never have too many tools to help you stay present and connected to your body! (Look up "body scan meditation" on YouTube for some examples to guide you at first.)

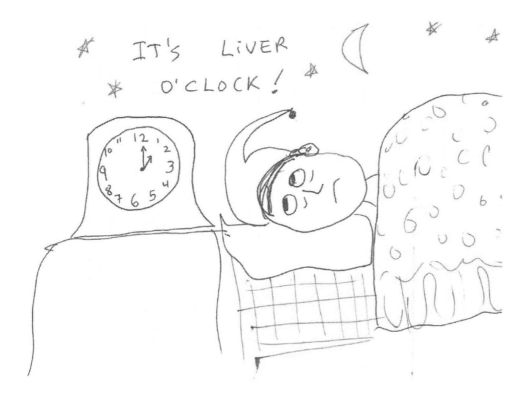

What the heck is "liver o'clock" and why should I care?! Well, in Chinese medicine (which is thousands of years old) there is a thing called the Body Clock. The idea is that different body systems are more active at different times of the day based on our natural circadian rhythm. This makes sense. After all, it makes sense that body would focus on things like processing and getting ready to eliminate waste at night, while we sleep. And doing things like making new blood cells and absorbing nutrients while we are awake and active, right? The Chinese body clock can be incredibly helpful when it comes to decoding hidden problems. For example, one of the most common problems that I see in the office is people waking up frequently at "liver time." This means between 1-3am. So, if you frequently wake up between 1-3am and have a hard time falling back asleep, there is a very good chance that there is something going on that is irritating your liver! The most common culprit is (surprise surprise) **alcohol**. You are probably drinking alcohol too close to bedtime or simply drinking more than your body can comfortably handle. The solutions? Well, yeah, stop drinking the alcohol! OR... stop drinking it earlier in the night. OR... drink a smaller volume of it. OR... take a good liver support supplement (such as Livaplex, by Standard Process) before and after your alcohol consumption. OR take my 30-day Liver Detox Challenge! The point is... you want to work on supporting the organ or system that is dominant during the recurring time that you keep experiencing symptoms. So, if it's between 1-3am all the time, then, that, my friends, is liver o'clock!

METAL O'CLOCK!

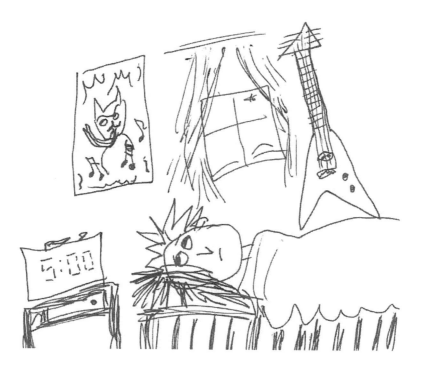

After "liver o'clock," the most common time that people come to me with problems about it "metal o'clock!" If we look again at our Chinese body clock, we see that the metal element (lung and large intestine) runs from 3-7am. Right where lung and large intestine connect in the middle of that time window - right around 5am - is where many people with challenges in the metal element wake up and then can't get back to sleep! If you are a "morning person" like me, you don't care, because you like to be up around 5am anyway! But most people are not looking to get up at 5, so this can be a problem. The good news is that if it's a metal element / body clock issue, then the solution is usually simple! For most people, the problem is eliminated by increasing intake of water and fiber for the large intestine and increasing water and breathing exercises for the lungs. Sometimes simply increasing water intake during the day it enough! For the breathing part, sometimes it's enough to just increase the intensity of exercises so that the lungs have to work hard, even if only for a short time, like doing a couple of short sprints!

RUN TOE → HEEL!
(NOT HEEL → TOE)

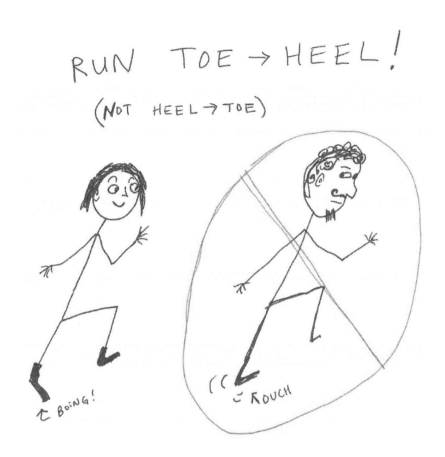

← BOING!

⌣ ᴿOUCH

As you may know... I'm not really a "fan" of running! I'm a little bit lazy, and running is so high-impact! <--especially on the city sidewalks! However... sometimes, you just gotta run!
For the bus 🚌

    for your life 💧

    whatevs! 🫳

So if/when you have to run once in a while, try to run toe-heel instead of heel-toe!
When we run by striking first on our heel, it's very jarring, and the impact travels right up to your knee and hips! This makes for faster and rougher wear-and-tear on the joints, which is something we want to try and avoid! Nobody wants to need a knee or hip replacement!
When you strike first on your toes (really, on the forefoot), you can feel that it's a much more "springy" sensation, the impact is dissipated, and it's gentle on the knees and hips.
Now, I'm talking about these short occasional runs that we do in life.
I'm **not** talking about marathons, long distance, etc.!
For **that** kind of running, it's a bit more nuanced (and "ideal" is more of a mid-foot strike), but in any case, you just don't want to ever do hard heel-striking!

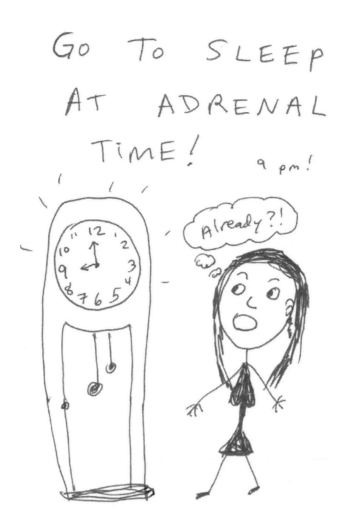

Yep, time for another trip to ye olde body clock! On the Chinese body clock, the time between 9-11pm is labeled as "triple heater" or "triple warmer." This is more of a concept than a physical location. It's a complicated concept, in my humble opinion, so I will just say that for our purposes, this is the time on the clock where the adrenal glands sit, and therefore, for us, it is "**adrenal time.**" This is when the adrenals glands (which made adrenaline, cortisol and all that good stuff) rest and refresh. By this time of day, you should be done with your fighting and flighting! Here's a strange thing about adrenal time. If you can get to sleep in this time window (closer to 9 than 11), then you will feel much more rested than if you get the same number of hours of sleep, but with a later bedtime! If you are resting/sleeping while the adrenals are trying to rest, too, it's just the best bang for your energy buck. In some times and cultures, people even go to sleep around 8 or 9, then wake up around midnight, get some work done, and then go to sleep again later! Seems really strange, but they, too, are harnessing the resting power of sleeping during that 9-11 time window!

p.s. I mention this, too, in my book, *The Issues are in the Tissues.*

TAKE A GROUP EXERCISE CLASS!

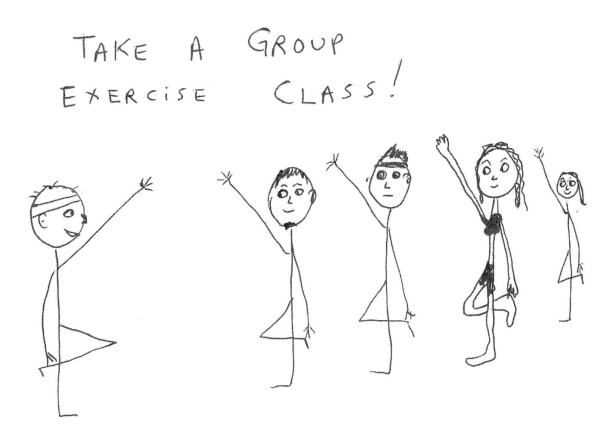

Is the world's biggest introvert telling you to take a **group** exercise class??? Yup. We don't have to review the benefits of exercise. **Exercise is good for you.** But group exercise classes come with some added benefits - even for us introverts! First of all, if you have signed up for a group class, you have some built-in positive social pressure to show up! Even though **everyone** knows it's important, it's still hard for most people to actually show up and **do** the exercising! It's also a simple human fact that we try harder and do better if other people are **looking** at us. Are the other people in the class **really** "watching" you? Probably not as much as you think. But the fact that you think they are makes you try harder! I know that this is very true for myself! Left alone to pursue any kind of endurance workout, I will wimp out much faster than if I am doing the identical workout in a group setting! Also, it's very healthy to have some kind of regular exposure to a group of people who share some of your values. When random people keep going to the same place and running into the same people over and over and over, that's how new friends are made! The digital and "work from home" era has made it harder and harder to make new friends in "the real world." Also, increased isolation tends to make us more fearful and suspicious of other people. A group exercise class can be an antidote. And finally - especially for the introverts! - it's a great chance to get out of your comfort zone! We can't grow without expanding our edges and moving out of our comfort zones.

PUSH YOUR pH TOWARDS ALKALINE (above 7.0)

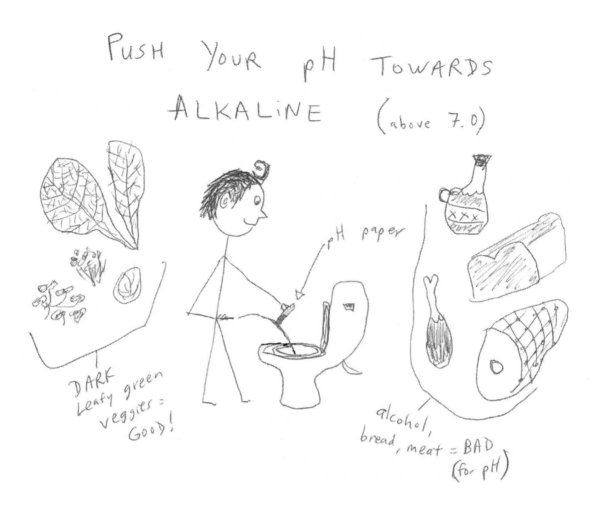

DARK Leafy green veggies = GOOD!

pH paper

alcohol, bread, meat = BAD (for pH)

I've been sitting on this nugget for a long time. I honestly just didn't know what to draw!

All I could think of was a person peeing on a piece of pH paper. 😳 👹

So, yeah, there's a guy peeing on a piece of pH paper!

You might remember pH paper from high school or junior high school (or college?) experiments on acidity and alkalinity.

Or you might use it to make sure the water in your aquarium is right for your fish!

Well, guess what?

It's a handy tool for helping to gauge your own body's acidity or alkalinity, too!

Why does it matter?

The body does a great job of regulating its chemistry, including the pH of most of its tissues.

Your blood, for example, holds steady in a very tight range of barely alkaline: 7.35 to 7.45 - almost perfectly neutral (7).

But when we eat certain foods or put ourselves into certain situations - especially stressful situations - it can drive our body chemistry towards acidity!

And since the blood has to stay in that very narrow range, what do you think the body does

232

to neutralize the acid?

Well, it does what you might do in the chemistry lab! It takes minerals, such as calcium, and uses it to neutralize the acid.

And... where do you suppose the body grabs that calcium from?

If it's not readily available from food, then it will pull it from your bones and muscles!

This is part of why heavy soda drinkers are at a higher risk for osteoporosis.

Because the body is pulling calcium from the bones to help neutralize the acid!

A "natural" healthy human diet, rich in green leafy vegetables, tends to push the body towards alkalinity.

A heavily processed diet pushes the body strongly towards acidity.

Since each individual's body chemistry varies according to their genetics, etc., it's really handy to check the pH of your urine first thing in the morning and pay attention to how it fluctuates based on your diet.

Most pH paper is yellow at first, and then will change color according to the pH.

Ideally, you want your pH paper to be in the green range.

Some people say "it should be the color of a leafy green vegetable."

One patient came to me and said, "This paper doesn't work. It never changes color at all."

Um... the paper wasn't defective. That guy was **very acidic!**

For me, I know that when I eat plenty of dark leafy greens, my pH stays in a healthy zone.

But if I forego the greens and eat some processed food, it jumps to acid. And if I have a cocktail, then it becomes **really** acidic! 💀

There are entire books available on this topic!

The simple thing is, get some pH paper. It's very inexpensive.

Test your pee first thing in the morning for a few days in a row.

See what your baseline appears to be.

Watch how it changes when your change your diet.

And see how you feel if you are able to keep it more alkaline than acidic!

If you're running acidic and you also feel like crap, well... now you have one more thing to aim for. 😳

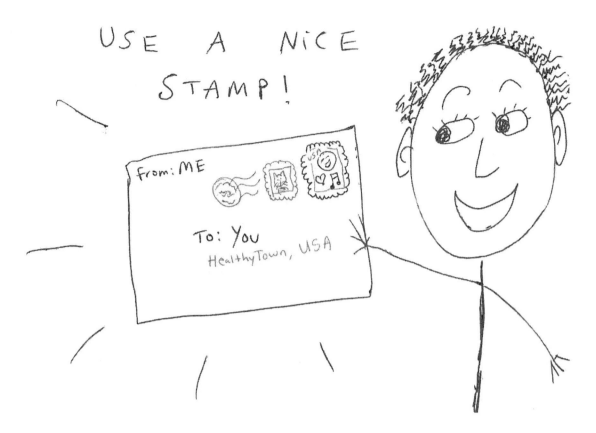

What does using a nice stamp have to do with health???

It's one of the easiest way to spread cheer (and thus increase dopamine and reduce cortisol) in a fellow human being!

It's exciting enough to receive mail (that's not a bill a scary legal notice) but a nice stamp just adds that extra special touch that says, "I like you!"

I can't believe how many people get all excited about a nice stamp.

Even my notoriously crabby mother recently wrote me and wanted to know where I got "all those beautiful stamps" from! (She is super religious so I cobbled together a bunch of old religious stamps onto a card that I sent her.)

Most post offices are shamefully lacking these days when it comes to stamp variety, so, I recommend ordering them online directly from the USPS!

And if you really want to go to town and get creative with your nice stamps, you can buy all sorts of old (unused) stamps off of eBay! That is where I get most of my old (but still usable) stamps. If you are patient and look around, you can often find them for face value or even less! But as long as the price is close, I'm not too picky. It's worth a few more cents to have some special stamps ready for a special occasion!

And if you lament that you have no one to mail things to, check out Postcrossing.com! Still the best way to ramp up your sending **and** receiving of cool snail mail, and probably the #1 best way for introverts to make new friends all around the world!

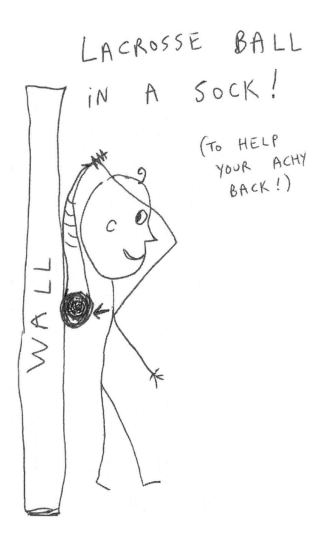

LACROSSE BALL iN A SOCK!

(TO HELP YOUR ACHY BACK!)

WALL

We talked about the benefits of using a lacrosse ball to roll out some tight muscles many nuggets ago, but it's worth repeating that it's a handy tool!

Also, I forgot to mention last time that the best way to use the lacrosse ball to work out some of the knots in your back is to put it into a long sock, like a tube sock, and use the sock to help guide it into place while you lean against a wall and gently move around, giving yourself a nice targeted massage!

While it's pretty awesome to get a professional to work on you periodically, don't forget that you **can** (and should!) give **yourself** some nice massage!

I know, tube socks sound kind of lame... but did you know that Prince always wore tube socks to bed?

Therefore, they are cool.

So, get some and a lacrosse ball, and feel better soon!

235

JUST NOTICE...

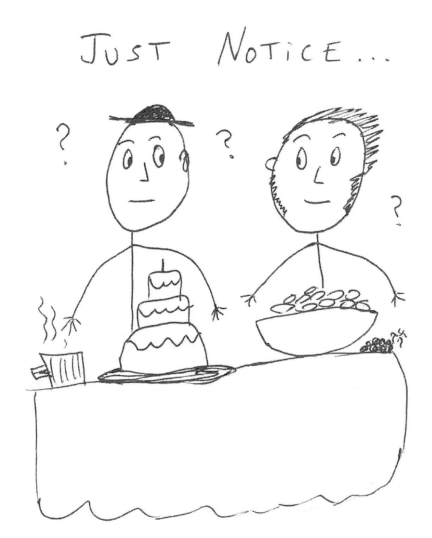

Just notice what? Mainly your body and your brain as you go about your day.

Pay special attention to what's going on when you are around food, movement, bedtime, drinks... anything potentially related to "health."

Just notice. Notice what you're thinking or feeling. Is anything tightening in your body? Does anything hurt? Does anything feel relaxed? Are you feeling numb? Are you feeling an emotion? Is there a dialogue in your head?

And what do you do once you notice?

Nothing! You just notice. You don't judge yourself or think "how can I fix this" or anything at all! Just notice. It's weird, but a lot of Mindfulness practice is about just noticing, without judgement. That's it!

TOWEL UNDER ONE SIDE BUTT MAY HELP SCIATICA

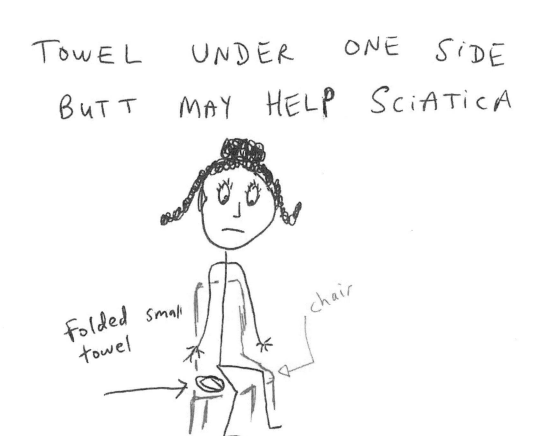

Sciatica is a painful condition where if feels like you're having electrical shooting pain down into your butt and leg!

There are many things that can cause it, and different things you can try to relieve the pain, but one of the simplest things to try is to fold a small towel and put it underneath one buttock while you are sitting in a chair.

(Man, it is hard to draw a chair for stick figures. I don't know why.!)

While it may seem that putting a little towel under one side is going to misalign your pelvis and make you lopsided, the idea is that if you have sciatica, you are already lopsided, and this technique might help to realign your pelvis!

If it makes it worse, then it's under te wrong butt cheek!

(I got this nugget from a little book called *Sciatica Exercises & Home Treatment*, by fellow chiropractor George F Best, D.C. - it is only around $4 on Kindle and has some great tips for sciatica relief!)

ENZYMES VS. PROBIOTICS

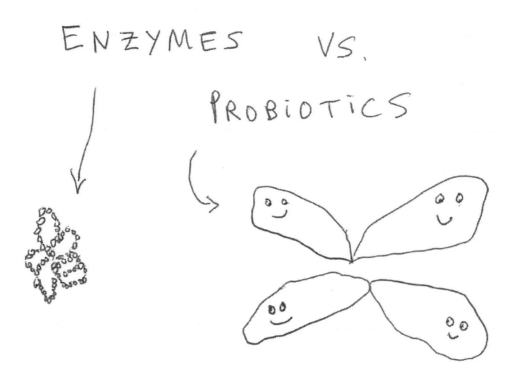

When someone comes to me with digestive trouble, one of the first things I ask is, "Do you take any enzymes?" And a lot of times, the answer is, "Yes, I take a probiotic."

Well, friends, I'm here to tell you that enzymes and probiotics are very different things! True, they are both good for your guts. But ... they're very different. First of all, enzymes are not alive! They are little substances produced **by** a living organism that work as a catalyst to help a chemical reaction happen. For example, the enzyme called lipase helps to break down lipids (or fats). The enzyme called protease helps to break down proteins. The enzyme lactase helps to break down lactose. If you have trouble digesting specific substances, then specific enzymes can help a lot! (The name of the product often lets you know that it's an enzyme type of product: Int**enzyme** Forte, Hydro**Zyme**, Multi**Zyme**, **Zy**pan, **Zy**me**x**, etc.) They are usually taken with food. Probiotics, on the other hand, are living creatures! They eat, reproduce, die, etc. These tiny critters are usually doing something nice for you. They produce substances that help to support digestion and immunity. They are the "good guys" that are living inside of your guts! (As opposed to the "bad guys" such as parasites or harmful bacteria.) In conclusion, I think it's a good idea to supplement with enzymes **and** probiotics, especially as you get older, and your body naturally produces a smaller volume of enzymes and also becomes more susceptible to weakening immunity!

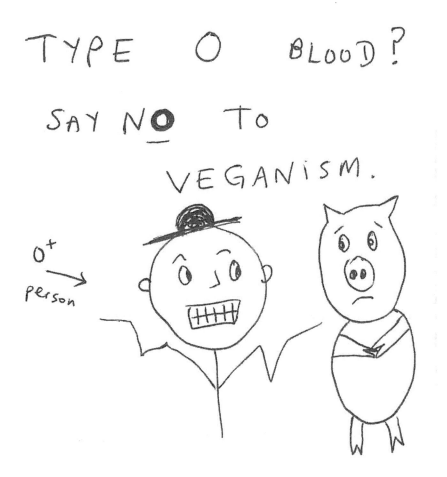

OK, here's another touchy subject... and I GET IT re: the philosophical, ethical, environmental, etc. pros of vegetarianism and veganism. I get it!!! And/but...

It sounds like a kooky theory, but I've seen it in action over and over and over again during the course of my entire practice: people with different blood types do **tend** to do better or worse with different diets. And the most dramatic seems to be the O type blood people, specifically when it comes to vegetarianism - and **especially** veganism. People with type O blood need **some** animal products (usually red meat) in their diet in order to feel really healthy. If you see (or if you are) a really sickly vegetarian with lots of weird health issues and you've been a vegetarian for a long time, **and** you have type O blood, then you may really want to consider adding some animal to your diet.

If you don't know your blood type, you can easily figure it out at home using an Eldon test kit. They are inexpensive and easy to find online.

There are lots of books and even apps for learning about and following "blood type diets," but I like Peter d'Adamo's books.

And don't worry too much for the pig in today's picture. Peter d'Adamo says that pig is not a very healthy meat for **any** of the blood type, so, that guy probably won't eat the pig...

WEAR SOCKS TO BED TO HELP YOU SLEEP?

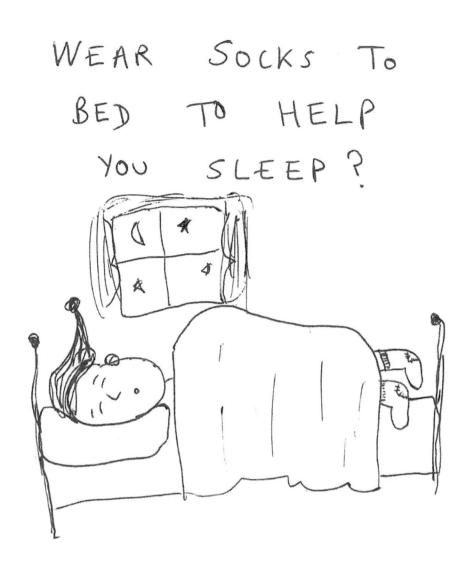

Does wearing socks to bed help you sleep better??

For some people, the answer is **YES!**

Loose, breathable socks (wool or cotton are best) can help the body to maintain a steady temperature, which is important for a nice deep sleep.

This is especially true if you are prone to cold feet at night!

(Maybe this is why Prince wore those tube socks to bed every night...)

Anyway, it's a very simple thing, so if you have trouble sleeping, then give it a try!

OLIVE OIL +
LEMON JUICE +
CAYENNE PEPPER =
LIVER ♡
Love

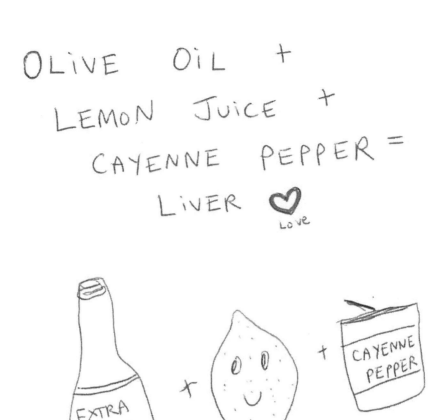

There are sooo many complicated cleanses, detoxes, etc. out there!

But you know, sometimes the old tried and true things still stand the test of time!

Here is an oldie but a goodie that is very helpful for the liver.

It's one of those "drink this first thing in the morning for about a week, before you eat or drink anything else" things.

The recipe is basically 1/2 ounce of extra virgin olive oil + 1/2 ounce of fresh lemon juice + a pinch of cayenne pepper. (Some recipes out there include a little bit of freshly pressed garlic.)

This concoction is a nice gentle liver tonic.

I don't think it delivers on the miraculous cure that some people tout, but... it does help, and you will feel noticeable results if liver congestion is something that you struggle with!

What kind of results can you expect? It will be things like improvement in mood, muscle tension, headaches, digestion...

MAKE INVISIBLE SNOW ANGELS ON YOUR FLOOR

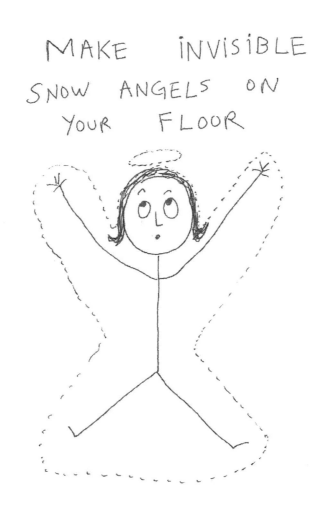

I know, this one sounds weird...but... it's good for you! You might not have enough space on your floor, depending on how big you are and how small your apartment or bedroom is... ...or how cluttered your floor is? Just lay down on your floor, take a few nice deep breaths, settle in your body, arms at your sides and feet together, and then slowly expand your arms and legs out and arms up, as if you're making a snow angel! Go slow if you are old and creaky or in any way limited! (Or if you're afraid of what you might bash into on the floor!) And when you get to the end of the range of motion then move back into the starting position. Just focus on breathing and going through the range of motion. You can look around your room from the floor vantage point and enjoy the weirdness. Do you feel like a tiny kid again? Do you feel like a crime scene victim? Just let your mind wander. This is a weird but good exercise for working on those expansive muscles while also resting while also shaking up your perspective. Enjoy!

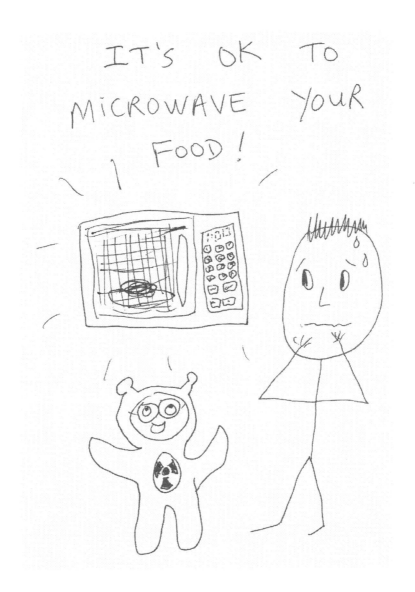

Yes! It's OK to microwave your food! (It doesn't always taste that great, but... 😵)
A lot of people in the holistic health world are still verrrry mistrustful of microwaves, and I guess it doesn't help that us children of the Cold War like(d) to call it "nuking" our food. Microwaving food does not have anything to do with radiation. It just jiggles water molecules really really fast which causes heat. **That said...** it **is** true that a lot of "microwaved foods" are indeed bad for you! But it's not because of the microwave ovens! It's because the foods themselves are ultra processed foods. Therefore... Hot Pockets are not a terrible "food" because of the microwave. They are a terrible "food" because they are ultra processed and... well... terrible. So have at it! Nuke that sweet potato with wild abandon, and... **enjoy!**

USE A TOWEL
OR ROPE TO HELP
YOU STRETCH!

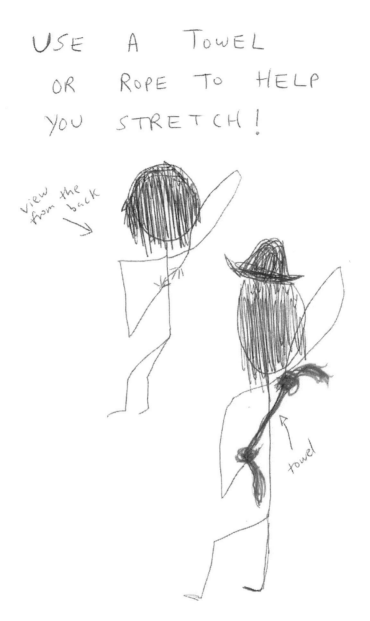

There is a great stretch that involves reaching behind your back from below with one arm and from above with the other, and then clasping your hands together. If you have full range of motion in your shoulders, then you should be able to do this on both sides! Once upon a time, I used to be able to do this. It was easier on one side, but I could do it! But... no more. So, what's a person to do? Well, one thing you can do to slowly improve your range of motion is to use a towel, rope or strap to help bridge the gap in your ability and very slowly and gently work on the stretch. Over time, it will get better and better.

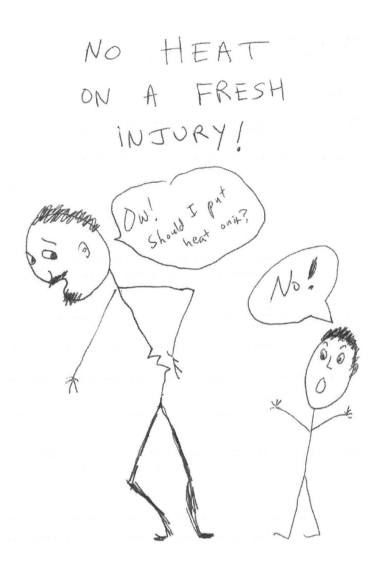

When you hurt yourself, it's sometimes hard to remember... do I put heat on it, or ice?!
Well, if it's a *fresh injury, don't put heat on it!* Heat brings more blood to an area, and that's
not what you want when an area is freshly injured and already starting to swell and become
inflamed! Sometimes, the injury is deep, like a strained back muscle.
How can you tell if it's inflamed if you can't tell whether it's swollen?
An area of inflammation is usually warmer than the areas around it.
So, if you feel a little warm spot on your back where the pain is, then that's inflammation!
And it doesn't need heat. If you have a fresh injury and there's some inflammation, then it's a
much better idea to ice it. Heat is best for chronic conditions (things that you've had for a
while) such as tight muscles and dull achy pain.

ICE MASSAGE
FOR BACK PAIN
(or shin splints, or ....)

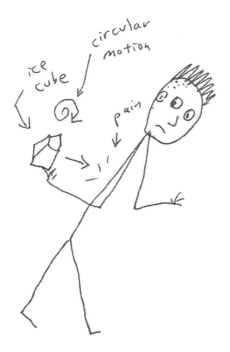

One of the rules of thumb when it comes to icing is, don't put the ice directly on your bare skin! You're supposed to always put a little towel or cloth between the ice and your skin - *except when it comes to ice cube massage or ice massage!* An ice cube is nice because it will melt in about the right amount of time for a short ice massage (about 5 minutes or less) but it's messy, too, so many people recommend freezing some water in a small paper cup and peeling off some of the bottom when you do the massage. Either way, put a towel under the area you're icing to catch the melted water.

The continuous movement of the ice is what makes it safe to put against the bare skin (as opposed to just leaving ice against the skin without moving it around), plus it's only for a short time. Ice massage helps with pain and inflammation.

NETi POT
FOR SiNUS RiNSE

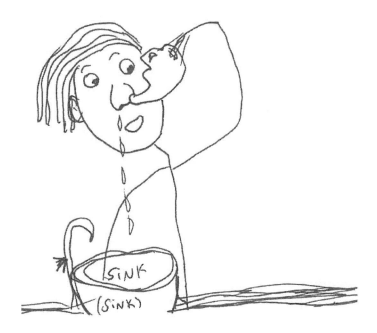

Once upon a time, I think that neti pots were mostly considered something that New Age people and hippies did, but now you can buy a basic neti pot at Walgreens!

The neti pot is a very simple tool that has been used for about 500 years in India to deliver a saline (salt water) rinse to the sinuses. This is great for allergies, colds and mild congestion. (It doesn't work if you are completely plugged up!)

The way it works is, you mix up some salt with very clean water (boiled and then cooled down or bottled / distilled), put it into the little pot, put the spout against one nostril, tilt over, and just let the water pour up into your sinuses on one side and out the other side of your nose while you breathe through your mouth!

Then, repeat on the other side.

It feels weird but oddly refreshing afterward!

You usually mix about 1 teaspoon of salt with about 1 pint of water.

note: people who have had sinus surgery or surgeries around the sinuses should NOT use a neti pot without consulting with a doctor!

SAFETY FIRST!

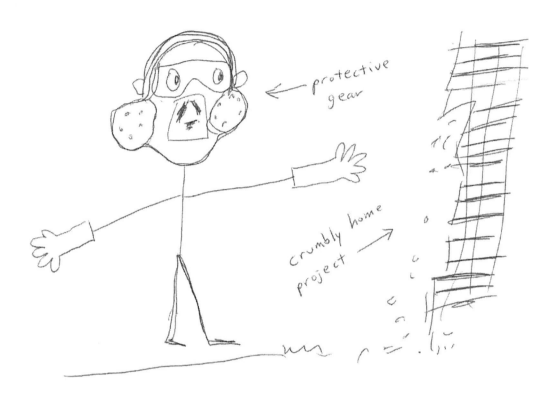

protective gear ←

crumbly home project →

Sometimes, it seems like a very American or manly thing to eschew protective gear, but... don't do it! I can't even begin to tell you how many people I come across who have developed serious health problems after choosing to forego protective gear during various home project situations!

Perhaps the worst offender, believe it or not, is sickness or trouble after ripping up old carpet and flooring without a mask! It's crazy what accumulates in and under old carpeting! Basically anything that kicks up tiny particles that you might breathe in means that you should be wearing some sort of mask.

And don't forget eye protection and gloves for handling chemicals!

In this case, an ounce of prevention is worth **far more** than a pound of cure!

(...especially when the consequences of certain kinds of chemical and particulate exposure don't have a good cure!)

Try Mindful Eating

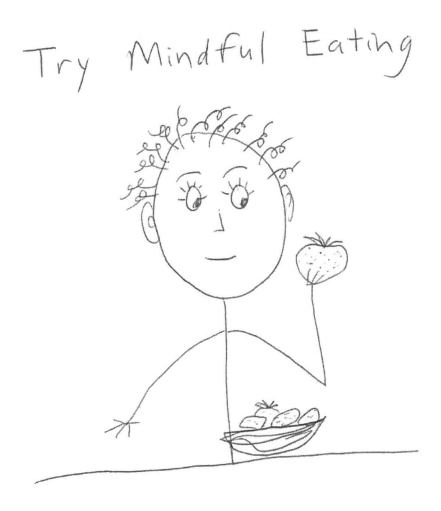

Mindful eating is not so much about **what** you eat as it is about **how** you eat.

I dunno that it's possible to be a "mindful eater" **all** the time... nobody's perfect!

But it's a great exercise that can help you enjoy your food more, and also can help with balancing portion control, whether you tend to over- **or** under-eat!

Mindful eating involves slowing down and taking in your food with all your senses and just noticing what's happening.

You start by just looking at the food. If it's practical, then pick it up and look at it from different angles, study the shape, color, textures. Really see the food in detail, and notice any thoughts or impressions that come to mind.

Then you can touch the food (unless it's something like yogurt or soup that you don't want to stick your hand into) and again, notice the texture. The firmness. The density.

Then you bring it up to your nose and smell it, and just notice the smell and any impressions that come to mind.

Before putting the food in your mouth, maybe just move it around your lips a little bit and notice if the sensation gives a different impression than when you were using your hands. Just notice the food and any thoughts that come along with it, and then finally put it in your mouth.

Before chewing it, pause and just notice again the texture and sensations of the food in your mouth and any thoughts or impressions that rise up.

And then when you start to chew, keep paying attention. What's going on in there? What does it feel like? Just notice all the sensations along your tongue, cheeks, gums, teeth, throat...

And finally swallow. And notice, how does your body feel about that?

After a few bites of mindful eating, you might not even be hungry anymore. Or you might be. Either way, it doesn't matter. The point of the exercise is just to notice.

I know, you probably could have eaten a whole hamburger in the time it took to just read the directions of how to mindfully consume one bite or piece of food!

Hey, I'm just the messenger.

Food is weird. We need it for survival, but it gets tangled up in so many complicated emotions and meanings beyond mere sustenance!

Next time you sit down to eat something (and if nobody's watching, I guess, if you're shy) try out the mindful eating exercise!

It's another great tool for your stress-reduction bag o' tricks.

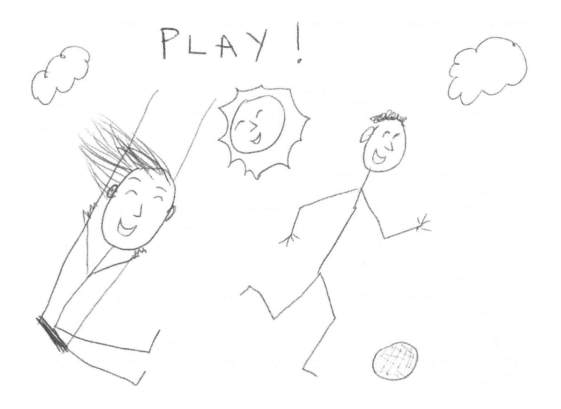

Yes, at any and all ages, **play** is an important part of health!

Play is something that can embody simple joy. Think of things you may have enjoyed as a child. They're things that you're not going to be evaluated on. Not a competition! Just something done for pure simple joy.

Maybe get a yo-yo and see if you can still do any of those tricks.

(I don't think I was ever able to do anything impressive with a yo-yo... but it was fun to try!)

Make a paper doll and some outfits for it.

Go play in the sand or dirt.

Play with an Etch-a-sketch.

Color.

It's totally up to you!

(Most of my play these days probably happens when I'm decorating postcards to send to a kid or to someone who likes stickers and stuff like that. Also, I do have an old set of Fisher Price Little People from the '70s in a shoe box that I take out once in a while!)

251

WHITE SPOTS ON FINGERNAILS = ZINC DEFICIENCY

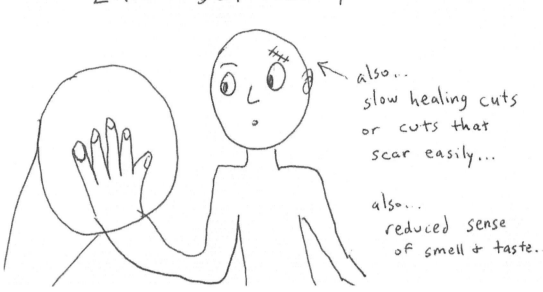

also...
slow healing cuts
or cuts that
scar easily...

also...
reduced sense
of smell & taste.

Gah! This sounded like such a simple and helpful nugget, but then I realized that you can't draw "white spots" on fingernails with a black pen! 😳 👻
Well, you get the idea...
Anyhoo... white spots on fingernails are generally caused by a zinc deficiency!
Simple zinc supplementation will take care of it.
Zinc is good for the immune system, but here are a few more things that zinc can help with: slow-healing cuts or cuts that scar easily, and also reduced sense of smell and taste.

Note: zinc supplements make some people nauseous if taken on an empty stomach. This is frequently the cause of the queasy feeling many people get when taking multivitamin/mineral supplements on an empty stomach. So take it with food!

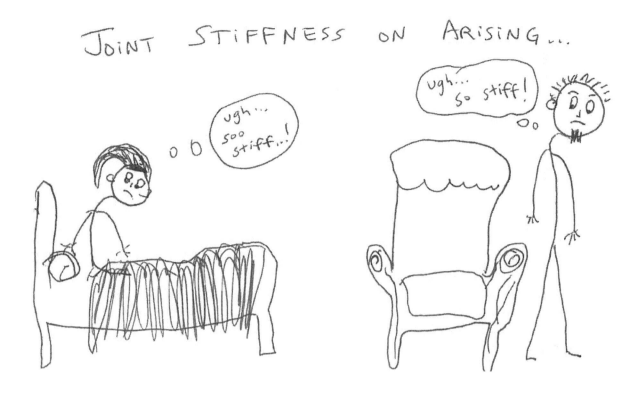

When we say joint stiffness "on arising," we are not just talking about rising out of bed! We are also talking about rising up from sitting down after a long time! (really, when rising up after being in any position for a long time.)

Can you guess the #1 more frequent cause for this?

Yes, it's our old frenemy, **dehydration!**

Usually it means you're not getting enough water.

But... if you have a terrible stiffness on rising after being in one position for a long time, and then it's OK again after you start moving around, then you might actually have a phosphorous deficiency!

This is the second most common reason for it, and it's especially true if your family has a history of arteriosclerosis (clogged arteries).

The fix for this is usually to start with a liquid phosphorous supplement (such as Phosphozyme Liquid, from Biotics Research) 1 dropper 2-3x/day until the stiffness subsides, and then switch to a lecithin supplement for long-term prevention and support.

POTASSIUM DEFICIENCY
COMMON SIGNS....

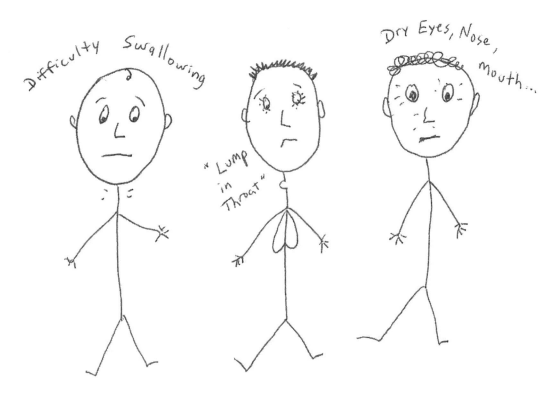

Did you know that some of the common symptoms of potassium deficiency are difficulty swallowing, a "lump in the throat" sensation, and dryness of the eyes, mouth and nose? How do you know if it's a potassium deficiency? Well, this one is pretty easy. You basically add some potassium to your diet and see what happens! In most cases, the problem is that you're not getting enough water or fruits and vegetables in your diet!

The easiest way to target an increase in potassium is to supplement with 1-2 teaspoons of apple cider vinegar (Bragg's or Spectrum brand) in water two or three times a day.

Also... in case you're wondering why so many old people seem to need potassium supplements, the answer is: dehydration!

Potassium is an essential mineral and electrolyte, and it a person is dehydrated, they tend to run low on minerals, which need water for proper absorption.

Potassium is really important for your muscles and your heart (which of course is a type of muscle). Yet another reason to keep on keeping on with the water!

DON'T "SHOULD" ON PEOPLE!

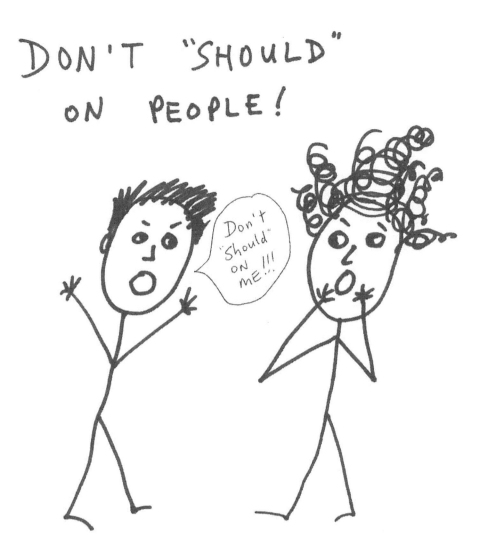

Today's nugget was inspired by a patient who came in today and told me about someone talking about all the "shoulds" that people throw his way and said, "Quit shoulding on me!" I thought that was hilarious, and also a great idea for a daily nugget! After all, anger is the most destructive emotion when it comes to health, and what causes anger? Anger comes from *unmet expectations.* Something did not happen the way it "should" have. Someone did not say or do what they "should" have! If we can ease off our expectations and let go of the "shoulds," then life can be more peaceful. Work to minimize or eliminate this word ("should") from your vocabulary! And if someone keeps shoulding on you, tell them, "Don't should on me!"

p.s. there is a little ditty from 1993 called "Don't Should on Me," by David Roth, that you can find on YouTube. "Don't should on me, and I won't should on you!"

255

STRONG CORE =
STRONG BACK

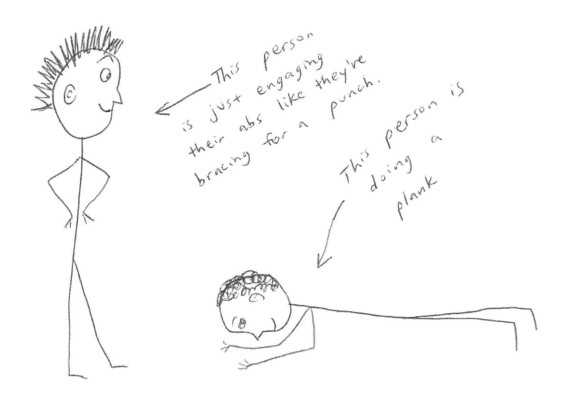

This person is just engaging their abs like they're bracing for a punch.

This person is doing a plank

When people feel like they have a "weak back," they often think about doing exercises to "strengthen" their back. This might be appropriate in some cases, but it's more common that people really have a **weak core!** You can strengthen your core by doing exercises such as the plank, or consciously engaging your core muscles as if you are bracing for a punch to the gut. (I started to try and draw someone about to punch someone else in the gut, but not in a mean way, just in a "training buddies way" but that seemed too complicated for stick figures, so now it just looks like one guy lording over the other guy who is doing a plank.)

The plank is one of my favorite core exercises. I never see people who injure themselves with this exercise! Anything's possible, but it's pretty rare. (As opposed to the overhead press, which injures people all the time!)

THE 8-MINUTE PHONE CALL

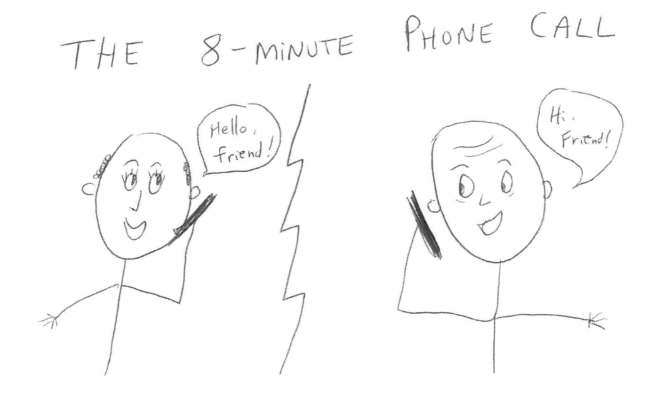

One of the top 5 regrets of the dying is, "I wish I had stayed in touch with my friends." Staying in touch seems like it should be easy, but it's hard!

The 8-minute phone call can help! 📞 🖩

The 8-minute phone call is exactly what it sounds like. You contact a friend and ask if you can schedule an 8-minute phone call.

This call should be exactly timed.

Why??

Because people are busy, and they are often hesitant to commit to an open-ended "let's catch up" kind of call!

Nobody wants to be an a-hole and say you're not worth catching up with, but.... life is life!

8 minutes is short enough that it feels easy and safe to commit to, yet it's longer than the impersonal "5 minute" call.

It's enough time to quickly catch up on the highlights and let each other know that you care!

Think of a friend you haven't connected with in a while and see if they will schedule an 8-minute phone call with you!

(I learned about the 8-minute phone call as part of the New York Times 7-Day Happiness Challenge.)

SIMPLE WARM INFUSION

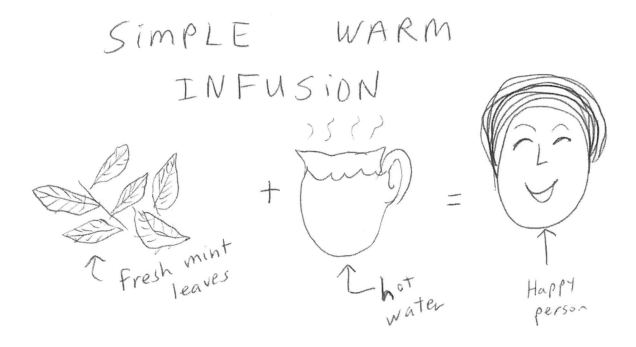

← fresh mint leaves

← hot water

Happy person

Sometimes a warm and refreshing beverage can be as simple as pouring hot water over a handful of mint leaves, letting it steep for a few minutes, and pouring it through a strainer!
I had a really delightful meeting with a colleague the other day, and that was exactly what we had for drinks.
I thought about adding a link to some fancy infusion recipes, but you know what? We're keepin' it real simple today!
Handful of mint leaves, water, smiles.

WET CLOTH ON WRISTS TO COOL DOWN

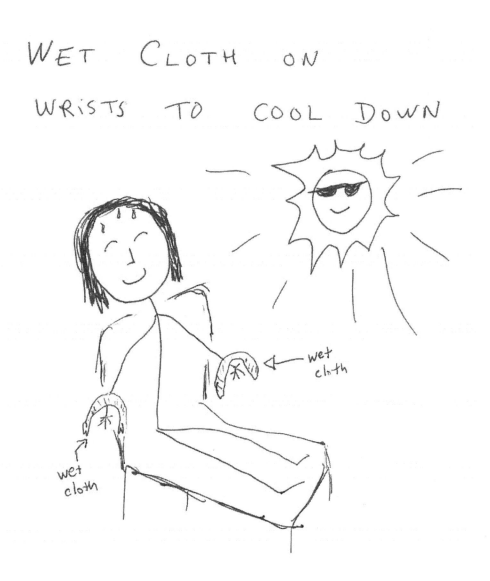

wet cloth

wet cloth

Here is a very simple trick to help cool off on a hot day.

Just put some wet pieces of cloth on your wrist(s)!

Why does this work?! It works because the blood vessels are close to the surface of the wrists, and the evaporation of the water on the cloth creates a cooling sensation, which passes to the blood and helps the body to feel cooler!

(This is also why some people put wet cloth on top of their head if they're trying to cool off!)

But the wrist method won't mess up your hair. (If you have hair. 😑🤖)

You can also use this same approach anywhere you can feel a pulse, since those are the places where the blood vessels are close to the surface of the skin.

BACK WHEN YOU WERE HEALTHY ....

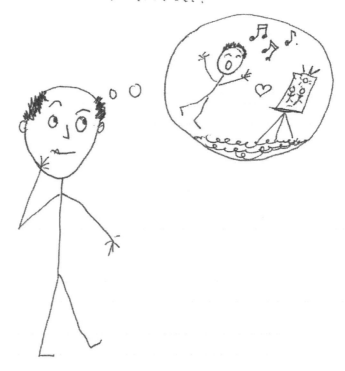

Think back to a time when you were healthy and feeling great. What were you doing? What were you eating? What were you listening to? It's true that you can't replicate everything from the past. Like, you can't have a 20-year-old body anymore if you're 60! (You can't have a 20-year-old body if you're *anything* but a 20-year-old!) But you can make it easier to (re?) adopt healthy eating and behavior patterns if you duplicate some of the elements from that time. The brain wants things to make sense. So, it will work to put things that go together together! If there was a hobby you were into, or a band that you listened to all the time, or a favorite food from back then, see if you can bring it back into your life. If you can recreate some of the good feelings from back when you were healthy, then it will be easier for your body to move towards other habits and practices that will put you closer to that state. If **now** is your healthiest time ever, well, good for you! AND, also, why not plant some seeds for future you to hang onto if they need to get healthy again? Use a new perfume or cologne, or learn to make a special dish, or listen to some special music, so that a very special scent or sound is associated with **this** special and healthy time of your life! Use your powers for good!

"TRAIN" FOR UPCOMING STRESSFUL EVENTS!

There is a funny meme that appears on my various feeds every so often.
It's usually titled something like "introverts getting ready to make a phone call" and it shows a sequence of people running, sweating, working out with a punching bag, etc.
It's funny because it's kind of true! And/but, even though I also drew a picture of a guy working out with weights (probably based on the meme) that's not exactly what I mean by "training for upcoming stressful events." Exercise certainly **can** be part of the training, but the idea is that whenever a big stressful event is coming up, it's going to be taxing on your body, and therefore it's smart to "get in shape" for it! I mean, isn't this why athletes train for events? Running a marathon or competing in a big tournament, etc. takes a lot out of the body! Athletes prepare for big events by watching their diets and modifying their exercise routines as needed. They make sure to get the right amount of sleep and water, and they minimize distractions! So, if you know you have a stressful event coming up - even a "good" stress event, such as a keynote that you've been invited to deliver, or a big wedding event or ..???
[fill in the blank of your stress] - it makes sense to prepare your body for it! Eat more veggies and drink more water in the days or week(s) leading up to it! Pay more attention to getting to bed on time, exercising and breathing mindfully. You will weather the stress storm much better, and you will also recover much faster than if you just head into it willy nilly!

FLAX SEED OIL INSTEAD OF FISH OIL (sometimes)

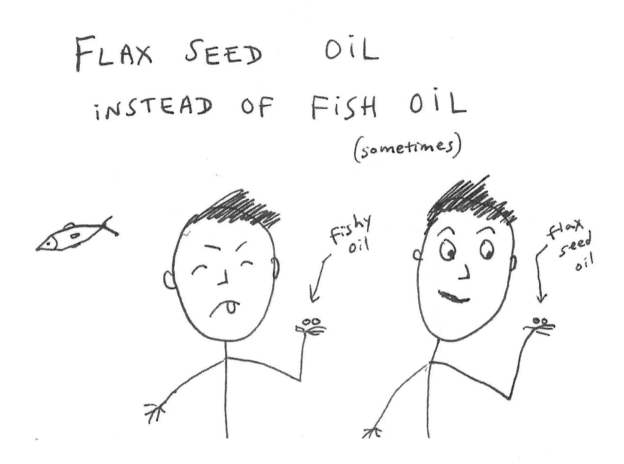

A good omega-3 fatty acid supplement is one of the basic supplements that most of us need to stay healthy.

For most people, the go-to in this department is fish oil.

Fish oil is fine and good (well... depending on the source...) but many people are not fans of the fishy taste and fishy burps that can accompany these supplements!

(If your fish oil supplement gives you bad fishy burps, then the oil is probably rancid and it's a bad quality of supplement!)

Well, good news: flaxseed oil is also a great source of omega-3 fatty acids!

Depending on your genetics and what's going on with your health, you may even do better with flax seed oil than with fish oil!

Feel free to alternate, too, and remember: the most helpful supplement is the one that you'll actually swallow!

GO TO BED AT THE SAME TIME EVERY NIGHT!

Go to bed at (more or less) the same time every night is an important part of sleep hygiene called sleep **regularity.**

Going to bed at around the same time helps your body to stay in a natural rhythm.

When your schedule is all over the place, it's hard for the body to relax and recuperate, even if you're still getting "enough" sleep hours!

(Although, let's be honest. If your schedule is all over the place, I'm pretty sure you're not getting enough hours.)

Little kids do better with a regular bedtime, and so do you! 😴

And yes, my bedtime really is 9:30, and/but that clock is also my tiny homage to the old 9:30 Club, in my hometown of Washington, DC. Little did I know that I would grow up to be a member of an entirely different 9:30 Club! 😴

TAKE A DAY
OFF....

What... that's it?? 😳

Yeah, pretty much. 🙂

There's lots of great reasons why!

But one of the overlooked reasons is that it can be a good reminder that *the world will keep turning, and people will figure out how to make do without you* once in a while!

And you can make do as well.

...or make something else...?

...or make nothing...

It's up to you - it's **your** day off!

But yes, take regular days off, and take a random day off periodically, too!

264

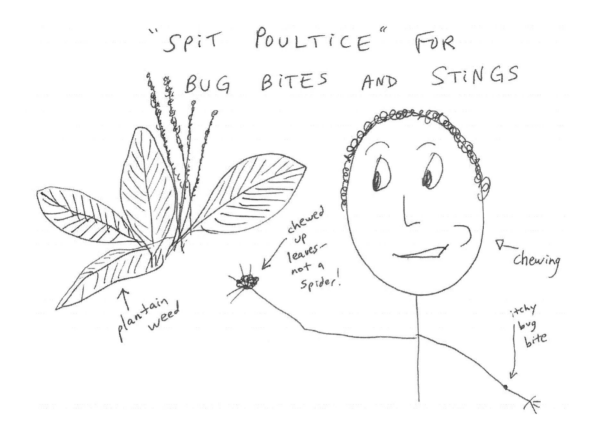

"SPIT POULTICE" FOR BUG BITES AND STINGS

plantain weed

chewed up leaves - not a spider!

chewing

itchy bug bite

OK, for this one, you can't really go by my drawing for the plant - which is supposed to be plantain weed! I'm about to go to the airport and scrambled to draw it from memory! 😳 🙊
This is a very common "weed" which is found throughout the United States but is native to Europe and parts of Asia.

If you've read my book, *The Issues are in the Tissues*, then you know that this is my favorite "weed." It is sooooooo useful and so easy to find! (And even **I** can grow it - and I have the black thumb!)

The short and sweet of it is this. All you do is find this plant (which is probably growing in your yard) and chew up some leaves and slap it down on that bug bite or sting, and it makes the pain and itch go away **fast!**

Yes, it's messy, because it's chewed up leaves!

But, mostly I am mentioning it as a very handy tip for you outdoorsy people who are getting bitten or stung far from the comfort of whatever commercial thing you would put on a bug bite!

Make friends with this super common plant! 💚

"LIVER MASSAGE"

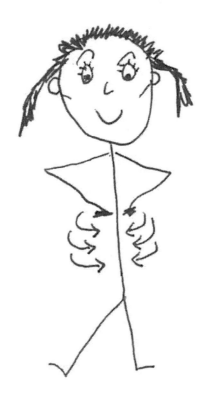

Here is a simple self-massage technique that I learned from an acupuncturist's video! (Thanks, Kat!)

The way you do this self-massage is, you take your hands and hold them flat, palms up, and go to the lowest part of your rib cage.

Massage along the edge of the rib cage using the "knife edge" (pinky side) of your hand, symmetrically, one hand on each side.

Slowly make your way down the abdomen, breathing deeply, and massaging up and down at an angle.

Technically, the liver is located behind the ribs, so you 're not directly massaging the liver, but this abdominal massage really helps to move the lymph and support circulation in the area.

It's great for getting the energy flowing!

SCARF ON THE PLANE

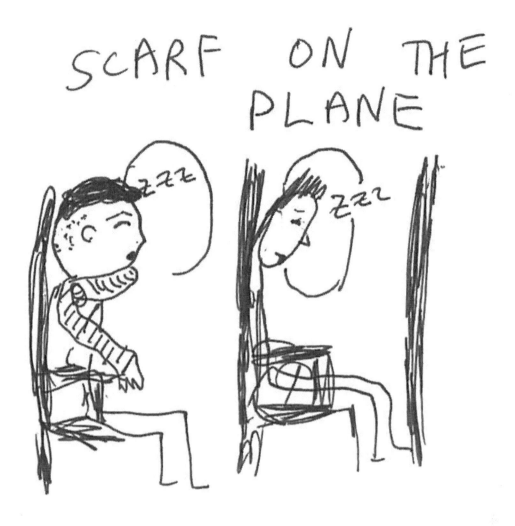

This one is mainly for people with neck issues who also tend to nod off during long plane rides.

I know those neck pillows can be a pain to pack, so if you don't want to bring a support like that, then bring a scarf!

Wrapping a scarf around your neck can help to keep it stable if/when you nod off.

It prevents your neck from going past the stable range of motion unintentionally and causing problems later!

People who have had whiplash injuries in the past are particularly vulnerable because they have ligament instability.

Ligaments are what hold your bones together!

Plus, planes can get weirdly chilly, and a good scarf is so cozy.

THERAPEUTIC DOSES VERSUS MAINTENANCE...

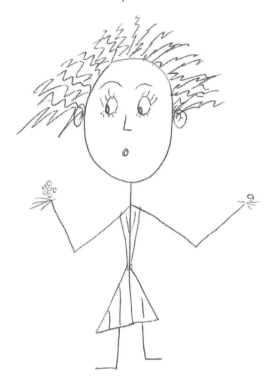

A lot of times, people are surprised when I tell them the dose they should be taking to get a therapeutic effect from certain supplements. Like, 7-10 *grams* of L-Lysine for certain viral outbreaks (which often translates to 14-20 tablets), as opposed to the daily preventative dose of just 1. Or 6-8 gel capsules of omega-3 oil for acute inflammation, as opposed to 1-2 for basic maintenance. Or 20-40 (?!) Cyruta Plus for bulging disc pain versus 3-6 for maintenance. You get the idea! Not ALL supplements work like that, but you should know that often, there is a big difference between the dose that you need to achieve a "therapeutic effect" (meaning that it works more like a drug) as opposed to a basic preventive or maintenance effect (where it works more like food).When you don't know the difference, that is where self-treating with supplements can be tricky! Unfortunately, Doctor Google is not much help in this department. So, if you're using nutritional supplements therapeutically, make sure you also have an experienced practitioner who can help to steer you in the right direction!

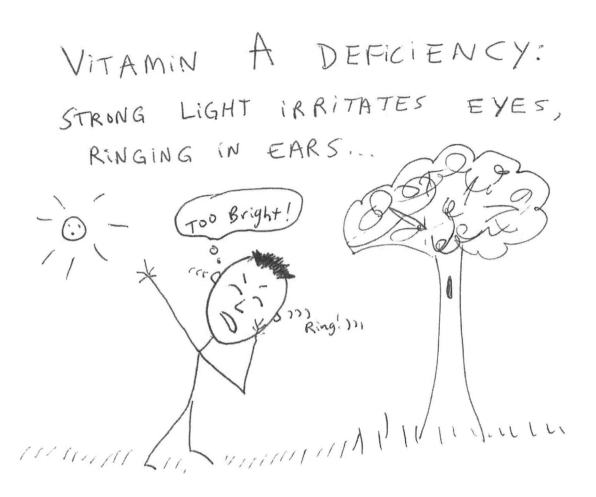

What do these symptoms have in common: strong lights irritate the eyes, noises in the head, and ringing in the ears?

They can all be symptoms of vitamin A deficiency!

Vitamin A is a fat-soluble vitamin, so you **can** take too much and end up with a toxicity problem!

So be careful when supplementing.

Also, there are a few other considerations if you have these symptoms...

The more common problem when strong light irritates the eyes is adrenal insufficiency, which is usually caused by too much unmanaged **stress**.

Also, if a person has high blood pressure **and** noises in the head or ringing in the ears, then the blood pressure should be addressed first!

If blood pressure is normal, then it's usually a vitamin A problem.

WATER FOR THE WIN (AGAIN)

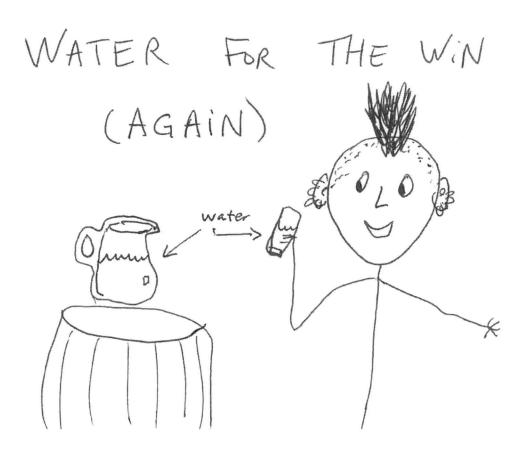

A colleague of mine recently posted on LinkedIn about his nerdy biohacking-obsessed friend who has been measuring every conceivable measurement and tracking every exercise, sleep method, wellness intervention, etc. to see how much he could intentionally optimize his health. He wanted to see which practices gave him the most health bang for his buck! Conclusion? There was **one** thing that made **by far** the biggest measurable difference to his health metrics. The winner?

WATER. 💦

Yep, good ol' fashioned plain ol' boring water was the winner.

Marketers gotta market, shiny object makers gotta shiny object.

Everybody needs to make a living.

But if you really want to stay healthy, then stay hydrated! 😊

Reminder: take your body weight in pounds, divide that number by 2, and aim for that many ounces a day. Get the first liter or quart down before noon and it will help a LOT with afternoon headaches or low energy! You can drink less water if you're ingesting hydrating foods, such as smoothies with chia seeds. But you should drink more if you are drinking dehydrating things like alcohol or coffees, and if you are losing water through sweating, etc.

ACCEPT THAT YOUR BRAIN is BOTH AMAZING AND RIDICULOUS!

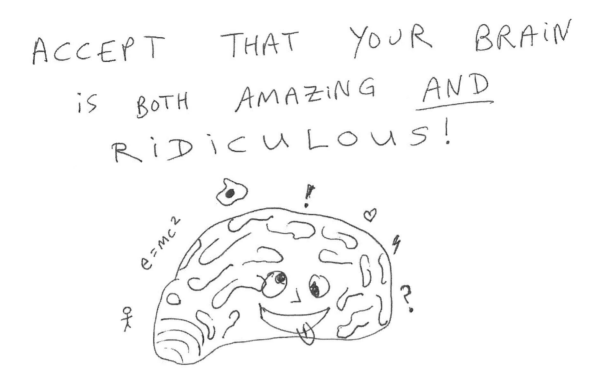

Accept that your brain is both Amazing **and** Ridiculous....

The brain is **amazing**.

We hear it all the time, and it's true!

But then why do we do stupid things? Why do we freak out when there's nothing to freak out about? Why does our own brain talk to us like a crazy person sometimes? Why why whyyy??? Because it's also ridiculous.

Well, it **seems** ridiculous, because we are working it in an environment that it was not designed to work in. Our brains evolved over millions of years to operate under certain fairly static and predictable conditions.

Our world is nuts. We did that. Oops.

Can it be "fixed?" Who knows?! I can say with certainty, "Not in our lifetimes!"

So stop, take a deep breath.

Accept that it's just the way it is.

Love and accept your amazing **and** ridiculous brain.

The more energy you can free up by letting go of the agonizing over whyyyyy your brain is doing what it does, the better!

My favorite ridiculous brain book is *Idiot Brain: What Your Head is Really Up To*. Check it out!

DREAM RECALL AND VITAMIN B6

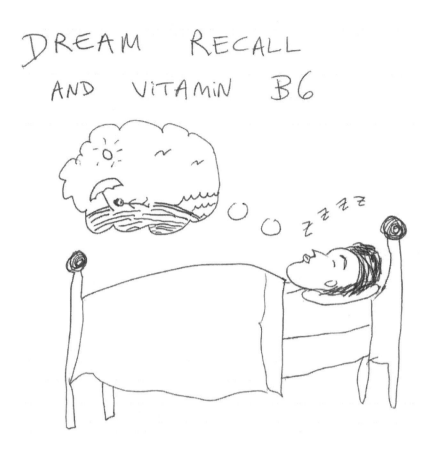

Do you remember your dreams?

Some people roll their eyes when I ask this question and they say, "I don't dream!"

Pretty sure that's not a thing. Well, it's not a healthy thing!

Dreaming is an important part of sleep and it's one of the ways that the body processes and learns! Usually, when people say, "I don't dream," the problem is that they are not sleeping well enough to get into the REM (dreaming) phase of sleep!

Supporting the adrenal glands and addressing big stressors is usually the first step to getting back to dreaming and dream recall!

A good quality vitamin B6 can be a huge help in this department!

B vitamins are water soluble, so they do not store up in the body.

And stress is notorious for depleting the B vitamins, especially B6!

I have always been an active dreamer, and it's what I love most about sleep!

But there was a dark and ominous period of about 2 years during chiropractic school where I wasn't dreaming. I was in an extremely stressful relationship, and my sleep was terrible. Once I got out of the relationship (and out of school!) my sleep came back to normal, and I was back to dreamland! 😴

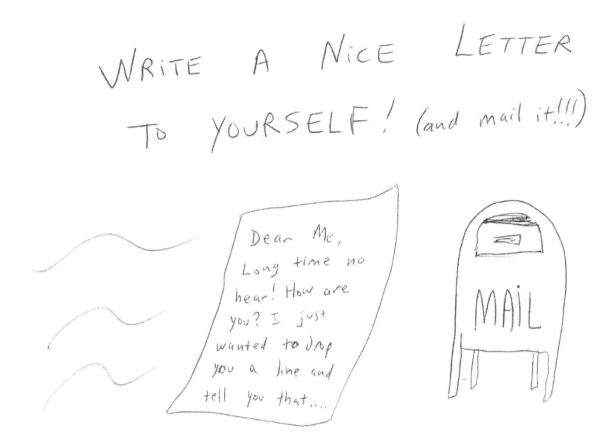

WRITE A NICE LETTER TO YOURSELF! (and mail it!!!)

Dear Me,
Long time no hear! How are you? I just wanted to drop you a line and tell you that....

MAIL

Remember that ridiculous brain of yours?

Well, it's not always a bad thing.

Sometimes, it's downright delightful!

Did you know that if you write yourself a nice letter, and then mail it to yourself, you will often feel delighted when it arrives and sometimes even forget that you are the one who wrote and sent it?!

For maximum effect, wait to mail it - or better yet, mail it to a friend who will mail it to you in about a month - and then you'll **REALLY** be surprised and delighted!

Everyone likes to receive a nice letter!

It's **OK** to send one to yourself!

273

ALTERNATING HOT & COLD SHOWERS!

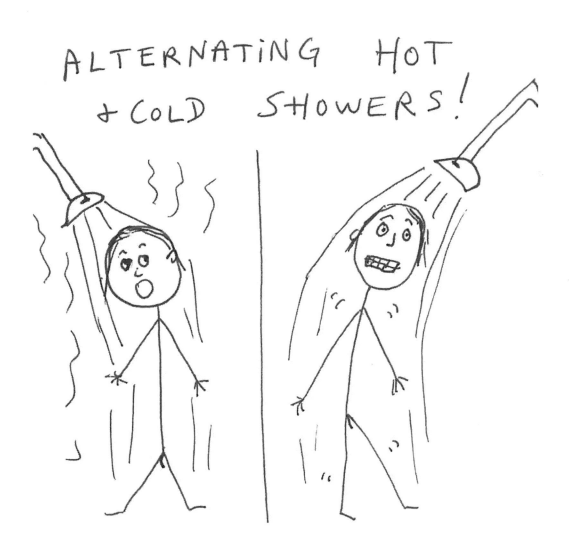

This is a great therapy that can help with depression.

It's basically what it sounds like: stand under a hot shower (about as hot as you can safely tolerate) for about 2-3 minutes and then switch over to cold shower for only about 15 seconds, and then repeat. Aim for 4 cycles.

It doesn't have to be sudden shocking changes! It's OK to ease your way up and down.

It doesn't sound too fun, I know - especially the cold part!

But you will be surprised at how good the mood boost feels!

For some people, it's such a great feeling that they come to *crave* the hot/cold alternating shower!

So give it a try! It can't be worse than the depression!!! 😳 🗿

EAT SEASONALLY AND LOCAL WHEN POSSIBLE

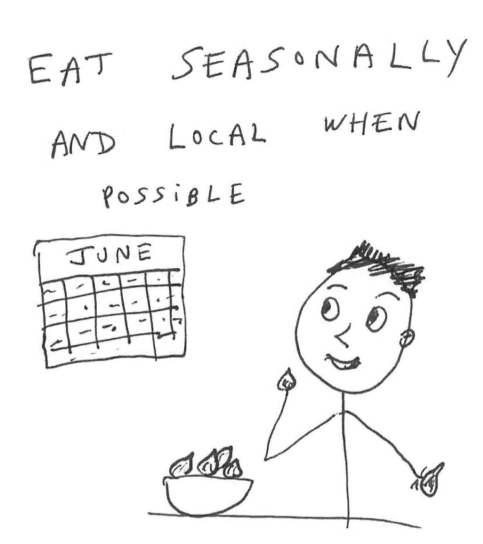

Depending on where you live, this one might be tough.

But, as much as possible, it's a good idea to eat seasonal and local food!

This gives you the best odds of nice fresh food with quality nutrients!

It's also healthier for the planet, as it cuts down on the costs of shipping foods from faraway places!

Our bodies were designed to live with certain rhythms, including seasonal rhythms.

Eating seasonally and locally helps with the dietary side of your health, and it also helps with peace of mind!

WARM YOUR HANDS TO WARM YOUR FEET!

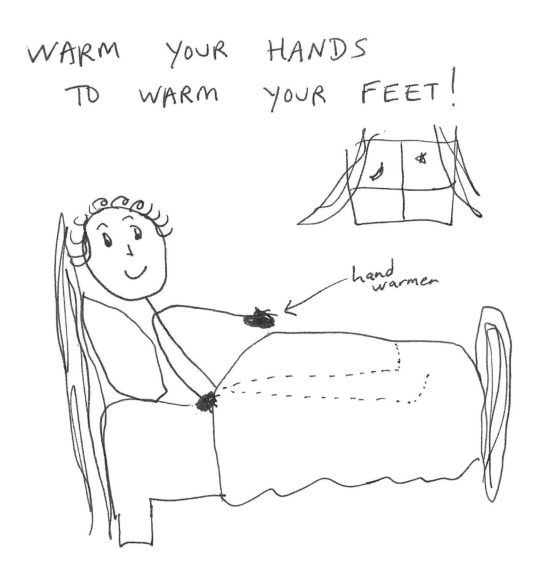

hand warmer

This one is similar to the cooling off one, but... for warming!

I know there are some cold-feet-in-bed people out there!

Well, did you know that if you warm your hands, then your feet will warm up, too?

It's all about warming the circulation, and it's a lot easier to hold warmers in your hand than it is to hold them on your feet!

There are some good rechargeable hand warmers out there that generate heat for hours! It's pretty crazy.

This will help you fall asleep faster (if the cold feet keep you up) and if you have a bedmate, they will certainly sleep better, too, without getting hit with your cold feet!

FOCUS ON THE SOLES... OF YOUR FEET!

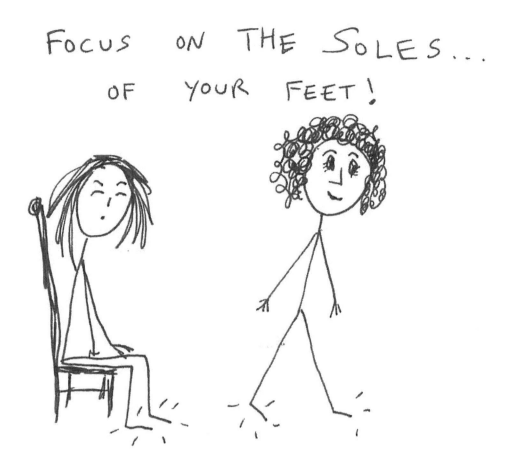

This is a simple Mindfulness practice that is just called the Soles of the Feet.

It's for use in a stressful situation where you need some help pulling yourself back in to the present moment! You can do this while sitting, standing or even walking!

If you're sitting, makes sure that you're comfortable, with both feet on the floor.

If you're standing, soften your knees and let your shoulders come down.

If you're walking, slow your pace and allow your arms and shoulerd to relax.

Next, move your attention to the soles of your feet. Feel your heels on the floor or inside of your shoes. Feel the curves of your arches (if you still have them!), the balls of your feet and your toes. Wiggle your toes if you like, to feel more present to the sensation.

Then, notice your thoughts and any body sensations. (Just notice, without judging or trying to change anything.) When you feel like you are a bit more settled than when you started, then you can return to your regularly scheduled life / activity! (And if you need more time getting present, just go back to paying attention to the sensations in the soles of your feet.)

PRESSURE TO RELEASE PRESSURE ON YOUR JAW

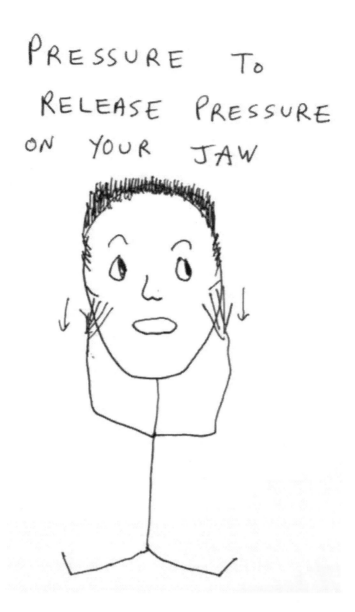

Your jaw contains the most powerful muscles in your body. This is great for biting stuff! And terrible for holding stress! If you hold a lot of tension in your jaw (clenching, grinding, etc.) then here's a simple thing you can add to your daily routine to slowly soften up those muscles. The simplest thing is just plain ol' pressure. Slide your fingertips down the sides of your cheekbones until they fall into that groove. Open and close your mouth to feel where the joint is. Now, just hold some pressure there - not too much - it shouldn't hurt! - and just take a few deep breaths. You can also do a gentle stroking type of massage by just firmly stroking the sides of your face, sliding down over the cheekbones and gliding over the jaw joint. Just a couple minutes of this consistently over a week or two will give you noticeable results! You'll feel more relaxed, and your teeth will thank you, too! (Especially your molars!)

BEANS, BEANS, THEY'RE GOOD FOR YOUR HEART...

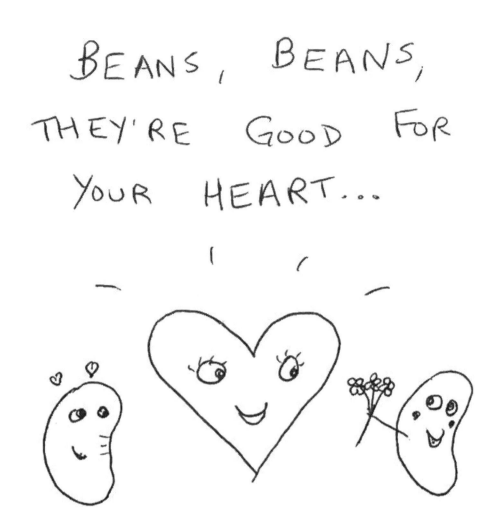

Beans, beans, they're good for your heart.
  The more you eat 'em, the more you fart!
The more you fart, the better you feel, so, eat your beans with every meal!

Ah, who didn't sing that little ditty in their youth?? 🐝 🤍 🐾
But did you know... that it's really true?
Beans ARE good for your heart!!!'

They are high in minerals and fiber and can help to lower unhealthy cholesterol levels.

The American Heart Association says so, too.
Beans and legumes are heart healthy foods!

.

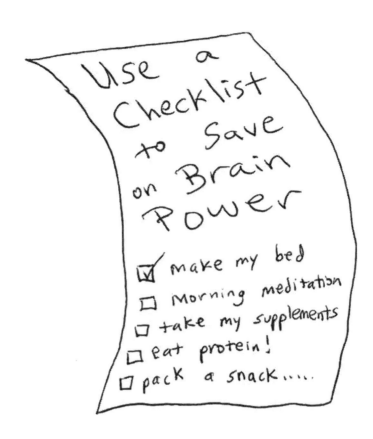

Checklists are not just for those people who seem to delight in checking things off of lists simply for the joy of it!

They are a simple and powerful tool for freeing up brainpower.

And what's so great about freeing up brainpower?

Everything!

Everyone is overloaded and stressed these days!

People are losing their minds because there's just too much noise.

It's impossible to remember everything, so things fall through the cracks.

Anything that is repetitive or predictable should get relegated to a checklist so that you don't have to think about it.

It doesn't matter how many times you've done it or if you think you "should know it by now."

Checklists save time, energy and stress.

I have a checklist for packing my suitcase, even though I've packed it countless times!

(When I don't use the checklist, I always forget something!)

THE YWTL STRETCH

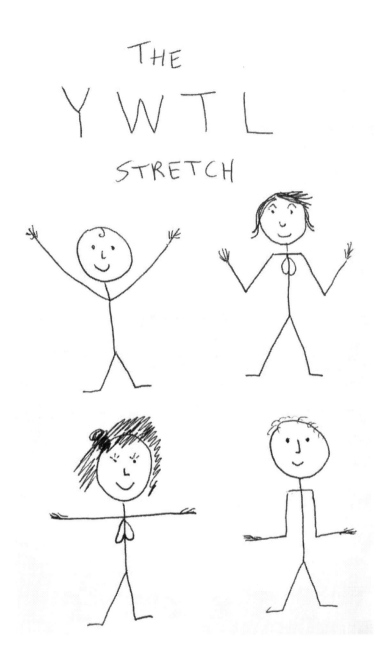

This is a simple and powerful series of stretches that help to open up the mid- and upper back. It's super helpful for people who spend a lot of time sitting, using a computer, or looking down at a cell phone. Sound like anyone you know? 😳 In this series, each pose is held for about 30 seconds, while you are breathing slowly and deeply, and keeping your head held up and shoulders pulled back. And it's exactly as I've drawn it. 😳

DO F.A.S.T.
in CHILD'S POSE

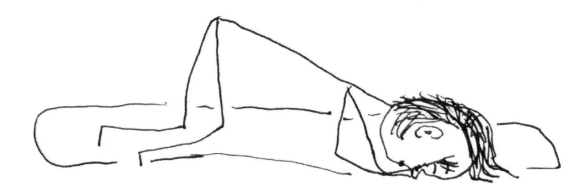

Everybody remembers FAST, right? 😳
First Aid Stress Tool? **www.firstaidstresstool.com**

Because we do it (almost) every day? 😳
It's a great and simple tool for reducing the intensity of stress!
It's also a great before-bedtime task to help process the stress of the day.
But one thing that can make FAST even more impactful is to do it in child's pose (or something approximating child's pose), by getting on your hands and knees, and then resting on your elbows while you hold the pulse points on your wrist with your open hand against your forehead. Why is this position sometimes more powerful than the usual sitting upright? It's because when you're on all-fours (what is also called the quadripedic position), the mammalian or emotional brain becomes more dominant. The neocortex - the "thinking brain" - becomes less dominant. This makes it easier to access deeper emotions and to process them more completely.

USE A BALANCE BIRD

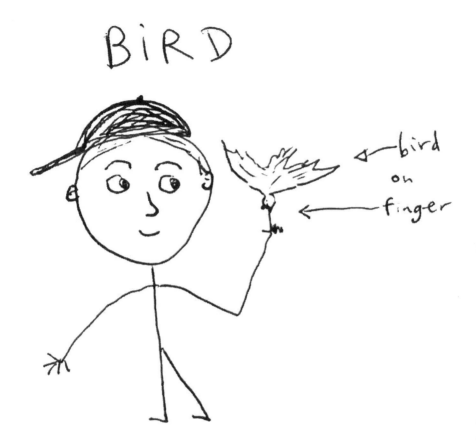

Meditation is one of the best things you can do to calm your mind.

And sometimes, it helps to have a simple small tool to help focus your energy.

One such simple small tool is called a balance bird!

It's exactly what it sounds like: a little bird that balances on a single point.

You just put it on your finger and let it balance there (usually on the tip of its beak) and breathe deeply and watch it, keeping it steady.

That's it! While your brain is focusing on one thing, it's really hard for it to focus on other things. So while you're focusing on the bird and your breathing, it's hard to focus on whatever you were stressing about a minute ago. They are just a couple of bucks if you buy them in the party packs. Great party favors for stressed pals! 😳 🤹

BALANCE BOARD

for balance!

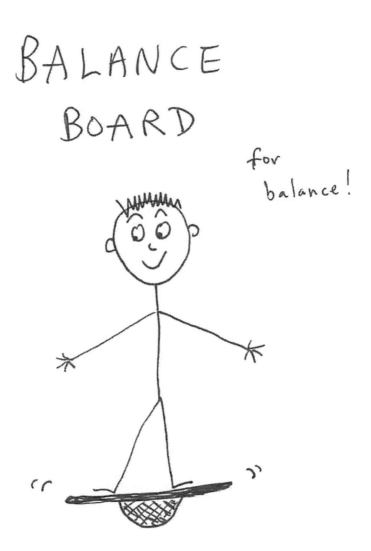

Yep. yesterday, we talked about using a balance bird, and today it's a balance board! The balance bird is to help with mindfulness and focus, and the balance board is for, well, balance! It's important to train your balance, just as you train for strength and agility. Balance is especially important to maintain as you get older. Falling down is more and more treacherous the older you get, so, make sure to train your balance while you can! There are some pretty fancy balance boards out there, like maze balance boards, but as with any piece of exercise equipment, *only get one if you'll really use it!* I like balance boards because they don't take up much space, and you can use them for more than one kind of exercise. Some people even stand on them at their standing desks or while waiting on hold!

VISUALIZE

TO BOOST YOUR MEMORY

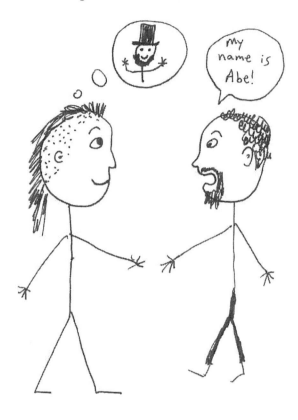

Creating a mental image of something that you want to remember helps to strengthen your memory by giving your brain another way to access the information! If you are "bad at remembering names," this will be a real game changer for you! When you are introduced to someone new and they tell you their name, quickly create a visual image of them that goes with something memorable. In our daily picture, our friend is imagining the new guy in an Abraham Lincoln hat and beard. Trust me, he will always remember that this guy's name is Abe. There is a guy I've only met like 3 times in my life (over the last 20 years or so) but he always remembers that my name is Kim! I wonder if he originally visualized my head on a jar of kimchi? Who knows?? Our capacity for remembering *images* was embedded in our DNA *much earlier* and is far more powerful than our capacity for remembering words! So, use it to your advantage! And make it weird. Memory champion Chester Santos - my favorite International Man of Memory - says that the weirder or more unusual the image is, the easier it is to remember.

3 - 2 - 1
METHOD FOR BETTER SLEEP!

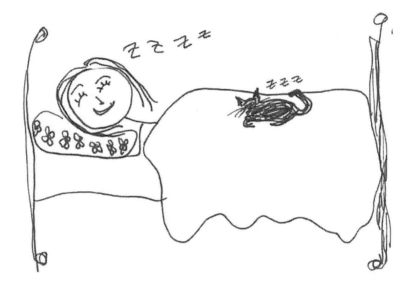

I was just listening to a short audio book called *The 6 Habits of Growth*, by Brendon Burchard, and came across a really simple method for getting better sleep.

He calls it the 3-2-1 method, and it's as simple as it sounds!

NO eating 3 hours before sleep.

NO working 2 hours before sleep.

NO screen time 1 hour before sleep.

Sounds too simple to be true - and also a little annoying, amiright?

But give it a solid go for 10 days in a row and see what happens!

(Noticeably better sleep is what happens! 😳 🐵)

This method obviously requires a defined bedtime.

Pro tip: set your bedtime such that you can get 8 hours of sleep if you need it!

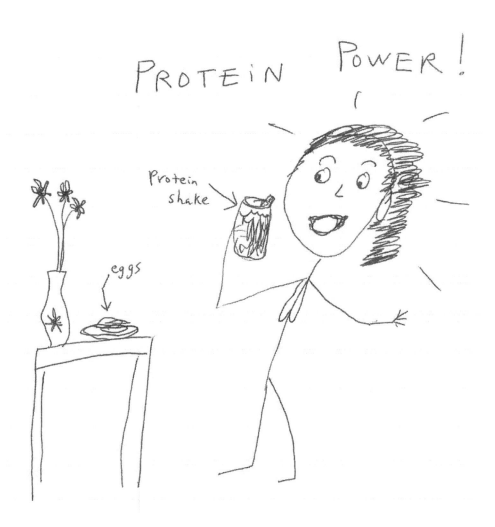

If you are feeling sluggish and low energy, you may not be getting enough protein in your diet! Eating good quality protein is like putting a nice log on the fire.

It will burn for a long time and give you good energy.

Eating carbs, on the other hand, is more like throwing newspaper on the fire.

It makes a bright light and looks great for a second, but it's gone quickly, and it doesn't give off much heat! Protein powders are a convenient way to supplement, but also incorporate more protein into your regular diet.

Animal-based foods are the best sources of complete protein (containing all of the essential amino acids): fish, eggs, poultry, meat, dairy.

Plant-based proteins are usually missing one or more essential amino acids, so it can be tricky. But if you're just trying to get more protein in your life, then don't sweat the details. Just eat more protein!

(and/but don't forget about the fiber!) 😵

POSTURE FEEDS EXPECTATIONS

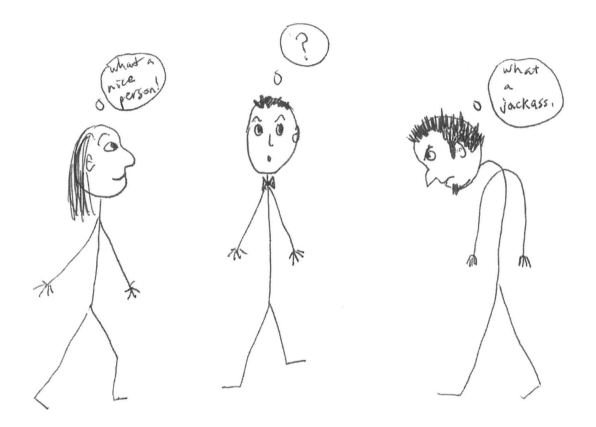

How you feel can determine your posture.

When you get some really bad news, you can feel your posture collapse instantly!

But your posture can also determine your expectations and how you feel about the world around you!

Here is a short exercise I recently experienced at a workshop given by the founders of DE-CRUIT, an organization that helps veterans work through trauma by way of Shakespeare and drama.

Stand up and turn your head slightly downward, tighten your jaw, clench your fists, and walk around stiffly, with shallow breathing.

You don't have to think about anything in particular, but keep that tight, downcast posture.

Then, look at someone - anyone!

What's your initial impression of that person?

How do you feel about them?

Now, try the opposite.

Stand up with your face pointed slightly upward, eyes also looking slightly upward, chest open, hands and shoulders relaxed, mouth relaxed and teeth apart, breathing slowly and deeply.

Walks around for just a little bit in this open relaxed posture, and again,

look at someone.

How do you feel about them?

No matter who the person is - even a random stranger - a strange thing happens.

With the downcast and negative posture, your impression of the person tends to be negative.

You might mistrust them, or dislike their stupid haircut, or wish they would move along, or...???

But in the open and upward facing posture, you are likely to have an inexplicably positive impression of the person. They seem like a nice person. It's easy to like that person.

But either way, you don't know anything about the person!

We think that our impressions and information about the world flow one way, through the sensory information-gathering apparatus of our bodies.

However... that's only part of the story.

We often paint the world in a certain light before we even set eyes on it.

Something as simple as our posture can change the way we experience the world.

Food for thought!

(And now straighten up and take some deep breaths!)

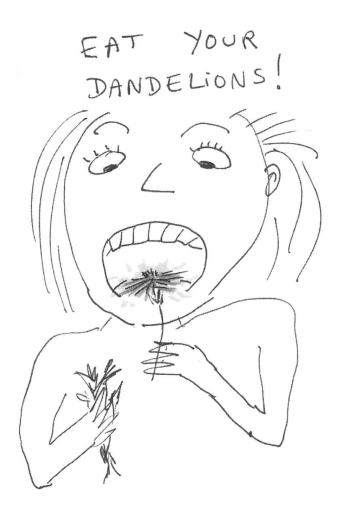

EAT YOUR DANDELIONS!

Well, I mean, don't eat them from your lawn if you use fertilizers and pesticides and all that mess... and don't eat them from other lawns and parks that probably also use chemicals and stuff... but if you can find some nice clean areas where they are growing, then eat 'em up! Dandelions are 100% edible, from the flowers to the leaves all the way down to the roots! They are very healthy, too. Dandelion leaves are excellent for the liver. The mature leaves are pretty bitter, so you may want to focus on eating the young tender leaves. The dried roots are popular as a tea, and the flowers are often eaten fried! One of the things I love best about edible weeds is that they are sooooo easy to grow! Because they're weeds!!! I can't grow much of anything with my black thumb, but can I get dandelions to grow? YES! You can even make dandelion wine from the flowers (kind of tastes like mead) but... it'll take you about 2 years to get your first jug ready to drink. So may as well stick to those salads, fried flowers, and tea!

TACO TUESDAY
TO THE RESCUE!

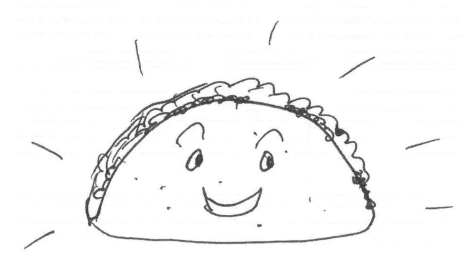

How can Taco Tuesday come to the rescue? Rescue what? Our minds! Sort of. You see, one of the things that stresses the brain is having to make decisions. Even a decision as simple as "what am I going to eat for dinner?" can be taxing and stressful! It's even worse if you (like me) are one of those people who doesn't love to cook in the first place! (And even if you do love to cook... a tired brain still doesn't like to make more decisions!) The solution is repetition. If you have default foods and meals for each day, then you don't have to think about it, and the brain can have a rest. That's where Taco Tuesday saves the day. What day is it? Tuesday! What are we having for dinner? Tacos! Done and done. I have a friend who makes a homemade pizza with his husband every Friday night. Friday night is pizza night at their home - always delicious and homemade. Simple and predictable and lovely. (Sounds more appetizing to me than Fish Friday!) So try choosing a default meal for each day of the week. You can go "off script" any time you want and prepare something else! It's not a contract! It's just a default thing to use whenever you can't think of anything else or are too tired. And if you pick something healthy as your default meal(s), then it will be that much easier to ease into healthier habits. We **rarely** make the "healthy choice" when choosing meals under duress, fatigue, stress, etc.!

WEIGHT-BEARING EXERCISE FOR OSTEOPOROSIS

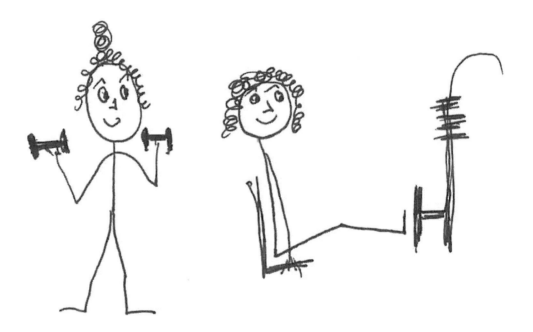

Unfortunately, loss of bone mass is a part of getting older.

But for some people, the loss becomes severe and results in a condition called osteoporosis, or brittle bones! Nobody wants that! And so, people turn to calcium supplements in their quest to strengthen their bones.

Calcium supplementation can help with many things (depending on what kind of calcium we are talking about), but you know what really helps to strengthen bones?

Weight-bearing exercise!

When weight-bearing exercise is completely removed from the picture (as with astronauts living in zero-gravity), bones start to lose density at an alarming rate! Extended stays on the Mir space station have resulted in bone loss of as much as 20%!

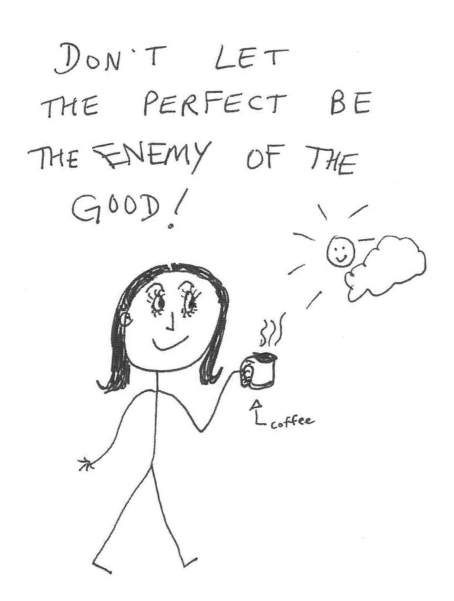

Sometimes, the more you know, the worse you feel! At least when it comes to what you "should" and "shouldn't" be doing. Sometimes, it makes you want to just give up all together! **Why bother** trying to be healthy? It's impossible! ...or is it? It's not impossible! *What's impossible is to be* **perfect**. Because, in fact, perfection doesn't really exist. It's an idea more than a real thing. Maybe you know that coffee is not the best thing for you. But it brings you great joy, and it helps you to get out the door and go for your nice long walks in the park. Then that's good! Maybe you know that most salad dressing is not very healthy. But it's the only way you will choke down fresh vegetables. Then that's good! Not perfect, but good. And you know what? Sometimes - often times - **good is good enough.**

IF YOU HAVE ANXIETY, THEN...
LESS CAFFEINE & MORE EXERCISE!

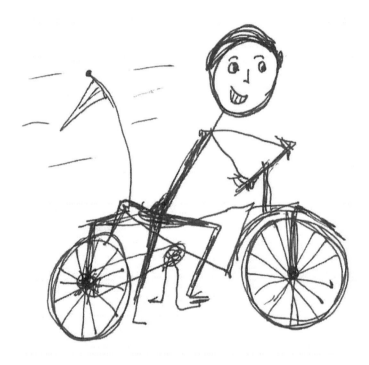

Oh boy. You wouldn't know it from that picture, but for many years, my primary form of transportation was my bicycle! I really do know how a bicycle works. I just can't draw one to save my life! Anyhoo. Sorry to be the bearer of bad news (again)! But...

If you have anxiety, and you're ingesting a bunch of caffeine... then you need to quit it! Caffeine and other stimulants mimic the symptoms of anxiety.

And if you already have anxiety, then it can make it even worse, with no real benefits in return! Exercise, on the other hand - especially heart-pumping aerobic exercise - **also** mimics some of the symptoms of anxiety (faster heartbeat, sweating, etc.) but it **does** give you lots of benefits, and your body feels much better for it! So, more exercise and less caffeine can go a long way towards reducing anxiety!

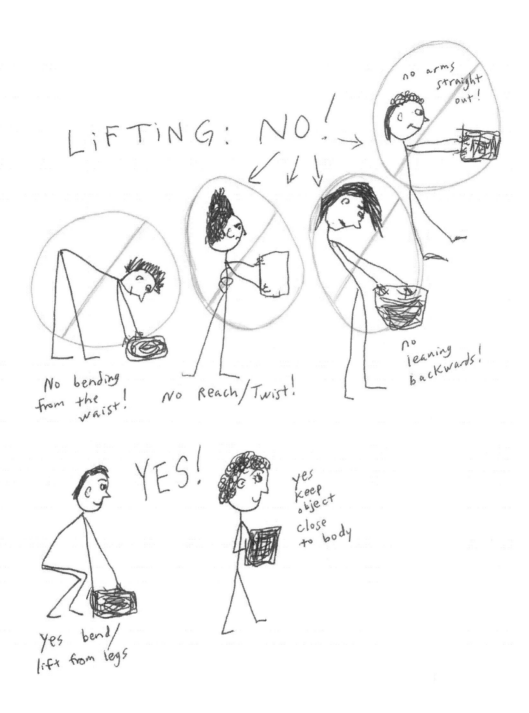

Today we're reviewing some of the basics of lifting!

The best way to lift is to **bend your legs and keep your head up when lifting**. Keep your spine as neutral as possible and hold the heavy object close to your body.

There are 4 examples of bad lifting above, but in my professional opinion, one of them is **the worst.**

The **worst** is the **reach/lift and twist!** *Reaching and twisting at the same time is just asking for trouble!* And if it's a reach/twist while attempting to pick up something? 😵 What is that thing the kids are saying these days? F*** around and find out? 😵

Also, don't lift while bending at the waist with straight legs - even if you think you're just pulling up a few weeds and that it doesn't really count at lifting. It does, and you will find out! Don't arch your back while lifting, and don't lift and carry heavy objects far away from your body! It's a recipe for injury.

DO WHAT YOU KNOW YOU SHOULD FOR THE NEXT WEEK!

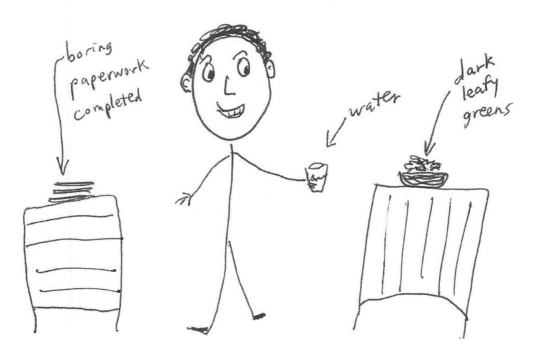

I know, I know... it seems like it was just a few nuggets ago when we said, "Don't should on me!" Buuut... today, we're talking about the kind of should that you **know** really is the voice of reason. 😑 On a recent episode of the Unf*ck Nation podcast, Gary John Bishop (one of my favorite "self-help" writers) posed this challenge: For the next week, **do** everything that you **know** you should be doing, and then observe the results. What kind of "shoulds" are we talking about here? Oh, you know. I really should get out of bed now. I really should drink more water. I really should exercise today. I really should choose the bitter greens instead of pie. I really should floss. I really should get to bed earlier. You're on your own when it comes to discernment and knowing which "shoulds" are reasonable and helpful and which ones are garbage. (Example of a garbage "should" would be something like, "I really should give up on my dumb life!") I know, sometimes it feels like you can't do it. But... but what if you could?? Just try it, one thing at a time. Just for a week.

NUTRITIONAL YEAST TO FIGHT BUG BITES?

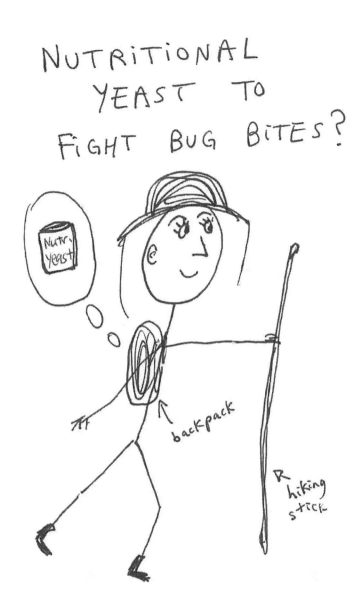

Have you ever heard that thing about how if you eat nutritional yeast, then you won't get bitten as much by bugs? The active ingredient is thiamine, so some people take vitamin B1 supplements or eat other thiamine-rich foods instead. Some of my nerdy hiking friends swear by it! But does it really work?? Kind of... By which I mean to say, no, not really (in terms of repelling). **However, it does work to decrease the itching!** So you won't be bothered as much by them. Just beware of using this strategy in mosquito-heavy areas. You want to actively avoid being bitten in the first place, since they are disease carriers! Also, as much as I hate to say it (as a person who prefers to dress in black)... if you want to avoid the mosquitos, it's a good idea to dress in white and light colors!

CRUNCHY FRESH FRUIT AND VEGGIES FOR YOUR GUMS

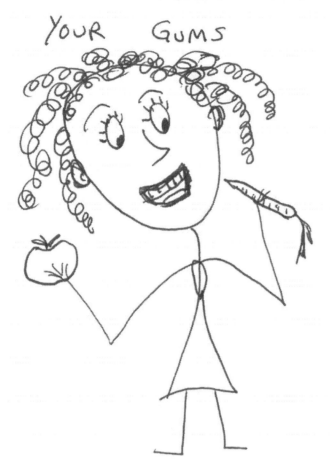

Crunchy fruits and veggies that are rich in fiber are also great for your gums!

They lower the risk of plaque build-up and help to keep your teeth nice and clean. 🦷 ✦

Dental care is expensive, even if you have insurance!

Sometimes, the positive motivation of "eating more fruits and vegetables is good for me" is not enough. Sometimes, you need the negative motivation of, "holy smokes, I cannot afford gum grafts and various huge dental expenses. I need to eat more crunchy fruits and vegetables!!!"

(How do you think I get myself to floss every day?? 😳)

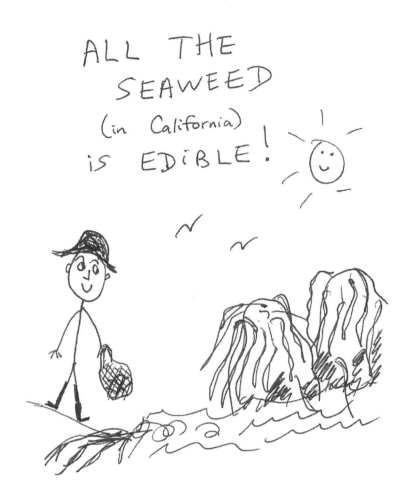

I wasn't sure about whether to include a California-specific nugget, but... why not? The majority of the Nuggeteers are from California, after all. So, guess what? ALL the seaweed native to California is edible! Yes, all of it! That's not to say that it all tastes good. Some of it tastes horrible, and some of it has a terrible texture. But all of it is technically edible, and none of it is poisonous. There are a lot of health benefits to eating seaweed! It's rich in iodine, minerals, vitamins and antioxidants. Does seaweed have a season? Yes. Even though it grows all year round, it is most abundant and best to harvest during the summer months (June through August) during the very low tides. Otherwise, it's impossible to safely get to a good harvest spot! To learn more about foraging for your own seaweed (and how to prepare it once you have it), look for seaweed foraging classes such as the ones offered through ForageSF. If you don't want to learn to forage, you can just buy some at the store! p.s. today's picture is supposed to be a guy foraging seaweed at low tide. Seaweed usually grows on rocks which are exposed at very low tide.

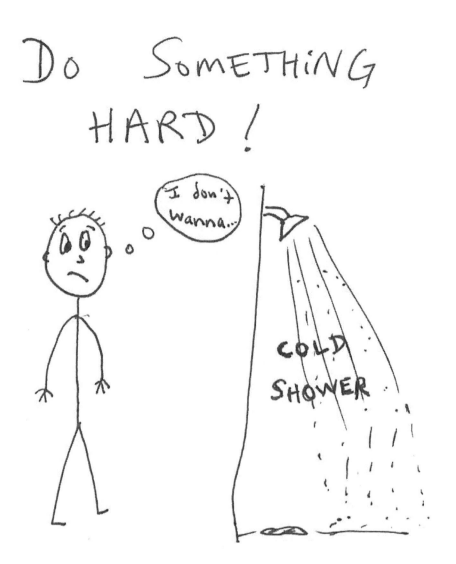

What's so great about doing something hard?

Well, the simplest answer is, it's great because it makes it easier to do *other* hard things!

Doing things to take care of ourselves can be so "simple," and at the same time, so "hard!"

They seem so hard because the most powerful parts of our brain are controlled by unconscious reflexes, reactions and trained responses.

These rarely have anything to do with logic or reason, and they don't respond to logical thinking, reasonable intentions, etc.

The good news is that we can *retrain* these responses and make it easier to do the things that we know we need to do for our health.

Like... take a cold shower.

You may recall there was a nugget some time ago that was about taking cold showers and how great it is for the vagus nerve.

Remember that one?

Well, in my lifetime, certainly I have taken a few cold showers, buuuut... it's never been a part of my daily health routine!

Why not?! Because I **love** hot showers.

Not just "I love a nice hot shower," but,

I... LOVE... MY... HOT...SHOWERS!!!!!

So... cold shower? Yeah, I'll think about it.

Put it on my "to do" list for when I am really desperate for a vagus nerve solution!

Well... let's just say, my vagus nerve got desperate, and I needed to whip out that solution.

So last night, I decided that I would do a quick workout first thing in the morning and then I would hop into that cold shower!

For **one minute!**

I went to sleep anxious about it, and I woke up **very** anxious about it!

Just thinking about that cold shower make me feel sweaty and paralyzed.

Anyone who knows me knows that I wake up early, get out of bed, and **go!**

But not today.

I just lay there under the blankets, lightly sweating and thinking about how much I did **not** want to take a cold shower!

I mentally dilly-dallied for a good hour and a half (!) before getting out of bed and doing my workout.

Then I went into the bathroom and turned on the water and just looked at it.

I stuck my hand under it and mentally complained, "COLD! COLD! Waahhh!"

I inched myself under it, internally whining and complaining until finally, I did it.

I probably stayed under it for a couple of minutes.

And then? Afterward?

Nothing! I felt *GOOD!*

So if you catch yourself thinking "why is this so hard?" then resolve to **do something hard**. It makes the other things easier.

(Side note: maybe it was a coincidence, but it really *was* easier today to avoid snack temptations and various other pitfalls that usually require a lot of willpower!)

Edit: It has been months now since I wrote this nugget. You may not believe it, but... I hardly take "hot showers" anymore! 😲 While I still don't love the initial getting into the cold shower, the results have been so nice that my body now craves them anyway! It is the weirdest thing, and I would not have believed it if I hadn't experienced it myself. 🐵 I'm 50 years old. I guess it's really never too late to change certain habits and preferences!

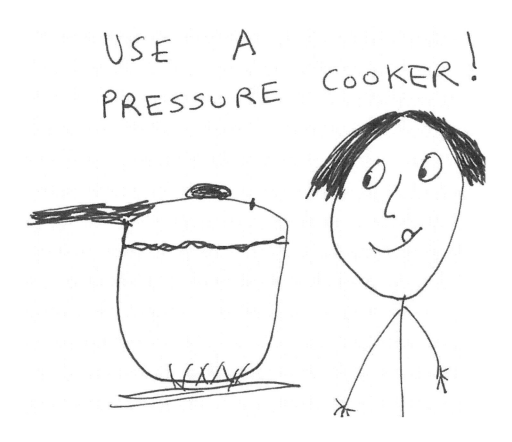

USE A PRESSURE COOKER!

I know, you were worried that this was going to be another stress nugget!

Nope, it's a cooking nugget.

If you haven't already made the pleasant acquaintance of a pressure cooker (or an Instant Pot), then get ready to make a new friend!

Pressure cookers can help you to save a lot of time when it comes to cooking, and yet you still retain a lot of flavor and nutrients.

They are especially handy when it comes to cooking things that traditionally take a long time to cook, such as artichokes, beans, etc.

I am a time-stingy and "challenged" cook (a-hem) and I love my pressure cooker.

The other day, I found a little bag of dry yellow beans in my cabinet and couldn't think of what to do with them. Then I found the easiest recipe ever. You put some water in the pressure cooker, the beans, an onion (peeled and cut in half but not even chopped!) and a couple of cloves of garlic (not even peeled!) and just go to town! 😆 Amazing. (And yes, it even tasted good!)

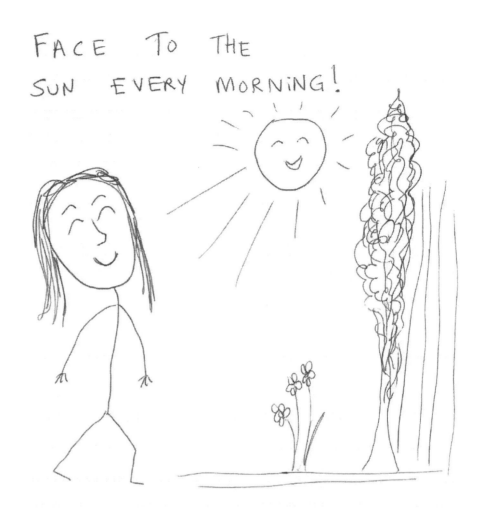

FACE TO THE SUN EVERY MORNING!

One of the best things you can do to help your circadian rhythm (the body's 24-hour cycle) is to get some direct sunlight on your face in the morning! Your body is most sensitive to sunlight about an hour after waking up in the morning and two hours before going to sleep. Sunlight in the morning directs your body to stop making cortisol (sometimes known as the "stress hormone") which it makes in the wee hours in anticipation of giving you the energy to wake up! If it keeps making too much cortisol even after you're awake, it can build up and lead you to feeling more stressed! About 30-45 minutes of direct exposure (as opposed to through a window) is best but do what you can! And don't forget to put on sunscreen, even though early morning sun is less intense than late morning and afternoon sun. It will protect you from the damaging components of the sun, but you will still get the benefits for your circadian rhythm! As for the 2 hours before sleep, getting sunlight at that time can keep you overly energized and can make it hard to fall asleep!

KEEP YOUR MOUTH MOIST!

A dry mouth is not only uncomfortable, but it can lead to some serious health problems! Gum disease, tooth decay and eventual tooth loss are some of the most direct and scary consequences of a chronically dry mouth! Some things that can dry out the mouth are obvious, such as smoking or eating really dry foods. But did you know that alcohol tends to dry the mouth? (Makes sense if you think about it...) Caffeinated beverages also tend to have a drying effect on the mouth, as do many common drugs and medications. So, what are some good ways to keep your mouth moist? Drinking plenty of water is the top and most obvious choice. (This is another reason why it's good to drink extra water after consuming alcoholic or caffeinated beverages.) Chewing sugarless gum helps to promote saliva production, which keeps the mouth moist. Most dentists recommend gum with xylitol in it, as xylitol tricks bad bacteria into eating it (thinking it's sugar) and then they starve to death! If you take a daily medication that makes your mouth dry, see if you can take it in the morning instead of at night, as dry mouth is easier to manage during the day and is more damaging to your health if it's happening while you sleep! Using a humidifier at night can also help. And there are even artificial saliva products (in rinse and spray forms) that can help to keep your mouth moist.

CHECK OUT THE ENNEAGRAM!

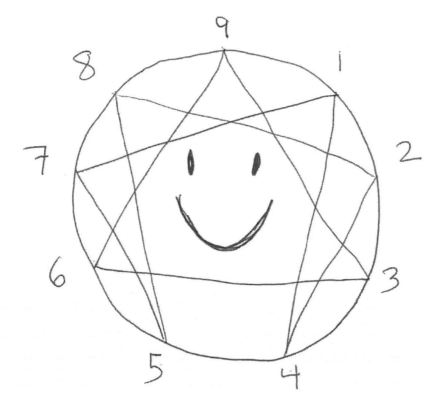

Although I think that the Enneagram is hugely helpful when it comes to navigating the worlds of stress and human relationships, I have hesitated to mention it as a daily nugget... Why? Because the nuggets are supposed to be simple things! And the Enneagram... well... it can be complicated. 😑 But worth the stretch! The Enneagram is basically a temperament classification system that helps us to understand the lenses through which we (humans) see the world. I like it because it's a dynamic system that recognizes that we are constantly changing and moving through healthier and less-healthy states of being. It also gives a roadmap towards growth and shows the red flags that warn when we're sliding down the path of destruction! At a glance, it looks like it puts people into 9 boxes or "types," but in fact, it encompasses more than 450 different "types" of people! So there's plenty of room for individuality, while still helping to understand oneself and the people around us in useful terms. The first hurdle when approaching the Enneagram is determining what your number is.

There are many tests online, and a lot of them are quite long!

Well, I'm here to tell you that there is an excellent "quick test" that is just 2 questions long! Yep, just 2 questions, and it's remarkably accurate.

It can be found in the beginning of the excellent Enneagram book, *The Wisdom of the Enneagram*, by Don Richard Riso and Russ Hudson.

For your convenience, I have included a version of this quiz in the Bonus Materials section of this book (page 409).

Once you find your type, I recommend typing "enneagram" and your type number into a Google search, and then clicking on the result that comes from the Enneagram Institute. This is probably going to be the top result. (For example, I would type "enneagram 5" into Google.)

Read through the description, and if it makes sense to you, then you will benefit from learning more about the Enneagram!

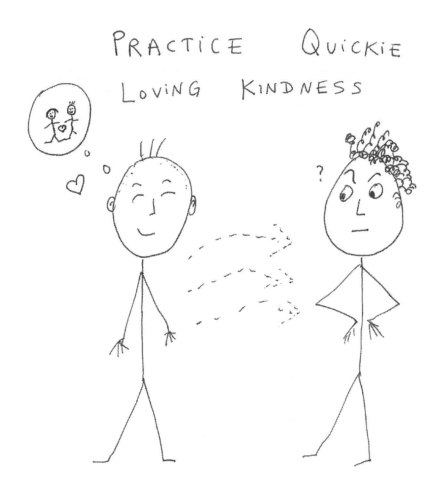

Darn, today's picture doesn't exactly tell the story like I'd hoped! It might look like someone is fantasizing that someone else is falling in love with them even though that someone doesn't like them at all! That's not what's happening there. What's happening is someone trying to practice "loving kindness" quickly when faced with a person who may be difficult to love! Here's how it's done. Picture someone who you love a lot, and who is very *easy* to love! We may love a lot of people who are ... complicated ... and are not always that easy to love, so don't pick someone like that! Pick someone - real or imaginary - who you find it very **easy** to just feel pure love for. And then just bask in that loving feeling for a few moments until you feel it warming your heart and soul. Then, picture that other person - the person who you *want to* feel more loving towards - and just project that loving feeling onto them, like laying an energetic blanket over them. You will find that it's much easier to feel loving kindness towards someone if you have just been feeling love for someone else! It only takes a few moments! And then you can be cranky again. But work on your loving kindness muscle, and it will get easier and easier.

DARK CIRCLES UNDER EYES = GUTS, WATER, SLEEP!

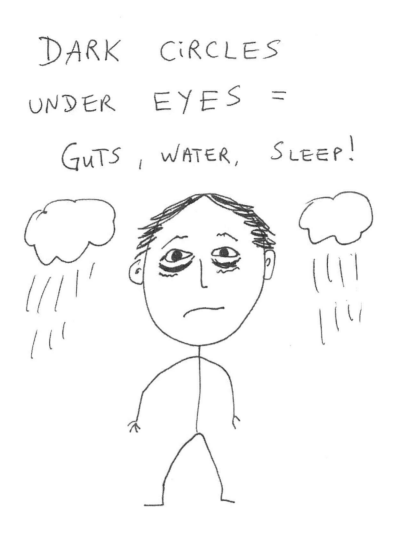

Dark circles under the eyes can come and go. Sometimes it's aging, sometimes it's genetic, sometimes it's lack of sleep, dehydration, or allergies. But if it seems to be more than just a bad night's sleep or allergies then it could be your guts! Various healing systems disagree on the exact point of trouble within the guts. Is it the stomach? Large intestine? Small intestine? Does it ultimately matter? The problem-solving steps are the same! What are you eating? What are you not eating? The most common problem is that food is not breaking down well and not enough **good** food is entering the system in the first place! The dark circles usually fade away after increasing water, healthy vegetable and fiber intake and supplementing with enzymes and probiotics.

(Anemia can also cause the dark circles, but this is not seen in the office nearly as often as people who are dehydrated, sleep-deprived and/or having gut trouble!)

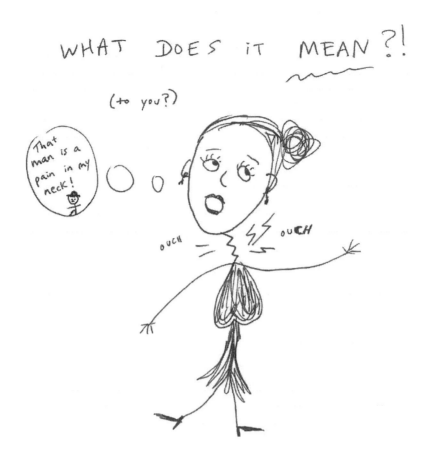

While doing some research to see what people are searching for online when it comes to mind-body health, I was surprised (but not surprised) to see that people are reeeally interested in body-emotion charts. They remind me of the classic Louise Hay book, *Heal Your Body*, which has the distinction of being "the most frequently stolen book" I've ever had in my offices! Maybe it would help you, maybe it wouldn't, to consult a chart or a book about what your body is trying to tell you. But chances are, you can find clues if you think about what the body part or pain *means to you*. Today's picture is inspired by my Gramma Blanche, who confided in me that the day my grandpa died, her chronic neck pain went away, too! She told me that she was afraid to say it out loud to anyone else, because they would think she was (1) mean and (2) crazy. But sure enough, she used to say (to herself) all the time that *that man was a pain in her neck!* And when he was gone, so was the pain in her neck. Do you develop mysterious shoulder pain that coincides with times when you feel that you are "shouldering a burden?" Does your sciatica kick in mysteriously whenever someone or something is a "pain in your ass?" Watch your language when it comes to your body and reflect on the meanings that you place on people, things and even other ideas. If you discover a misplaced meaning, work to replace it with another meaning or perspective. Your body will follow along.

310

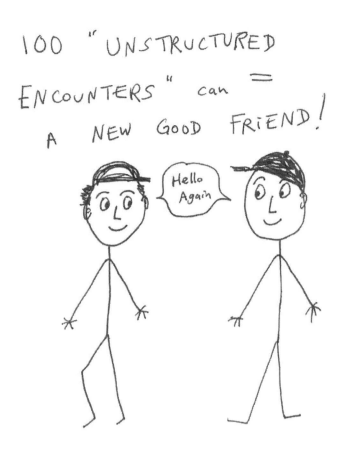

Why does it seem so much harder to make new close friends as an adult?? With certain childhood friends, you can reconnect after decades and suddenly feel like best friends again! Are those bonds strong just because we were young when we made them? Maybe... But scientists have also determined that there is something special about repetitive "unstructured encounters" that are conducive to forming close bonds. This unstructured time would be like those precious few minutes in between classes when you quickly caught up with friends or got into minor mischief. It was the time before school started or the time after, or during lunch breaks or the times when you were sneaking away from school. As a kid - assuming you went to a school other than home school - there were many opportunities for these unstructured encounters. Even if they were short, there were an awful lot of them! But as adults, we don't have nearly as many opportunities to experience frequent unstructured encounters with people. It's easier if you join a group - such as a church or volunteer organization - where you go to events regularly and have free time to socialize before or after the events. Having a good friend is an important part of your health! If you need a new good friend, start thinking about what you can do that will give you chances for unstructured social encounters!

SIT ON YOUR HAND TO GET A BETTER TRAPEZIUS STRETCH!

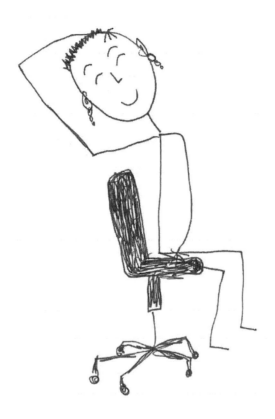

This is an easy one, but it took me a long time to get around to drawing it because... well... as you can see, it's hard to draw sitting on your hand with a stick figure without making it look like something else is going on there! 😵 🙉 Anyhoo... Tight traps are a big problem! Traps = trapezius = a large, paired muscle that connects to your lower thoracic spine, shoulder blades and the base of your skull. A simple trapezius stretch is to reach over the top of your head and gently pull it to the side. To stretch different areas of the muscle, keep pulling to the side with your arm, but slowly tilt your head forward, and you will feel the stretch move. If you sit on your other hand while doing this stretch, you will get an even better stretch! You can do this stretch while standing up, too, if you have a table or similar surface to hold onto as an anchor.

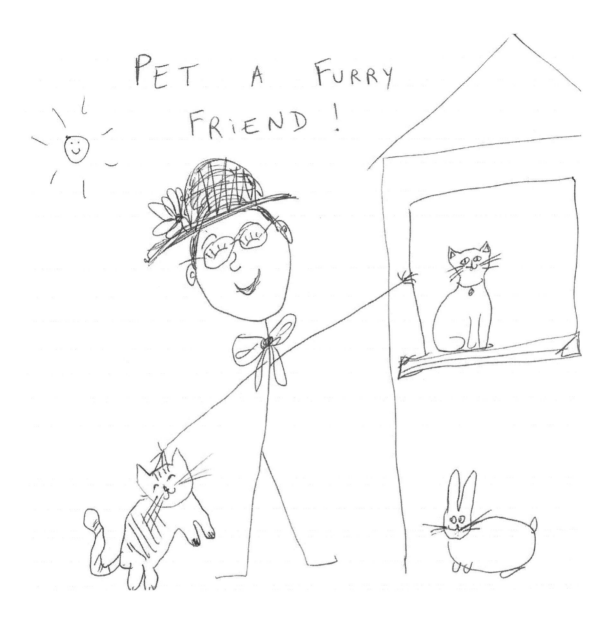

PET A FURRY FRIEND!

You know, petting a soft furry creature is just one of those things that we humans are hard-wired to enjoy! So, whether it's a cat, dog, bunny, rat, guinea pig, goat, horse, otter or bear (you know - the domestic type!)... pet a furry critter today! It will help to boost your general happiness score and may even work to extend your life. Pets can help you live longer, and petting animals helps to boost both dopamine **and** serotonin. I was going to say something snarky about how it's just furry animals and not, say, fishes, but... Jim Abernathy, photographer and conservationist, gives and gets plenty of dopamine and serotonin with his displays of shark affection! He completely changed my perspective on sharks! (That said, I will stick to mostly petting cats!)

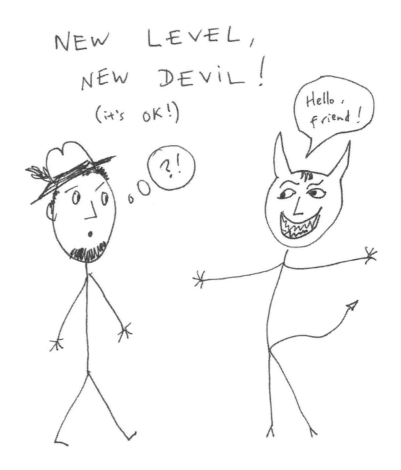

Whenever we're stuck in a big problem, it's easy to think that we'd be *sooooo* much happier if only we could just get past *this one thing!* And hey, sometimes it's true! And it always feels good to overcome a challenge! But then... when we get to the next level... ***there's another problem!*** What the hell! What the hell is right. **New level, new devil!** One of my mentors, Dr. Kerby Landis, used to say, "Do you think you'll have more problems or less problems when you're more successful? **More problems!** What do you think?! But you know what? You grow as a person, and you can handle them!" Gary John Bishop says a similar thing. "You go into a Starbucks, and it smells like coffee. You want to be successful? You know what success smells like? It smells like stress!" That's just the way it is! The point of today's nugget is, don't be surprised - and don't let it bother you - when you run into new problems and challenges as you grow and move forward in life! There's no such thing as a sustained "coasting" phase where there are no challenges and no stress. We're not even designed for that! Even the lack of stress can become stressful over time thanks to our annoying brains. We do best when we have a certain amount of stress, accompanied by periods of rest and recovery. So, if it's new problems that are showing up in your new level, then just take a few breaths and relax. "New level, new devil." You got this! (But if it's the same *old* problem that just keeps looping around over and over and over and you don't know how to shake it, then it might be time for some NET!)

314

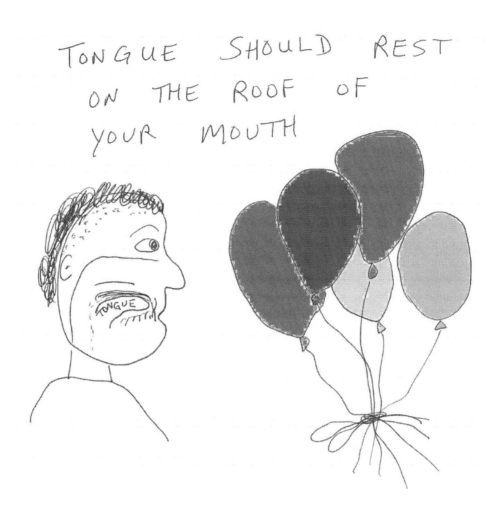

TONGUE SHOULD REST ON THE ROOF OF YOUR MOUTH

TL;DR version:

When at rest, where should my tongue be?

Your tongue should be fully in contact with your upper palate,

lifting with 1-6 lbs of pressure.

Lips together.

Keep your tongue suctioned to the roof of your mouth.

The tip of your tongue should be resting on your upper palate, just behind your front teeth.

It is trickier to get the back of the tongue to put the upward lifting pressure on the palate!

Swallowing is a great way to practice rear tongue lift!

OK and now here's the longer rambly part of today's nugget.

I know, you're a little confused, maybe horrified, and also delighted.

What the what is going on with today's drawing?!

And what does it have to do with those cute balloons?!

Well, to be 100% honest, I didn't even finish drawing my drawing. It was just too gross and difficult. Stick figure type people are just not right when it comes to trying to draw cross sections of a head! Also, clearly, I am no Alex Grey.

I meant to draw "the right way" on the left, and "the wrong way" on the right.

But the "right way" drawing was going so badly that I thought, heck, I will just call it a day and draw some balloons to cheer people up!

You can find a much better illustration of what we're talking about here, in a recent edition of Active Isolated Stretching specialist Diane Waye's newsletter. (You can find Diane at www.stretchingbythebay.com)

Diane reminded me on the importance of this basic concept. Where your tongue rests in your mouth has a big impact on how well you breathe, and it can also affect your neck and your posture!

(It's also part of why it is so helpful to release tongue ties in small kids, as the natural pressure of the tongue against the soft palate contributes to normal cranial development.)

(And yes, Diane gave me permission to share this info and her newsletter with you! She is an amazing resource when it comes to structural functionality of the body!)

On a related side-note... the opposite can happen, too.

That is, you can have something happening in the neck and then notice that for some reason, your tongue's position in your mouth feels off!

One person described it as feeling like their tongue goes "a little bit sideways" when they are out of alignment.

So, practice resting your tongue against your palate!

Six Packs Are Made In The Kitchen!

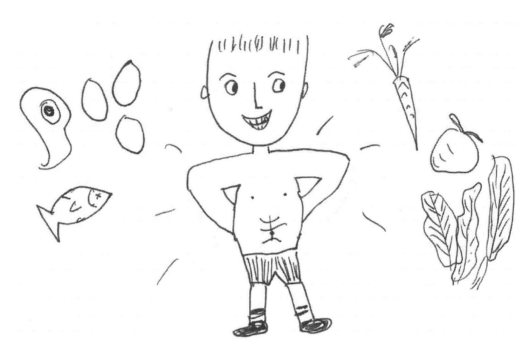

I was listening to an episode of my trainer's excellent podcast, Move Better, Feel Great with Ace Morgan, and something he said really stuck in my head! In this episode, he was answering some common questions that he gets. One of the common questions was, "How do I get a six-pack?" And Ace's answer was, "Six-packs are made in the kitchen." followed by: "...aand it takes about 2 years." While I'm not advocating for everyone to aim for six-pack abs - I'll certainly never have them! - it's important to remember that body changes usually start in the kitchen **and take time**.

So, don't get fooled by crazy ab-worker machines, gadgets, etc.!

Sure, you still have to exercise your body if you're aiming to get some of that muscle definition!

But the basics are the basics forever.

Eat good lean protein, more vegetables than fruits, and cut waaaay back on simple and refined carbs!

317

Go BANANAS!

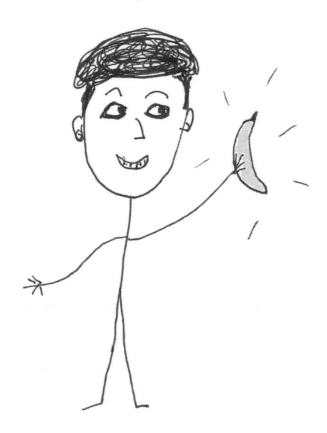

The humble banana is a great snack!

They have lots of potassium, magnesium, manganese, vitamin B6, vitamin C, antioxidants, and fiber.

Sometimes people avoid them because they are worried about the sugar content.

Well, guess what? If you are looking for less sugar content, then pick a greener banana!

Green bananas have a low glycemic index - around 30 - compared to ripe bananas, which rank around 60.

Is it possible to overdo it on the bananas?

Of course, it's possible to overdo anything!

If you're getting farty and bloated from too many bananas, then that's too many bananas.

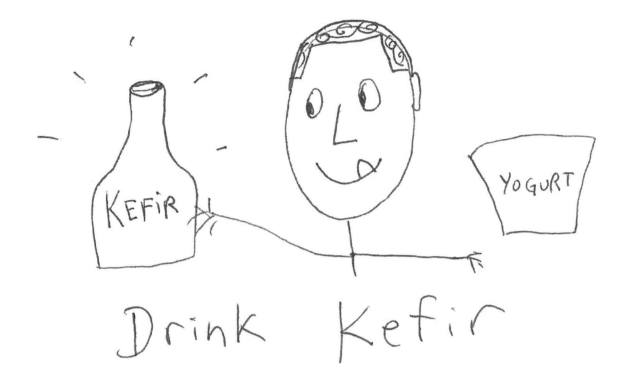

Drink Kefir

I used to think that kefir was just a fancy way to say, "yogurt drink."
But it's not!
Kefir is indeed much more of a liquid than yogurt, but nutritionally, it packs a much more powerful punch!
If you are looking to boost your gut probiotics, then kefir is the way to go, as it contains about 20 times the probiotic content of the same volume of yogurt!
It also contains more nutrients overall.
By the way, there's nothing wrong with yogurt (unless you're sensitive to dairy)!
It's just that people seem to always mention that they're eating it for the probiotic benefit, and I'm just here to tell you that kefir is a better way to go if that's your goal.

EAT YER SPINACH!

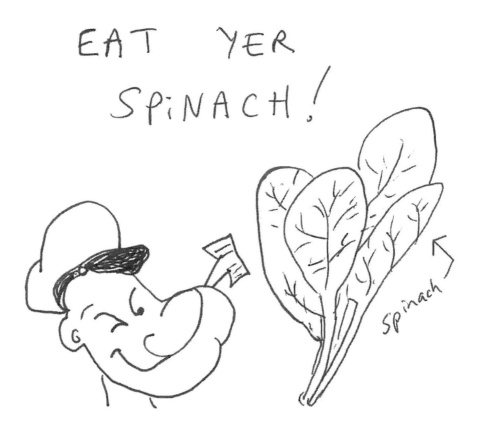

Spinach

I think that Popeye and his spinach thing was funny because it seemed so ridiculous that canned spinach could make someone so strong!
(Or was it just a way to get kids to eat their spinach in the old days??)
Spinach may not give you big muscles, but it is one of the most nutritious greens out there! Spinach is rich in antioxidants and minerals like calcium, iron, and magnesium (when cooked). There are many ways to prepare it, and it's easy to mix with other foods or eat alone. One of my favorite "easy smoothies" is just a bunch of spinach blended with water, mint leaves and a pear! It's so simple, but it's a great energy booster. Maybe a little like Popeye, after all...? 😳 👾
NOTE / **caution**: for some people, there is a downside to spinach! People on blood thinning medication should not eat large amounts, since it is rich in vitamin K (which helps to support blood clotting) and people who are prone to kidney stones should also limit their spinach intake, since spinach is rich in both calcium and oxalates, and many kidney stones are made of calcium oxalate.

GET COMFORTABLE WITH DISCOMFORT

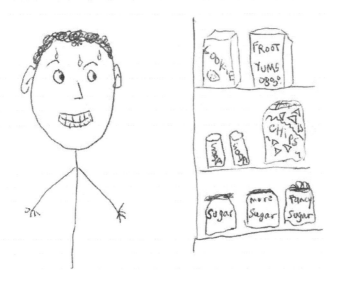

Here's another annoying factoid about human design. We're not really designed to be "happy" - or even satisfied - for a sustained amount of time! What's worse, it turns out, we seem to be built to favor a certain level of **dis**comfort! This is because dissatisfaction helped us to continue to strive and innovate, as a species. Unfortunately, yes, once again, we have really done a number on our own selves..! These days, we are surrounded with ways to push for a dopamine rush and get a shot of some "feel good" chemistry! (You're probably holding a dopamine-delivery device in your hands right now!) 😵 We can't change the world, and we certainly can't change the way we've evolved up to this point! What we *can* do is to train ourselves to become more comfortable with discomfort. What is the point of that?? It helps to improve your tolerance for discomfort, so that you are less likely to impulsively go for things that give you a quick (usually unhealthy) fix. **This has big benefits for your health!** It also has big benefits for your bank account, your productivity and probably your relationships, too! So, next time you are starting to feel uncomfortable and want to go do something that you know is counterproductive but might make you "feel better" (like eating a sugary snack, scrolling on social media, checking the news headlines, posting memes, etc.) just stop, take a few breaths, and feel the discomfort. Just pay attention to the feeling and keep breathing. You can even set a timer for 10 minutes and see if you still have the impulse after that time. You'll be surprised at how often the urge passes if you simply put a waiting period on it!

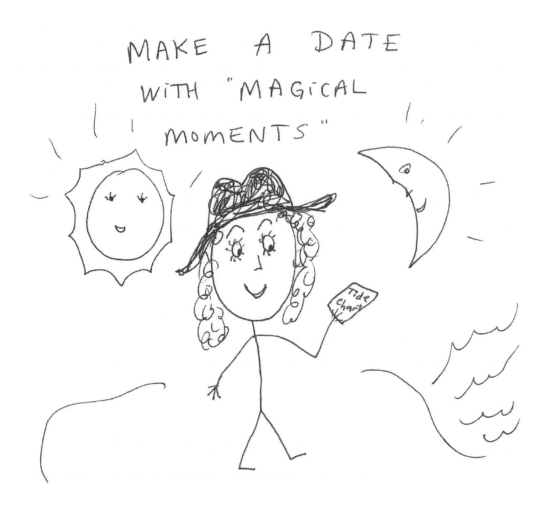

People think that I am unusually lucky with all the cool pictures that I capture on a near-daily basis down at the beach (or wherever).

(You can see them on my personal Instagram @_kimakoi_)

Sure, it's totally luck as to whether or not I will stumble upon a certain configuration of clouds or a particular shell or an interesting character.

But it's not luck at all that the light is usually beautiful or that I seem to catch a lot of full moons reflecting over the water, etc.!

You see, a lot of magical moments are predictable!

In this context, I mean things like moonsets, sunrises, exceptionally low tides, magical lighting, etc.

There is even a thing that photographers *call the magic hour* or the golden hour. It's that hour right before sunset, and the hour right around sunrise.

It's considered the best time to take photographs outside because the light is so beautiful and magical!

322

Fishing enthusiasts, boaters, etc. love to use tide charts to plan their adventures.

But they are a great tool for people just looking to catch some magical moments outside.

Instead of randomly being surprised to see a nice moonrise or moonset, you can look up what time (and from which direction) the big fat glorious full moon will rise, and when it will set! You can see on the chart if it's going to be one of those cool days when moonrise matches sunset (or vice versa) and plan to stand at a cool spot where you can see both!

Of course, clouds and rain can always ruin that plan.

But your odds of catching a beautiful sight are much better if you know ahead of time when it is happening.

(Same with things like searching for sand dollars on the beach. So much easier at low tide!)

The main website I use to look at this kind of info is tides4fishing.com

But lots of websites have charts for golden hour / magic hour times for photography, too!

You might be stuck at work during many of these times, but since they are so predictable, you can plan to enjoy them sometime!

Not all magic is random.

Make it happen!

TAP ON YOUR FACE FOR PAIN RELIEF

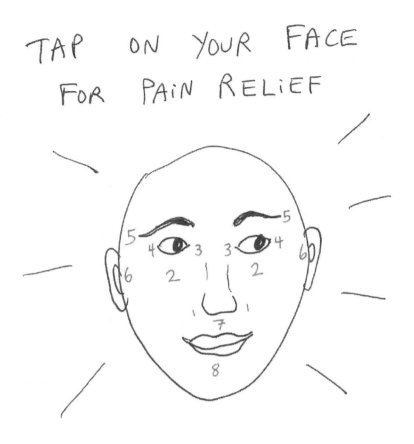

OK, this one is a little strange... and it doesn't always work... but sometimes it does, and for that, it's worth trying! This is an acupressure approach to relieving pain. It's like an acupressure aspirin. It can relieve the pain in the meantime, but ultimately you will still have to figure out what is causing your pain and get to the bottom of it! Today's drawing shows the points on the face that will be tapped. Which one(s) and how many taps are we talking about here? Well, 50-150 taps before you get a sense of whether it's working for you.

I know, it sounds like a lot! But it's not that bad. Tap fast! And which one(s)? It depends on where the pain is located! There is a little series of charts (on pages 411-413) that match each zone of the body with a number, and that number corresponds to the place on your face where you tap. For example, if your hips are hurting, then that goes with zone #4, so you tap the bony area just outside your eyes. If your lower back is hurting, then that goes with zone #7, and you would tap that spot just between your upper lip and your nose. If the top/front of your shoulder is hurting, then that's zone #1, and you tap just below and outside the edge of your nose. You can also find these charts online at https://drkimsf.com/paintapping which was a forgotten page of my website for many years!

Whoops.

WATER = THE ANTIDOTE TO AFTERNOON ENERGY DROP

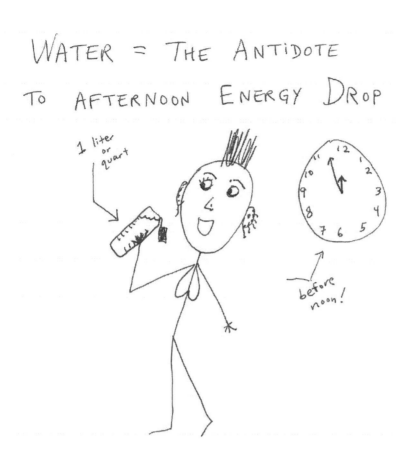

1 liter or quart

before noon!

Pretty sure I've said it before, but it always bears repeating... Water is the antidote to that afternoon low energy! But it's not always that helpful after the fact. You have to be proactive! That means, you have to drink **at least 1 liter or quart of water before noon** in order to get the benefit! Sometimes people tell me that they do drink about that much water before noon, but they still get the afternoon drowsies... but then they mention that, oh, they also drink coffee in the morning. Well... guess what, folks? Coffee may be a liquid, but it's not a good source of hydration! In fact, coffee is a net **de**hydrator. If drinking water is like adding money to the hydration bank, then drinking coffee is like making a withdrawal from the hydration bank! So, if you're drinking coffee in the morning, then add another cup of water to that liter before noon! (or even more if you are drinking more than one cup of coffee!) Same for if you're drinking alcohol in the morning! But if you're drinking alcohol in the morning, then you have a bigger problem than dehydration. 😑 Just sayin'...

BE CAREFUL WITH THE DIRTY DOZEN

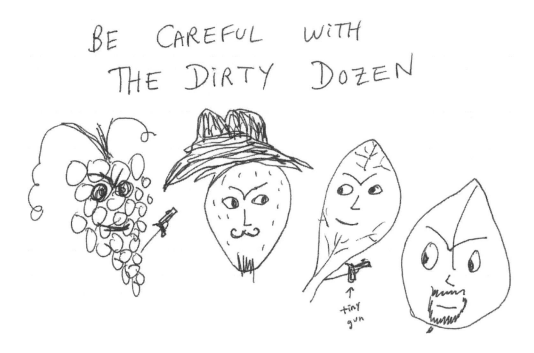

tiny gun

Every year, the Shopper's guide to Pesticides in Produce releases a list of The Dirty Dozen, which are the 12 most-contaminated fruits and vegetables, based on an analysis of data from the USDA (U.S. Department of Agriculture). This year, a total of 210 pesticides (?!?!) were found on the top 12 foods! 💀 Here they are, ranking from most to least contaminated:
* Strawberries
* Spinach
* Kale, collard and mustard greens
* Peaches
* Pears
* Nectarines
* Apples
* Grapes
* Bell and hot peppers
* Cherries
* Blueberries
* Green beans

And yes, some of those foods are really healthy! Cue the sad trombone... So... should you just stop eating these foods? Nope. The benefits (probably) outweigh the risks, **but...** these are the foods where you will want to choose the organic versus the non-organic options (even though they are more expensive) **and** these are the foods that you want to pay extra close attention to when it comes to washing!

MAKE FRIENDS WITH THE CLEAN FIFTEEN!

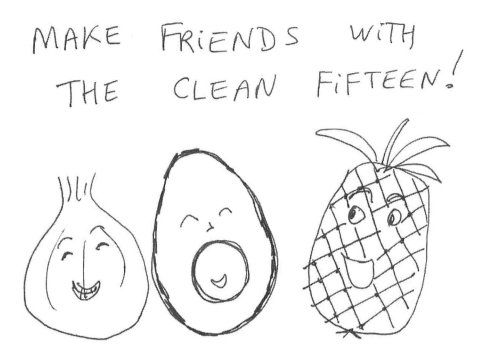

The Clean Fifteen

Yesterday, we talked about the dirty dozen. Well, good news - meet The Clean Fifteen!

The same organization that analyzes the data from the **USDA** to determine which fruits and vegetables are the most contaminated with pesticides also determines the opposite!

So here are the 15 **least** contaminated fruits and vegetables, listed from least to most contaminated:

* Avocados
* Sweet corn
* Pineapple
* Onions
* Papaya
* Frozen sweet peas
* Asparagus
* Honeydew melon
* Kiwi
* Cabbage
* Mushrooms
* Mangoes
* Sweet potatoes
* Watermelon
* Carrots

So go to town Charlie Brown and enjoy the clean 15 with an extra bit of relief!

DON'T LET YOUR OILS GO RANCID!

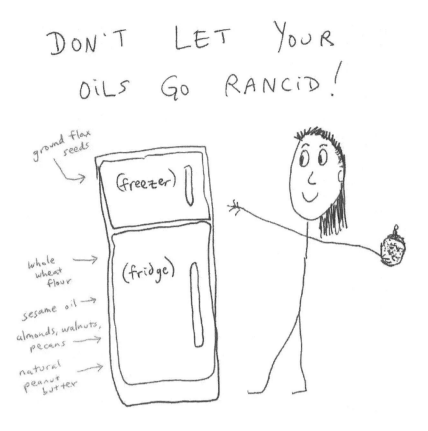

ground flax seeds →

(freezer)

whole wheat flour →

sesame oil →

almonds, walnuts, pecans →

natural peanut butter →

(fridge)

Rancid might be a pretty good punk band, but... it's not good for your food! Rancid oils don't just taste bad. They are bad for your health! When oils go rancid, they break down, and sometimes break down into toxic components. This won't usually make you sick on the spot (like eating meat or fish that's gone bad) but it will contribute to long-term health consequences. For example, one of the toxic components of rancid oils are free radicals, which can contribute to scary things like the development of cancer! ☠ Heat and light exposure are the main things that tend to speed up an oil's breakdown, so keep your oils stored in a cool dark space! Ground flax seeds will go rancid pretty fast, so store them in the freezer, and still aim to use them up within a month or so. Don't grind them up in large batches! If you have whole wheat flour, that should be stored in the refrigerator (for up to 2 months) or the freezer (for up to 8 months). Almonds, walnuts, pecans, natural peanut butter, sesame seeds and sesame oil should all be stored in the refrigerator as well. (Nuts will last a couple of years in the freezer, but... don't buy them in the first place if you're not planning on eating them a lot sooner than that! sheesh!) I know, that might sound like a lot of stuff to add to your refrigerator. Where will you find the room?! Well, you can take the hot sauce, onions, garlic, tomatoes and coffee beans out of the fridge. They don't belong there! Anyway... I'm not ageist much, but... consume your oils when they are young and fresh! 😊

COUCHES ARE FOR SHORT SOCIALIZING. NOT FOR "WORKING"

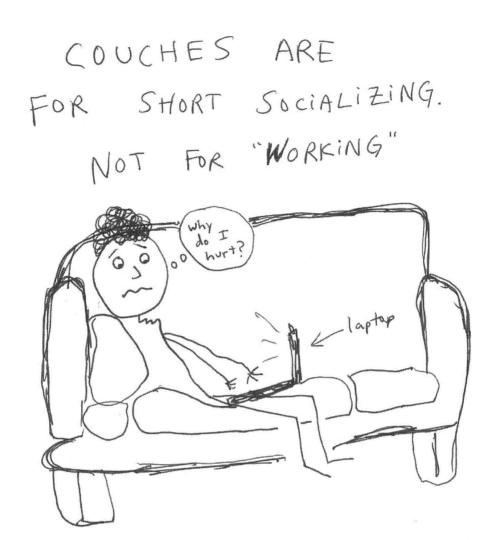

People think that I hate couches. Well... they're not wrong? I thought of captioning the picture as, "Couches are for making out, not for 'working!'" but I wasn't sure if that would be uncouth or inappropriate or what? (Besides which, I think my couch-make-out-days are over!) Anyhoo... Couches always **look** inviting, but they're just not designed for sitting in for long periods of time (unless you want to essentially become one with the seat).

They're usually not designed for anyone's body in particular, and therefore almost certainly not for yours! People constantly develop chronic back and neck problems when they start spending too much time on the couch. This was especially common during the pandemic, when so many people were working from home - often from their couches! Just don't do it! Also, couches are terrible for napping and sleeping. "Couch neck" is a thing that all chiropractors are familiar with! So, don't spend too much time on your couch, unless it's in short friendly bursts.

FEELING CRAZY?
CHECK YOUR HORMONES!

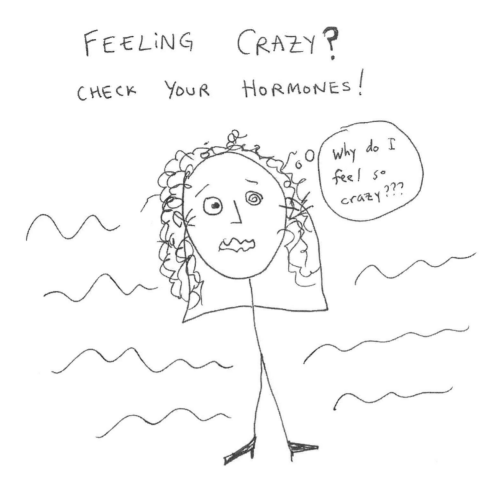

Hormones are something we don't think of too often, but boy do they have a huge impact on how we feel! There are all sorts of hormones in the body, but the ones we think of the most are the sex hormones: estrogen and testosterone. These levels change throughout our lives and tend to drop as we get older. They're worth checking out if you are feeling mysteriously out of sorts, low energy, etc. Thyroid hormones are also worth checking because they also affect things like energy levels, weight, mood, etc. Some functional medicine practitioners go all out and check the hormones from every possible angle. While this can be super cool from a nerd perspective, it's not necessary for the average person to look that closely under the hood! It's a good idea to get your basic blood work done about once a year anyway, so while you're at it. ask to take a look at your basic hormones, too! Being able to rule in or out a hormonal imbalance for your symptoms is a big help and potentially a big time saver, too! Your primary health practitioner will be able to order the labs for you. (And in many states - including California - even your chiropractor can do this!) While the blood work won't tell you what to **do** about a hormonal imbalance, it gives you a hint on where to start and a baseline for measuring results!

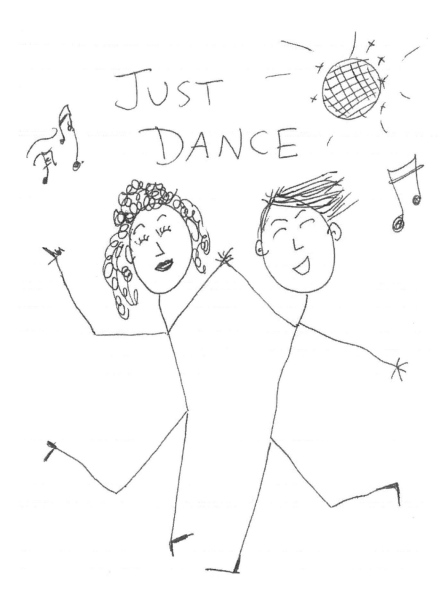

I never thought that I - the world's biggest introvert - would be advising people to **dance** - *with other people* - but here we are! *sigh* Yeah. It turns out that dancing with other people is one of the best things you can do to protect your brain against the ravages of dementia, Alzheimer's, etc.! Social dancing combines multiple protective factors into one activity.

* It's a good form of physical exercise.

* It forces you to learn new things (new dance steps).

* It keeps you engaged with a social group.

* It fosters close physical contact with other humans.

So, put on your dancing shoes and start dancin'!

(Or... like me... think about how in the world I'm going to find some kind of goth line-dancing club for aging gen-Xers?? Stay tuned - we might have to make it happen ourselves in the Sacramento back building!)

SCHEDULE YOUR "WORRY TIME"

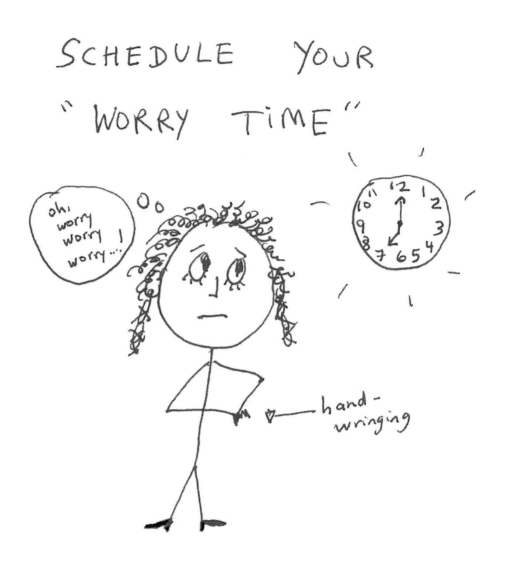

Yep, you read that right. Schedule time to worry! Like... how much time are we talking about here? I dunno, how many worries have you got? Call it an easy 30 minutes to start? Every Wednesday from 7 to 7:30pm, just go off into your room and **worry like crazy!** If your brain tries to worry at another time, let it know that it's not TIME to worry - to hold off until Wednesday at 7pm, then let 'er rip! Scheduling a time to worry can ease some of the stress by taking away some of its power, while also giving yourself a chance to "worry." You will probably come away from it thinking, OK, that was silly... and then maybe scheduling less time for it next week.

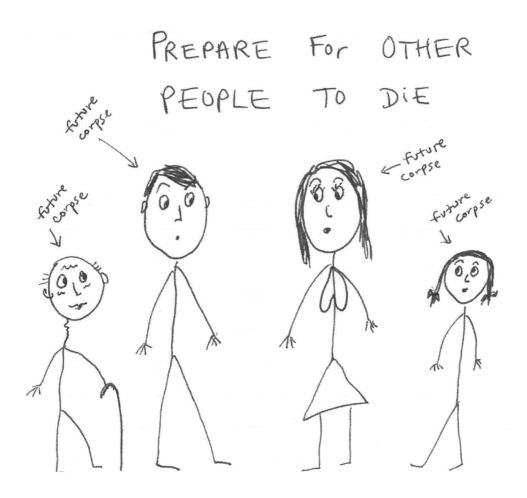

OK, so... a while ago, we had a Daily Nugget that was about preparing to die. As in, **you** preparing for **your** eventual demise! This one is about preparing for **other** people to die. On the one hand, you can't really be prepared, can you? Death can come any day (or night), any time, without warning! Nevertheless, since it comes to **everyone**, it's worth preparing for as best you can. When people don't prepare for it, it can become overwhelming. (It can be overwhelming even if you thought you did prepare!) But as with all scary things, preparing can help to reduce the fear and help to cope. If you are lucky (?) enough to live a long life, then guess what? Almost everyone you knew or loved when you were young will be dead. A great book for facing this topic is called *Advice for Future Corpses (and Those Who Love Them)* by Sallie Tisdale. It is an excellent book that explores all angles of the topic (grief, what happens to the body, what happens as death draws near, etc.) from a very practical perspective and a Buddhist philosophical angle. Striving for a healthy life also includes developing a healthy relationship with death! 💀 ♡

"DRESS UP" TO GO TO THE AIRPORT

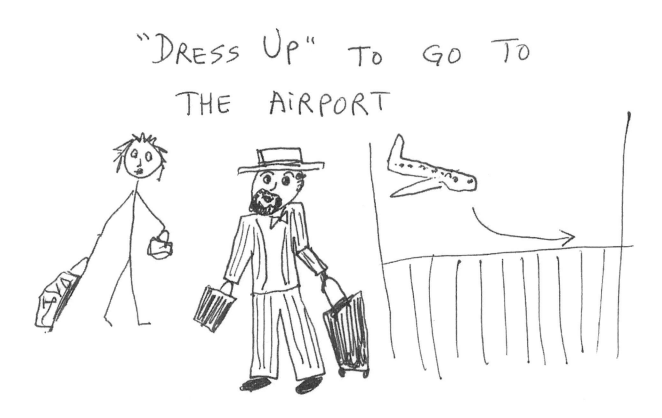

Do you ever hear oldish people complain about how people used to dress up to go to the airport? "Now look at them! I tell ya..." blah blah blah

I used to hate that. The whole dressing up for the airport! I had to do that when I was a kid. I hated it because "dressed up" meant "church clothes" which meant **so uncomfortable**! And I'm all about comfort. But... turns out... there is something about dressing up for the airport. First of all, if **you** are one of those people that pines for the days when people dressed up to go to the airport, then **you** should dress up to go to the airport! *Be the change you want to see in the world*, and all that jazz! Recently, I was "forced" to go to the airport all dressed up. I was taking a same-day flight to my cousin's wedding up in Portland, so I just wore my nice suit to the airport. It was not a business suit, of course. It was a tailored seersucker suit, which I guess is unusual anyway these days. And boy, did I get a lot of (positive) attention that day, especially from the (older) ladies! Turns out, dude bros really like my tuxedo t-shirts, but the ladies like a **real** suit! Anyway, on that day, I realized that everyone is so frazzled and anxious at the airport, it brings a bit of sparkle and adventure when someone is unexpectedly well put together. It makes you wonder, where is **that** person going, all dressed up like that? It turns out that it was kind of fun. If you really hate "dressing up," then, forget about it. But if "dressing up" is something that makes you happy anyway and if you like to spread random joy, then try dressing up the next time you go to the airport. You will be surprised!

334

WEAR SUPPORTIVE SHOES!

(or wear supports in your shoes!)

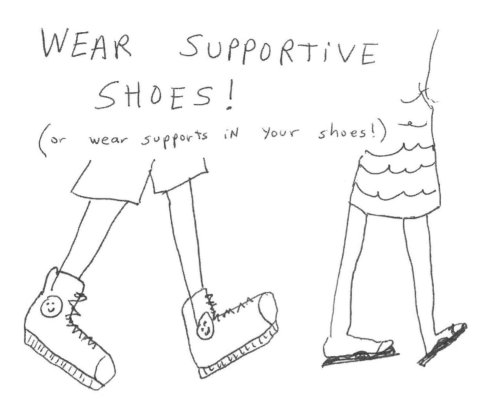

I can't believe it took me this long to say to wear supportive shoes! I guess I thought it was self-evident. Seriously, though... the shoes you wear have a huge impact on the biomechanics of your whole body! They obviously affect your feet, but they also directly impact your knees, hips and back! Remember, everything is connected to everything! Supportive shoes means that they support the arches of your feet and have enough cushioning to protect you from the impacts of whatever you're walking on. If you're walking on sand and natural dirt, then you don't need as much cushioning because of the natural give of the earth. But if you're walking around on concrete all day, then you really need good cushioning! Some shoes have lots of cushioning already built in. Yes, that's why I've grudgingly become a big fan of the world's fugliest shoes: Crocs. They are just so dang comfortable...! But some shoes have basically no cushioning at all, and this is a problem. If you have shoes that you love (hello fashion people and classic Converse high-top wearers!) then you need to invest in some good inserts. If your feet are fairly standard and symmetrical, then you can get away with off-the-shelf inserts such as SuperFeet. But if your feet are unusual or if one foot is really different from the other, then you need to spring for some custom orthotics for the best results! (And yes, you can even get really thin custom orthotics for dress shoes - even open-toe shoes with heels - and you can also find custom-made sandals and flip-flops. But the main thing is, make sure that you have good support in your shoes!

GET A COACH

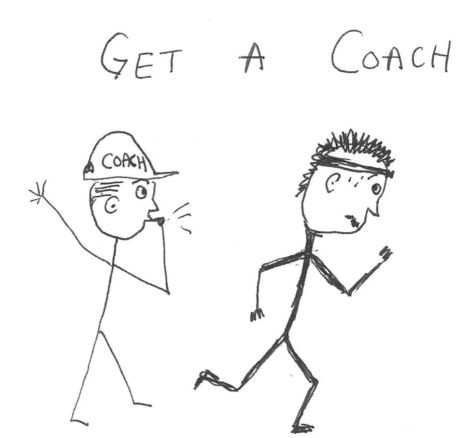

Get a coach.

For what?

For whatever it is that you really want to take to the next level. Somewhere along the way, we got it in our heads that we have to do everything all the time all by ourselves! But this is crazy. We can't do that. Or at least, we can't do it very well. It's also crazy to go to the other extreme and think we can have a coach for everything. But there's usually **something** that you really wish you could take to the next level. Maybe it's developing a more muscular body. Maybe it's growing your business. Maybe it's rekindling your relationship. Maybe it's writing your book. Maybe it's getting your nutrition on track. Maybe it's bowling. Whatever it is, there's a coach out there for it! A good coach is someone who knows the game and knows how to win it. A good coach is also someone whose methods you will respond to and follow! It's not always easy to find the right fit - especially now when it seems like **everyone** is trying to be some kind of coach!!! You don't have to work with the same coach forever! There are different seasons of life and different needs and different coaches for different problems. But if there's something that you've been stuck on and that you really wish you could excel with... then find a coach!

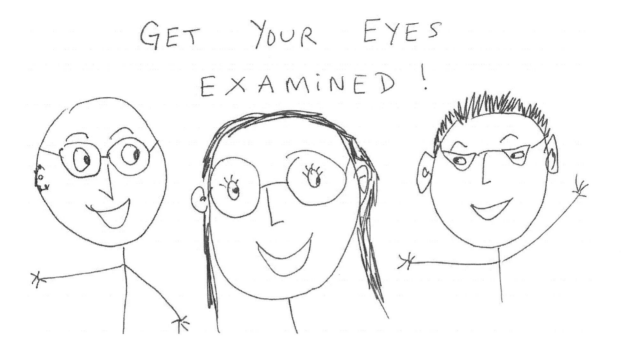

GET YOUR EYES EXAMINED !

OK, here is another one that seems "obvious."

But I wouldn't say it if it didn't need saying!

Get your eyes examined regularly!

Regularly means about every 2 years if you are under 65 years old and then every year after that.

Seeing clearly is the most obvious benefit (as well as screening for things like glaucoma), but I have seen many cases over the years where people have developed severe mystery headaches that ultimately turned out to be a result of their needing to wear glasses!

Often, they weren't even aware that anything was particularly amiss with their vision. It's amazing what the body can get used to!

And if you have young children who are just starting school, make sure to get their eyes examined, too! So many kids who need glasses aren't aware that they have a problem, and it can result in lots of stressful learning problems in school.

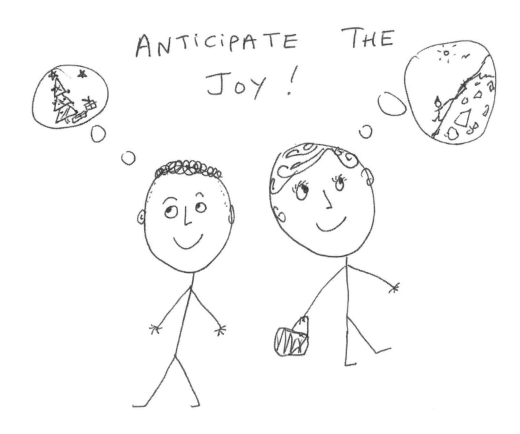

There is a thing called "anticipatory joy" that you can use to help to maintain a good mood. It's pretty much what it sounds like. When you are looking forward to something, it makes you feel good! The weird thing is, the thing itself (once you experience it) is often **less** joyful than the anticipation of it! This is because reality usually falls short of expectations.

But that doesn't mean it isn't worth harnessing the joy of anticipation! Unhappy times often correlate with times when we feel we have nothing to look forward to. Happy times usually correlate with times when we feel like we do have something to look forward to! Even if there are genuinely distressing things happening in our lives, it's helpful to find something to look forward to. We can feel more than one thing at a time! It doesn't have to be a big thing, like a vacation or a major holiday. It can be looking forward to seeing a movie over the weekend, or looking forward to trying out a new place for lunch, or looking forward to a warm bubble bath with a good book. The idea is to put some good things on your calendar so that you always have something to look forward to! My favorite things to look forward to involve travel, but I also get a lot of joy from really low tides, moonsets that happen just before dawn, the release of certain cool stamps and film festivals!

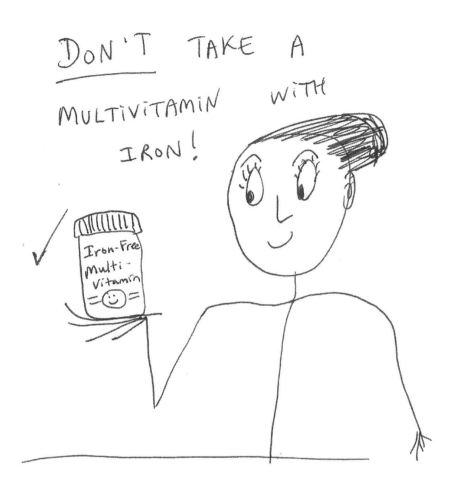

DON'T TAKE A MULTIVITAMIN WITH IRON!

Iron-Free Multi-Vitamin

Unless you have been specifically diagnosed with iron-deficiency, there is no reason to take an iron supplement!

If you end up with too much iron, the only way to get rid of it is to lose blood, which can be pretty inconvenient!

Even women who are menstruating do not usually need to take an iron supplement unless they tend to have extremely heavy periods.

Too much iron can lead to inflammation of the joints, liver, heart, and brain!

Also, not all anemias are caused by iron deficiencies! They can be caused by poor diet, medication side-effects and gut inflammation.

So, when you are looking for a multivitamin, choose the "iron free" option.

TAKE A NAP

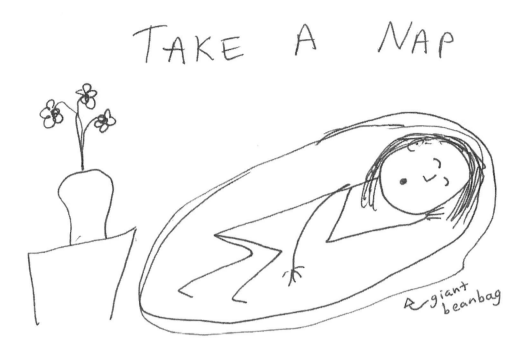

a giant beanbag

Taking a short nap (between 10-20 minutes) can be a great way to give your brain and body a quick break!

Naps have been shown to improve mood, increase alertness, reduce fatigue, and even improve memory. 😄 🤗

To get the most benefit from napping, make sure to keep it short (between 10-20 minutes) and don't nap after 3pm, as late naps can make it harder to fall asleep at night.

That said, napping is not for everyone! If you have a hard time sleeping at night, then napping at any time during the day might make it harder to sleep at night!

As a general rule, naps are best done in a comfortable, dark, quiet space.

Some people incorporate naps into their daily routine, and other people use them when they are anticipating sleep loss (such as with a long work shift) or a big energy loss (such as having to host a big event).

If you are drawn to the magic of napping, then you might love SARK, who I consider The Queen of Naps. She is an artist who has built her career out of her passion for napping! Check her out if you love bright colors and positivity with complete permission to nap!

REVISIT SOMETHING YOU "DON'T LIKE"

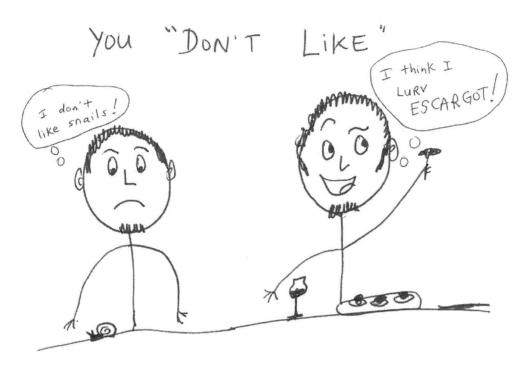

There are lots of reasons to like or not like something. But sometimes, we decide that we don't like something, and that's that! We never revisit the subject or give a thing another chance. And this can potentially mean missing out on a lot of enjoyment in life! Because we change over time. Our tastes and perspectives change with age and experience.

Are there foods that you decided a long time ago that you just DON'T LIKE? When is the last time you gave them another chance? Recently, I was having dinner with some friends when one of the dishes came out with LIMA BEANS. I grimaced. As a kid, lima beans were my MOST HATED FOOD! I would swallow them whole, like pills, without chewing, so that I would not have to taste them! But I'm an adult now, and I was with other adults, so I just ate them. Chewed up those lima beans! And you know what? I enjoyed them! They were good! (Maybe because as a kid I'd only been served them out of a generic frozen veggie mix bag with no seasoning?) Same with music. Do you think you hate country music? Or opera? When's the last time you gave it a chance? What are you sure that you don't like or would never like? Give it a try and see if you surprise yourself! (Full disclosure: it doesn't always work out so great. I tried, and with great certainty confirmed, that I still do NOT like anchovies on pizza! Blech! ✜))

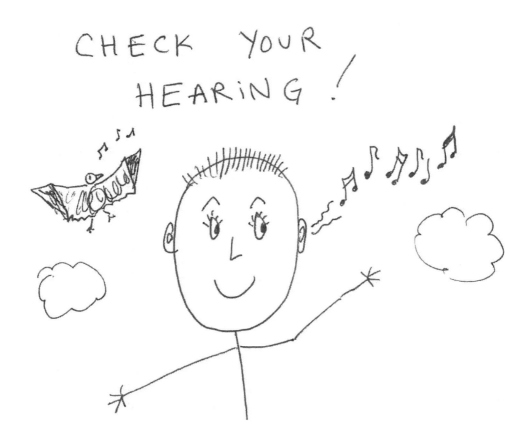

Have you heard the news? Turns out, people with hearing loss are up to 5 times more likely to develop dementia than those without it. However, **the use of hearing aids can cut that risk in half!** Hearing was one of several modifiable risk factors for dementia identified in 2020 by the medical journal The Lancet. We have all experienced the healing effects of music, but sound itself stimulates and supports healthy brain cells, too. A lot of my aging musician friends have experienced some hearing loss, and some of them have started to wear hearing aids. I always dreaded that possibility, and I still envision those gigantic flesh-colored things that old people wore on their ears back when I was a kid! Well, one of my friends recently showed off his amazing new hearing aids that can be controlled by an app on his phone, and I gotta say... hearing aid technology is **much** more advanced (and much cooler!) than it was back in the day! It's nothing to be afraid of anymore. So, make sure to get your hearing checked, especially as you get older. And **especially** if you keep asking people, "What did you say?"

GIVE BLOOD!

Giving blood is obviously good for *other* people, but it can also be good for *you!*

If you have a tendency towards high hemoglobin or high iron in your blood, then giving blood is the best way to get those numbers down, which can help to lower your risk for things like blood clots, heart attacks and strokes!

Men often have more trouble with this than women, since women lose some blood every month while menstruating.

Donating blood can also help to lower blood pressure.

Also. you get snacks afterward!

And don't worry about the calories if they offer you cookies and juice. It takes about 500 calories to replace the blood you just loss anyway, so it's a wash!

And great breaking news: the FDA has finally relaxed restrictions on gay and bisexual men donating blood! The questionnaires will now check for "individual risk-based questions" regardless of gender or sexual orientation. This makes a lot more sense than the old guidelines!

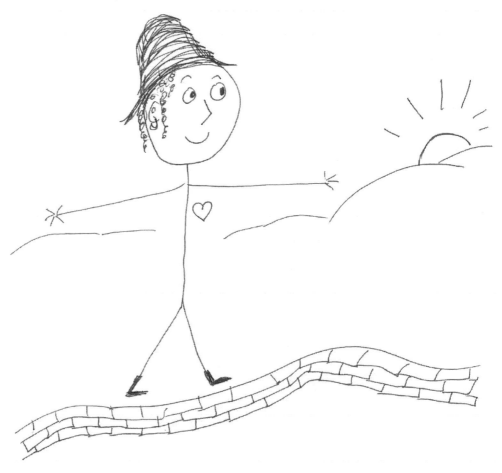

OPEN SPACE + EYES UP =
FEEL GOOD CHEMISTRY!

Here is a really simple one, if you have access to some nice open space outside...
If you need a quick dopamine boost (aka some "feel good chemistry") then just step outside
where you can get a sense of spaciousness and raise your eyes up towards the horizon!
(If you are perched up somewhere such that looking at the horizon involves looking down,
then just lift your eyes upwards anyway, towards a nice patch of sky. You will get the same
effect!)
This is something we are just wired to feel good doing.
Simple!

CLOSURE = GOOD

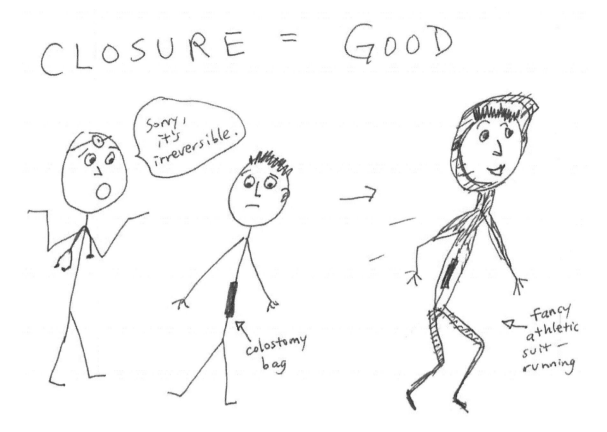

OK, here is a strange one that won't sound very good at first, but... it's good! So, there was this strange study concerning people who had gone through surgeries and ended up with colostomy bags. In half of the cases, the surgery was potentially reversible, depending on if and how well the patient's underlying condition healed. However, in the other half, the procedure was non-reversible, and all those people for sure would have to have the bag for the rest of their lives. The researchers wanted to see if there was a difference in the outcomes around how well the people adapted to life with a bag. The results were surprising.

Guess which group did better? The group with the **permanent** bag did much better than the group with the "potentially reversible" situation, even though both groups faced exactly the same day-to-day challenges! The conclusion? The finality of the situation for the second group made it much easier for them to move on and figure out how to live their lives.

The first group had a much harder time committing to their new life situation because there was always a "what if..." part of their mind that clung to being able to go "back to the normal." This principle can apply to many situations. So, when faced with a harsh challenge that might be "forever," remember that sometimes it really is better to have the certainty that what's done is done, and to move on. Clinging to certain types of hope can cause more harm than good.

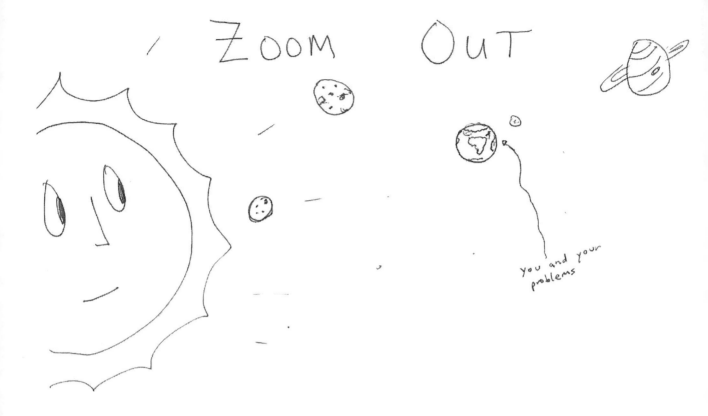

When we're bathing in our problems, they can seem so huge and engulfing.

It's hard to get perspective!

So, it can help to zoom out.

Zoom your lens out further and further.

See your town, and your state, and your country, and the continent, and the planet, and just keep zooming out further and further, and see the unending hugeness of the universe.

For some people, this can be terrifying, as we realize that we're just a tiny speck!

But for many people, this can be relaxing, to see that our problems are the tiniest blips in a huge and magnificent universe!

All these things will pass.

And that's OK!

It reminds me of the classic Carl Sagan video, Pale Blue Dot, which you can find on YouTube.

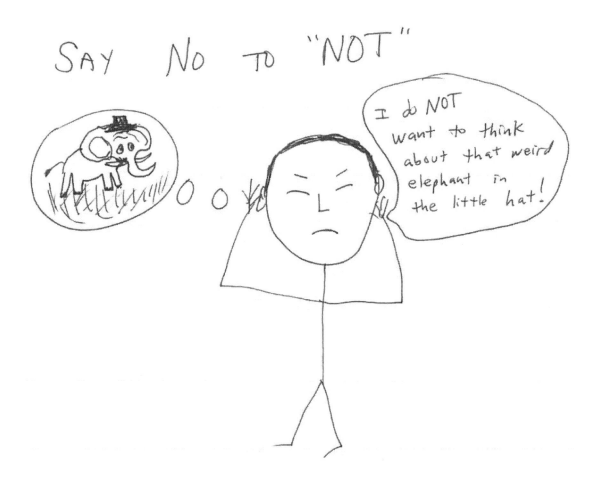

In NET, we are trained to avoid using the word "not" when crafting our "OK statements." So, that's why when we are testing both sides of an issue, we may say something like "I'm OK winning" and then "I'm OK even if I lose" versus "I'm OK winning" and "I'm OK not winning." Why is that? I was told that it's because the brain doesn't see or hear the word "not." I don't think that's exactly true. So here is **my** theory! I think it's because the mind is a powerful visualizer, and when we use the word "not," the picture formed in our head is basically the same as the picture that is formed when we don't use it! For example. if you say, "I hope it rains," then inside of your mind, you can probably see a rainy day! But then if you say, "I hope it does **not** rain," then what do you see in your mind? Still the vision of a rainy day! You can't help it. So, if you want to focus on sun, then you would say, "I sure hope it's a sunny day!" And now you know why we try to avoid saying "not" in NET. Getting rid of the word "not" can be a big help in your day-to-day life, too. We tend to gravitate towards what we can see in our mind's eye. So be careful with your language, and when you want something then choose affirmative words that paint the picture that you want!

DEEP SQUATS
FOR SO MUCH GOOD

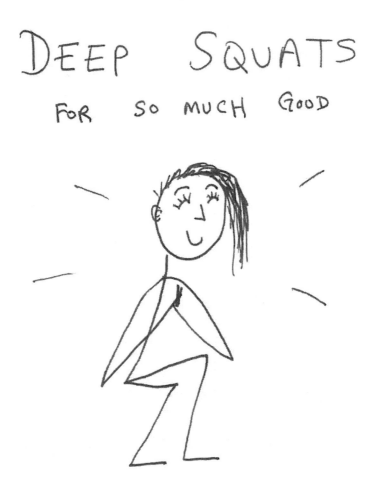

A lot of people do squats in the gym, but not as many people work on doing their ***deep*** squats. Deep squats are a thing that people around the world do every day throughout their lives because (believe it or not) it is a natural resting position for humans!

I know, I know, if it's so darn natural and restful then why can't I do it?!

Well. most of us Nuggeteers are living modern western lives where we're sitting down most of the day. And even if we aren't sitting most of the day, we do sit down when we are looking to rest. **very** few of us settle into a deep squat when it's time to rest.

The problem with chair life is that when we sit in a chair, the position causes the muscles in the back of the legs to shorten. It causes stiffening in the hip flexor muscles and contributes to low back pain. hip pain and a weak core. If you can't do a full deep squat, don't feel bad - I can't either! - but it's worth working towards. And if you can do one, then it is a skill worth keeping!

GET HELP!

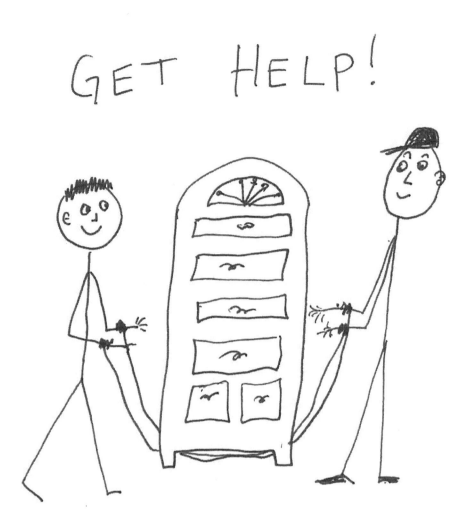

What's happening in our picture today? It's 2 people using forearm straps to safely move a heavy piece of furniture! Today's nugget is about asking for help when you need to do something that you *could* do by yourself, but that you also might hurt yourself... by doing it by yourself. This is especially true of moving heavy objects! It's so easy to get injured, and depending on your age and physical condition, it can take a really long time to heal. Always ask someone for help, and if you're not sure what the best way to do something might be, go ask YouTube! There is a video for everything out there, and there is always someone demonstrating a better way to do something.

Also, yes, I am aware that the guy on the right looks like he has feather dusters for hands!

p.s. this nugget also applies if you are facing a heavy lift mentally or emotionally!

It's not "weak" to ask for help. It's efficient and smart!

LIGHT COLORED CLOTHES OUTDOORS DURING MOSQUITO SEASON!

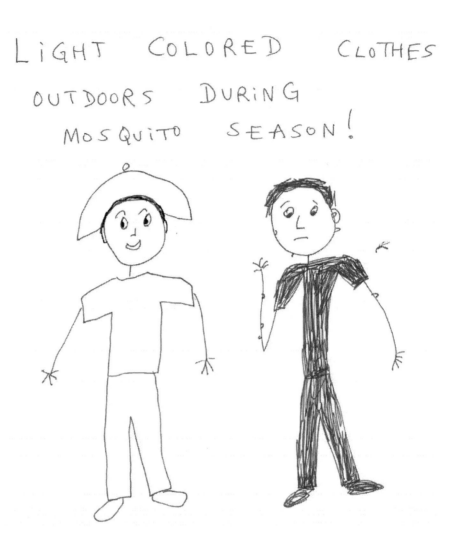

You know it's serious when **I** am advocating the wearing of light-colored clothing (for health purposes)! Well, mosquitoes are disease-carrying troublemakers, so, you have to do what you have to do! One of the things you can do to deter them is to wear white or light-colored clothing when you are working outside during mosquito season. They tend to be drawn to movement and dark colors, because dark-colored shapes in motion tend to be animals full of delicious blood! They instinctively know that they are more likely to evade detection against a dark background and that they are more likely to be seen and swatted against a light-colored background! I guess that is why traditional gardening clothing tends to be light-colored, and that goth gardening isn't much of a thing... (except for the Goth Gardening group on Facebook...) They are also drawn to people who smell like stinky cheese. So... I guess don't eat stinky cheese if you're going outside during mosquito season! And yes, I can explain what the white shirt person is wearing on their head in today's illustration. It's supposed to be a garden chapeau.

HOLD A ROCK

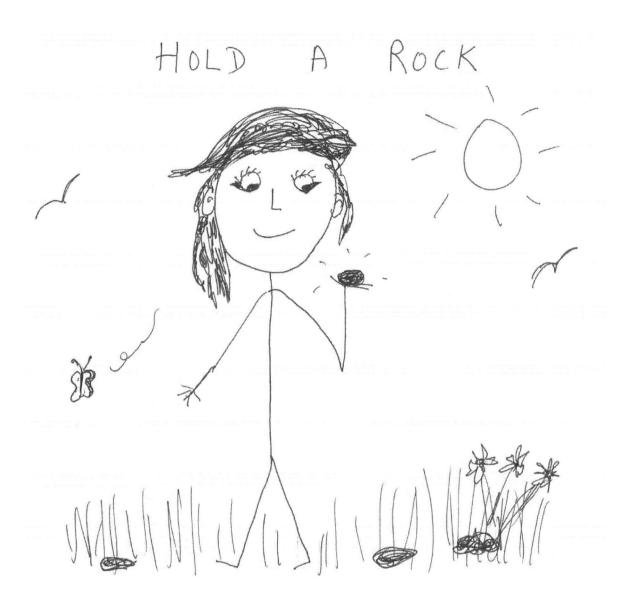

These days, we could all use a bit more grounding, and there's nothing like a good rock to help reconnect you to the power of the Earth!

You can hold a nice rock any time you need to feel grounded and reconnected.

I'm a big fan of smooth beach rocks because they also carry the imprint of the water that has shaped them and the fire in which they were forged.

So in your hand, you can hold the power of earth, water, and fire!

The element of air you carry with you as long as you breathe.

So breathe nice and deep while you hold your rock!

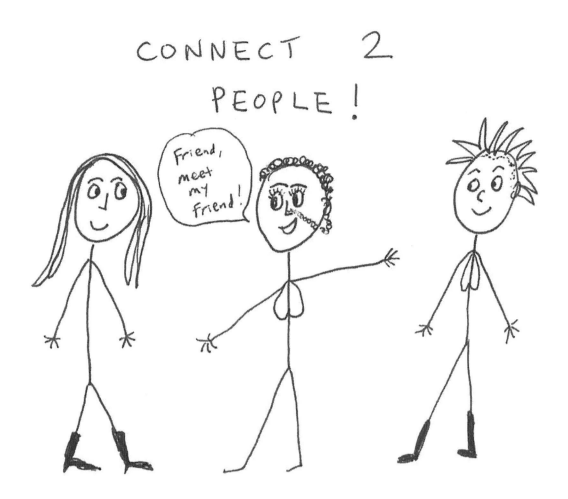

Today's nugget is great for your social health, which of course is important for your overall health!

Connect someone you know to someone else you know, who you think should know that someone!

It can be hard to meet new people - especially for us introverts - and it's always nice when someone can make a warm introduction.

I know, this is probably starting to sound like a business networking tip... 😳🤖

But it's really just about connecting people to people.

And that's how communities are formed!

MAKE YOUR OWN CUSTOM YOGURT

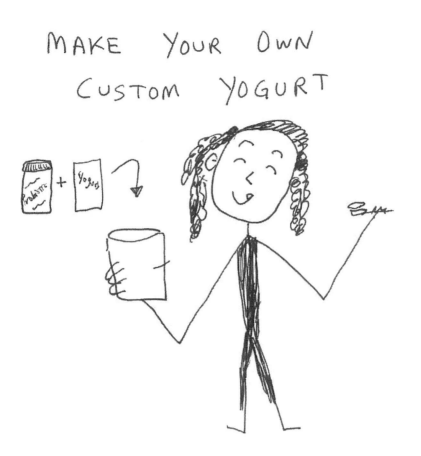

This nugget is about more than just making homemade yogurt, which can be a healthy and fun thing, like making any fermented food. Making yogurt is pretty simple, especially if you have a yogurt maker! The standard way is to buy a small container of yogurt, and then use a spoonful to inoculate the milk that will eventually become your new batch of yogurt. Once you have a thing going, then you just save a little bit from that batch to inoculate the next batch, and the process goes on and on for as long as you like! But what is a "custom yogurt?" This is a yogurt that has been inoculated with very specific probiotics that have been chosen for a specific reason. In his book *Super Gut*, Dr. William Davis goes into depth about the most common helpful probiotics and how to experiment with them and with making custom yogurts to improve your gut health. The custom yogurt making process basically involves taking a couple of capsules of your favorite probiotic supplement, mixing it into your yogurt-to-be, and then waiting for the magic to happen! And then once you've got it going, then you're going to save a lot of money on that particular probiotic. 😄

You will become a small-time probiotic farmer!

Seriously, though, you will get the most benefit from probiotics if they are tailored to what works best for **you**.

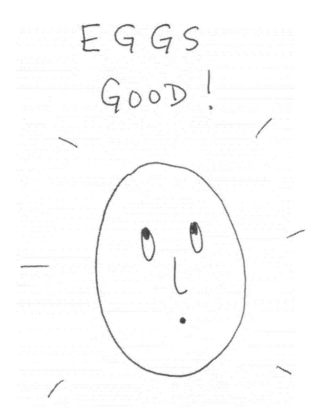

EGGS GOOD!

How in the world did I get to 330 nuggets without doing one on eggs?!

If you're allergic to them, well, I guess today's nugget is a dud.

But if you're not allergic and you're wondering whether they are a good food or bad, I'm here to say that eggs are a **good** food.

They are a complete protein, containing all of the essential amino acids (meaning amino acids that we have to get from food directly, since our body can't manufacture them).

Eggs got a bad rap some time ago because they contain cholesterol, and of course nobody wants high cholesterol!

The thing is, only a small percentage of our cholesterol comes from food sources.

Most of the cholesterol in our blood is manufactured by the liver!

It's actually an anti-inflammatory that is made *in response to* high intake of saturated and trans fats from foods like red meat, pastries/pies, etc.

Of course, like any good thing, there is such a thing as too much.

The standard recommendation is about 1 egg a day (6 a week).

I know that body builders eat them by the dozen, but... bodybuilding is a thing unto itself!

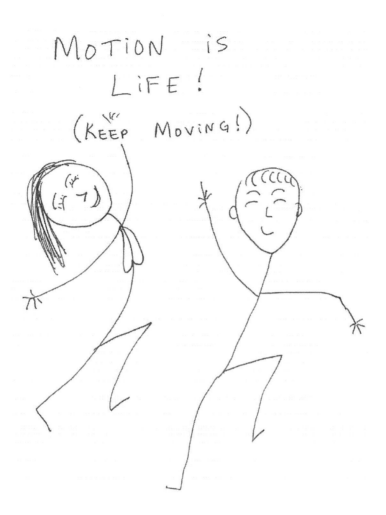

The first chiropractor I ever worked with would always make a pronouncement after delivering an adjustment. One that he used a lot was this: "Motion is life!" And it is! When you think of being vibrant and full of life, you imagine yourself in motion! And when you think of the diminishing of life, you imagine slowing and stiffening until one day... all motion stops. 😵 💀 So when you are just sitting in a lump, staring at a screen, remember that *motion is life*. Get moving! On a similar note... I was watching an interview recently (yeah yeah, sitting in a lump, staring at a screen) with Ville Valo (one of my favorite musicians) and he was asked if he had any advice for people who might be struggling with depression. Here was his answer: "Keep moving. It's harder to hit a moving target." Indeed! So... keep moving and remember that motion is life!

THINK NEW THOUGHTS

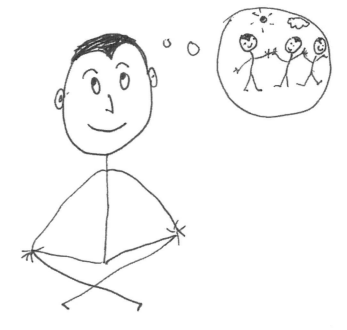

Think new thoughts, eh? What's this about?

This is about thoughts being the start of the chain of events that goes from thoughts to choices to actions to outcomes. If you keep thinking the same thoughts, then you'll keep making the same choices, which will lead you to take the same actions, which will lead to the same experiences and outcomes! In short... if you keep thinking the same thoughts, you're likely to keep living the same day over and over again. Yep, like that movie, Groundhog Day. If you're delighted with your current life and day-to-day experiences, then by all means - keep thinking the same thoughts!!! But if you could use an upgrade in your health, wealth, relationships, peace of mind, etc., then the place to begin is to start thinking some new thoughts. At first, it will feel "fake." The thoughts you're already thinking feel "real."

But where did those thoughts come from? You weren't born with them! Once, they were new thoughts, too. Now you're a grown-up. You can choose to create new thoughts and new thought habits. Where do you start? What's a counterproductive thought that creeps into your mind frequently? One of mine was "People suck." This is counterproductive to many things - not least of which being my attempt to grow a business around taking care of **people!**

So, I had to replace it with something like "People are doing the best they can. 😑"

It may not be perfect, but it's better, and it's getting me better results, too.

As the old timers used to say, "No more stinkin' thinkin'!"

MONITOR YOUR BLOOD PRESSURE

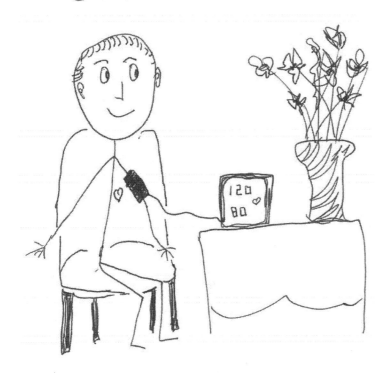

Don't rely on that annual physical (if you even go annually) to look at your blood pressure! Blood pressure is one of the easiest things to monitor on your own, and it's one of the most important indicators of heart health. When I was growing up, 120/80 was considered to be "normal" blood pressure. Now, they have revised the number to 110/70. There are various theories as to "why" that is, but you know what? Close enough! If you're in that ballpark, you are doing fine. If you start creeping up, then you will want to figure out why it's happening and make some changes! When I was young and cynical, I used to think, who cares if I have high blood pressure? I'd rather die fast of a heart attack anyway! Well, now that I'm older, I know that high blood pressure doesn't always result in a quick merciful heart attack. Sometimes it gives you terrible kidney disease, or causes a stroke, which can be a slow and debilitating way to go. Sure, we all have to go somehow, but... don't make it any dumber than it needs to be! What about abnormally low blood pressure? Well, that's a problem, too! When your blood pressure drops below normal, you should contact your doctor if you are also having symptoms such as fatigue, inability to focus, difficulty concentrating, fainting, blurred vision, or vomiting. I know, I know - it's hard to seek medical attention if you've fainted! Anyhoo... just check it periodically, especially if you are over 40! Blood pressure monitors are inexpensive and easy to find!

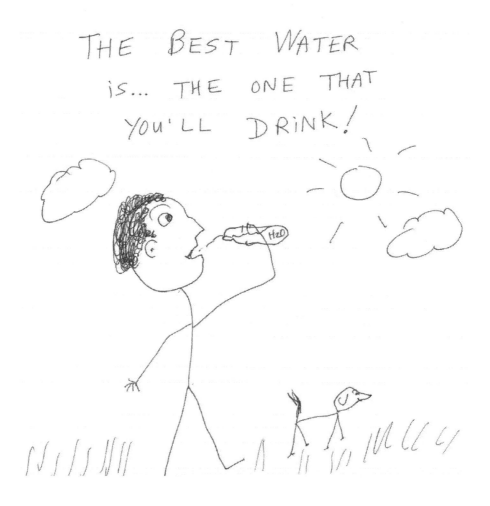

THE BEST WATER is... THE ONE THAT YOU'LL DRINK!

There are so many different kinds of water out there, and people always ask, "What is the best water to drink?" Well, obviously, you want your water to be clean. It should be as free from toxins, etc. as possible! It should have a neutral-to-alkaline pH if possible. But when it comes down to it, *the best water is the one that you'll actually DRINK!* Believe it or not, many people avoid drinking water if they feel like it's not the "right" water. Well, I'm here to tell you that it's better to drink a good amount of less-than-perfect water than it is to drink too little water in your quest to find the "best" one. Different waters do taste different, so, if you're struggling to increase your water intake, then try some different ones! You may find that you really like one. Don't get hung up on the idea that you'll only drink that one forever. Think of it as "water training wheels." Just get it and drink lots of it until you are accustomed to drinking plenty of water. Eventually, your body will crave the hydration and it will not be as much of a struggle to find water that you'll really drink.

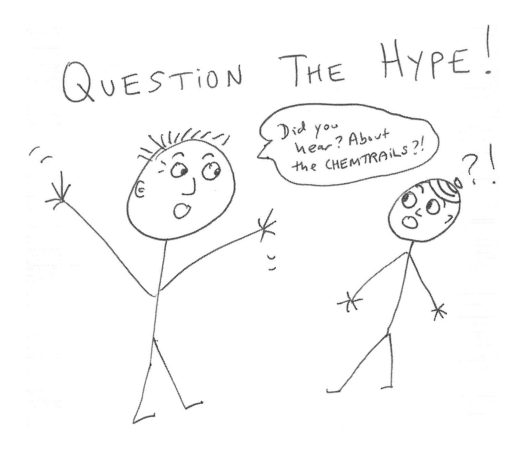

Yes, question the hype! Which hype? ALL the hype! --especially when it comes to health stuff. Miracle cures, miracle gadgets, fast fixes for terrifying new threats, the latest, the greatest... I'm not saying that innovation doesn't happen or isn't real. Of course, it happens and is real! But not everything that is hyped up is all that it's hyped up to be... It's harder and harder to tell these days, thanks to psychology-driven marketing, beautiful media and now AI! The good news is, the basics are the basics are the basics forever.

It's always going to be a healthy move to drink more (clean) water.

It's always going to be a healthy move to improve your ability to take a nice slow deep breath.

It's always going to be a healthy move to treat people with kindness and respect (including yourself!).

It's always going to be a healthy move to get about 7-9 hours a of sleep per night.

It's always going to be a healthy move to keep your body moving throughout the day and to work up a sweat once in a while!

You get the idea!

So, when you feel emotionally pulled towards some shiny new health thing or idea, take a deep breath, pause, and question it.

GROUP F.A.S.T.

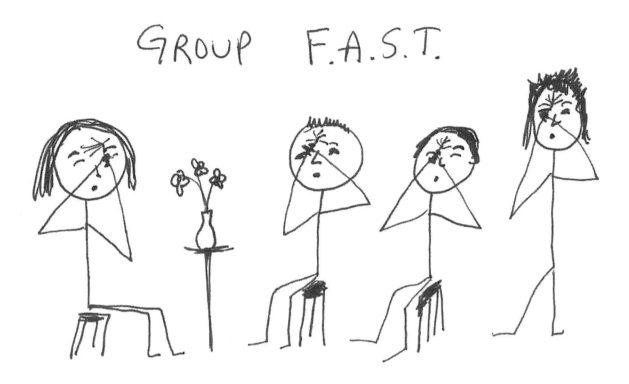

I think that FAST (the First Aid Stress Tool) and drinking water are probably the health nuggets that get the most repeating here in the Daily Nuggets. Why? Because they are so darn simple, accessible, and powerful! And, therefore, forgettable. That's why you need a reminder! So, what's this about "group FAST?" Are we joining a cult now? No, but...

Doing anything in a group tends to amplify its effects, since humans tend to mirror each other. When you do FAST in a group setting, it helps everyone to de-stress and relax. When might you do FAST as a group? Teachers can lead their classrooms through it to help settle down the energy and improve focus. Families can do it if there's been a conflict and people feel tense. Coworkers can do it before or after a meeting. I demonstrated it once during a party - not even a stressful event - and people said that they felt noticeably more grounded and relaxed afterward! You don't need to be in active distress to de-stress! (Unfortunately, most of us are walking around stressed already and we don't even know it!)

When doing group FAST, it is even more powerful if everyone is focusing on a particular theme. For example, if someone is feeling stressed because of a bully, then everyone can hold their points and breathe deeply, focusing on a time when they were bullied. It helps to synchronize the healing energy.

Experiment with it!

You can always go to www.firstaidstresstool.com for a refresher on how to do it!

MASSAGE YOUR ILEOCECAL VALVE

What's your ileocecal valve and why should you massage it? The ileocecal valve is the connector between your small and large intestine. It opens when it's time to allow digested food into the large intestine for water reclamation and elimination, and then it closes again. Sometimes, it gets stuck in the open position, and waste material flows backward into the small intestine! Sometimes, it gets stuck in the closed position, causing a backup. It can get inflamed and cause referred pain in the low back which can mimic the pain of a herniated disc. It can even cause sciatica! The ileocecal valve is located on the right side of your body in the lower abdomen. To find it, touch the front of your "hip bone" (which is really your ASIS, I know, but that's what most people call that bone) with one hand and your belly button with the other, and draw an imaginary line between those 2 points. At the center of the 2 points, go just a little below that line and press in. You might need to press in deeply and move your hands around. If your ileocecal valve needs some loving, then you will find a tender spot or a hard spot that feels kind of like a muscle knot that needs to be worked out. That's the spot! Massage that spot gently in circles. Clockwise works for most people, but listen to your body, and if your body says counter-clockwise then counter-clockwise it is! Most people who do have problems with the ileocecal valve (or ICV) have a problem with the valve sticking in the open position (usually due to inflammation) so it can be helpful to pull slightly in a diagonal direction towards your left shoulder.

TAP INTO THE FEELING OF WHAT YOU WANT

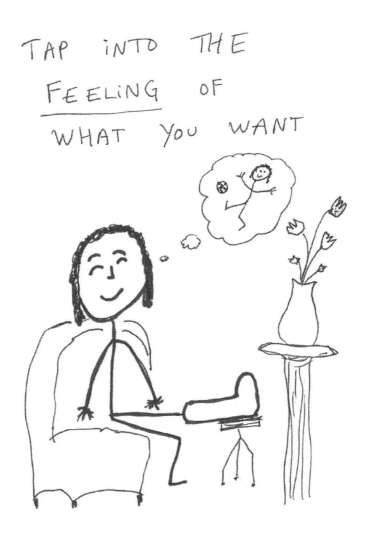

People talk about visualizations and affirmation for manifesting the thing you want, but you know what the most important part of the equation is? It's tapping into the *feeling* of having the desired outcome! The **feeling** is the emotional juice that feeds the most powerful parts of the nervous system. If you just visualize the thing you want, but you have a weak or negative feeling that goes with it (such as the feeling of "yeah but how the heck am I ever going to get *that?*) then it sends mixed messages to your nervous system, and you're likely to stay just where you are. So forget about the "how" or "when" and all those details. Just picture the outcome and most of all *feel the feeling* of what being in the picture will be like. Are you excited? Do you feel relaxed? Are you breathing deeply? What does it feel like? This technique is not just good for helping you to achieve your goals, but it's also great for helping to heal your body!

There are some great books about this. The first one I ever read was *Excuse Me, Your Life is Waiting* by Lynn Grabhorn. Dr. Joe Dispenza also has some great books expanding on this principle.

BRUSH OR SCRAPE YOUR TONGUE!

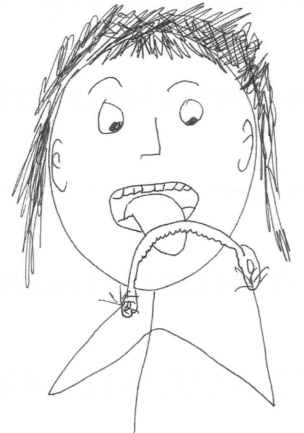

Did you know that scraping your tongue can help reduce plaque buildup on your teeth? It's also great for preventing bad breath and getting rid of gross morning breath!

There's not much to say about it other than that. 😬

Some people just use their toothbrush to brush their tongue.

I find that it's much more effective to use a tongue scraper.

There are several different types out there, so just find one you like!

TYPE A BLOOD =
THE NATURAL VEGETARIAN*

*pescatarian

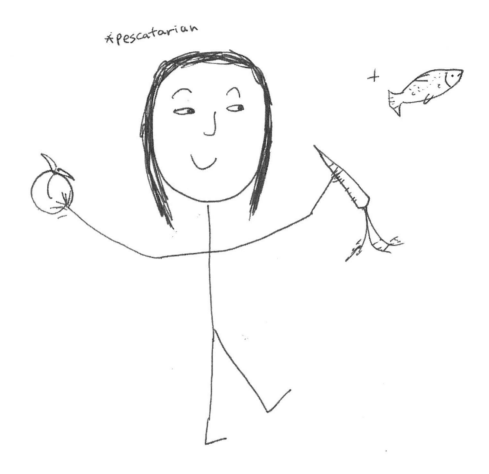

Remember how we said that people with type O blood tend to need some red meat and hard exercise to be really healthy? Well, people with type A blood tend to do really well with a mostly vegetarian* diet and exercises that are more relaxing and energetically nourishing, such as tai chi. I put the * next to vegetarian because type A blood people still tend to need *some* animal protein and do well with fish. If you still don't know your blood type, you can get order a home blood typing kit and figure it out! They are inexpensive and easy to use. Peter D'Adamo's classic books are still great if you are interested in learning more about blood type diets.

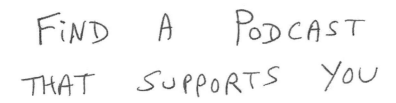

FIND A PODCAST THAT SUPPORTS YOU

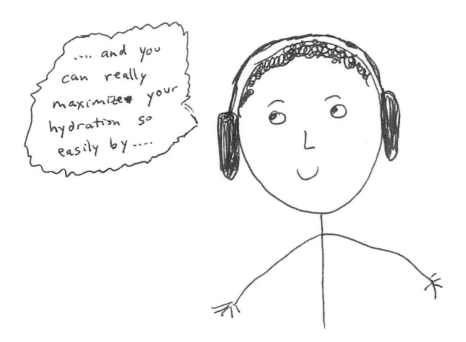

Podcasts are an amazing resource!

There are so many great podcasts that you can access for free.

When you find one (or many) that you feel really supports you on your healing journey, then make note of it and return to it whenever you need an extra boost! Sometimes you're riding high and you're in your groove and everything feels just fine! And sometimes you feel like a pancake that fell onto the floor. A wise Lyft driver once told me, "Sometimes you're the hammer, and sometimes you're the nail." Having good go-to podcasts that help to shift your mood and your mindset are important tools in your self-care toolbox! I really enjoy the Snap Judgement and Spooked! podcasts, which are both produced by Glynn Washington. I love his engaging style and his ability to bring people's stories to life! A healthy podcast doesn't have to focus on the particulars of your physical health - nutrition, exercise, chiropractic, etc. - in order to be healthy! Remember, a huge part of being healthy is having a healthy mindset and a sense of peace and wellbeing when it comes to coexisting with our fellow human beings. We're stuck with each other. May as well find ways to get comfortable!

365

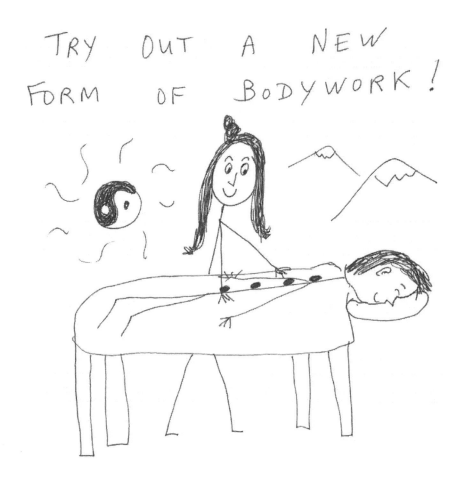

TRY OUT A NEW FORM OF BODYWORK!

There are so many great types of bodywork out there! How do you know which one to pick?! The best way to know is to just explore. Try something you've never tried before. Once you get an idea of how your body responds to a particular approach, then you'll have a better idea of when it might be just the thing you need! If you have plenty of time and money, then this - trying out new types of bodywork - is easy peasy! If you don't, then... get creative. Sometimes you can find schools or training academies that offer low-cost treatments so that the trainees can get practice. Many bodyworkers are also open to trade or barter, depending on what you've got! Over the course of my career, I have enjoyed many mutually beneficial barter relationships. I have bartered for meals, opera tickets, bodywork, minor home repairs, and haircuts (back when I had hair)! No one approach handles everything, so explore as best you can. Your body will thank you!

PAY YOURSELF ENERGETICALLY FIRST !

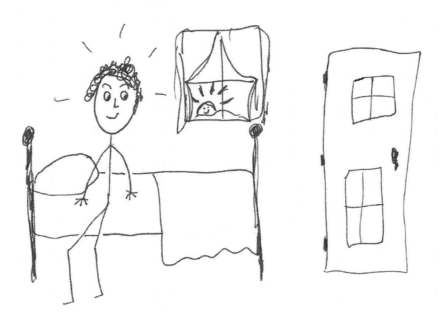

There is a classic business book called *Profit First*, by Mike Michalowicz, where he talks about how the only way to really make a profit in business is to take your profit first - off the top - and then make it (the business) work with whatever is left! The other approach - figuring your profit will come out of "whatever is left" - is a losing strategy. Why? *Because there's never anything left!* The same is true of your energy. If you wait "until everything else is done" before you dedicate some time to yourself, then, guess what? That means never. Because "everything else" is *never* done! Your best and most useful energy is usually found in the window of time shortly after you wake up.

What you do with this time sets the tone for the whole day!

What are you doing with this time?

Don't waste it on the news, social media, worry, etc.!

Use it for **you**!

Use it to meditate, journal, quietly exercise or engage in a hobby or activity that lights you up.

Don't wait until you're exhausted and cranky to try and do the things that nourish you.

You deserve the best of your energy - the creamy goodness on top! - not the sad dregs on the bottom.

So pay yourself (energetically) first thing in the morning!

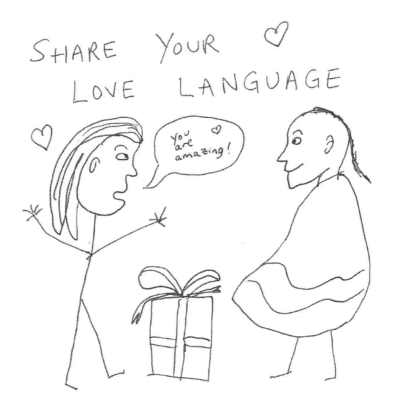

I know, the whole "love language" thing is becoming almost an eye-rolling meme-worthy thing these days, but... there's still some value and truth to it! In case you don't know what a "love language" is, it is the way that people give and receive love. According to the book *The Five Love Languages*, there are 5 main ways in which people give and receive love:
Words of Affirmation, Acts of Service, Gifts, Quality Time, Physical Touch.
While everyone may enjoy any or all of those things, there is usually one that **really** stands out when it comes to feeling *loved*. For example, if your "love language" is words of affirmation, then you will not really *feel loved* unless someone **says loving words** to you. Sometimes your giving and receiving languages may be different. For example, you may need words of affirmation to feel loved, but you may be a gift-giver when it comes to expressing your love. So, what is today's nugget about? I guess the first step is to figure out your own love language. But the nugget is about sharing it with the people you love - especially if you have a partner - because guess what? People are not psychic, and people assume that other people share the same love language that they do!
When relationships fall apart, it's often because of something stupid. One of those stupid things could be as simple as not loving the other person in the way that **they** need to feel loved! So, be a grown up and communicate clearly what your love language is to the people who should know that information! And, be mindful of others, and consider *asking them what their love language is.*

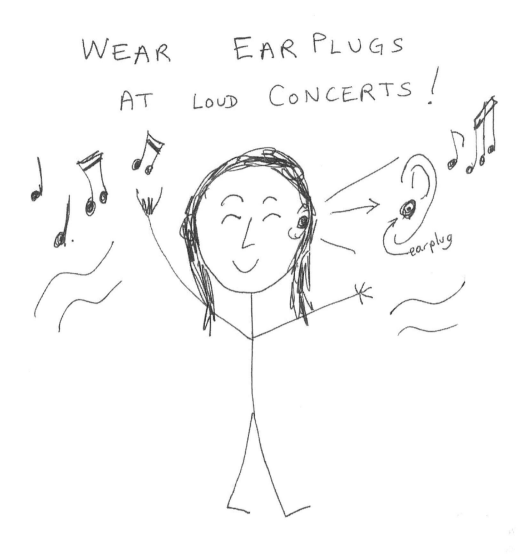

This one should be so obvious, and yet...

I'm surprised at how many people still don't use ear protection at loud concerts!

Concert earplug technology has come a long way since those squishy foam earplugs!

With the new ones, you can still hear the music clearly - not muffled - and you are preserving your hearing for the future.

You can even get a decent pair for under $20.

Even though hearing aid technology is pretty awesome these days, it's even better if you can preserve your hearing for as long as possible!

So protect your ears at concerts! (and other really loud places...)

DELETE SOCIAL MEDIA APPS FROM YOUR PHONE!

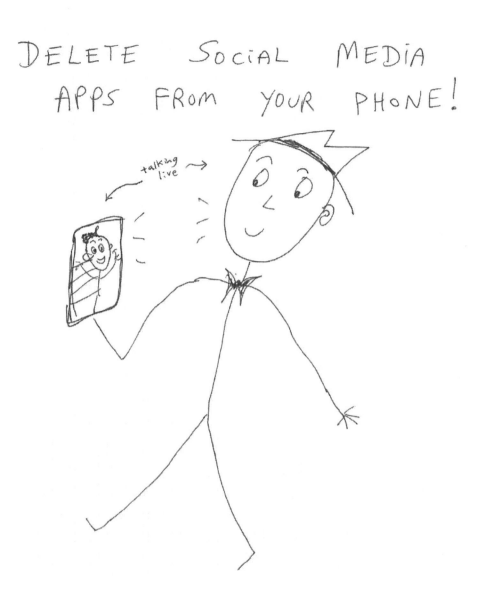

talking live →

Yep, I said it.

Delete social media apps from your phone! This is not to say that you can or should never use them. They can be great! But... they can also be a **COLOSSAL WASTE OF TIME.** By deleting them from your phone, you will not be so tempted to "just take a look..." or scroll aimlessly throughout the day. It will be a lot easier to schedule a defined set of time to look at them on your computer or laptop sometime! And guess what? Even if you do delete the apps from your phone, it's not that hard to reinstall them any time you do want to use them! Sounds like a pain? Yeah, that's the idea! It doesn't even take a minute to reinstall an app... but it's just inconvenient enough that you're not going to do it for those impulse scrolls! Give it a shot. It will improve your mental health!

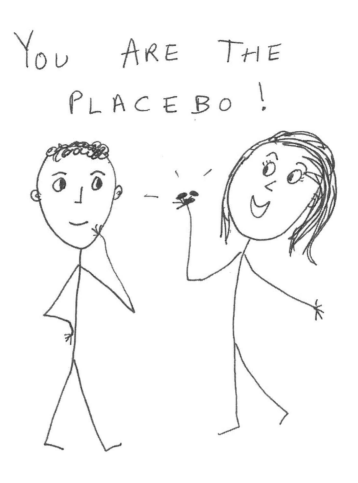

It has always bugged me when people wave off the placebo effect as no big deal. Are you kidding me? It's incredible! A placebo is a substance - such as a sugar pill - that has no therapeutic value, and it is used in experiments to compare to the "real" drug, etc. to test for efficiency. The weird thing is, a certain percentage of people - often a lot of people! - do show positive effects when taking the placebo, as compared to people who took nothing. It's a testament to the incredible healing power that we already have within ourselves! Our bodies can produce a surprising array of substances - including opioid pain relievers - if only it receives the right signals from the brain. There is a great book by Dr. Joe Dispenza called You Are the Placebo: Making Your Mind Matter that goes into more detail on the amazing healing power of the placebo effect and how **you** are, in fact, the placebo! I recommend checking it out. And, knowing how powerful it is, there is nothing wrong with actively using placebos for yourself. There are studies that show that people taking sugar pills out of a bottle that is even labeled PLACEBO still get the benefits, because there is a part of the brain that doesn't notice the writing, but just knows that a pill probably does something! (I think that this is how a lot of homeopathy probably works.) Anyway, don't knock the placebo!

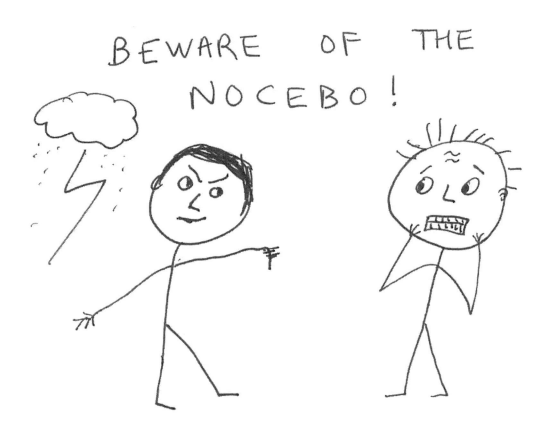

Everyone's heard of the placebo,

but do you know about its evil twin, the nocebo?

The nocebo effect is when you get sick due to a negative prediction or proclamation!

People have even died after receiving a false diagnosis of a fatal condition!

That's pretty extreme, but milder examples happen allll the time.

Take "flu season," for example.

Ever notice how many people get the flu as soon as they hear that it's "flu season" or "this is a really bad flu season!" ?

I suppose it's *possible* that most of those people would have caught it with or without the belief, but... I dunno... I'm very suspicious.

People have also been shown to exhibit false "side effects" of fake medications (sugar pills) after being told that they would experience the side effects.

So be careful when people give you negative predictions about your health!

Your body has incredible powers to heal you OR to make you sick!

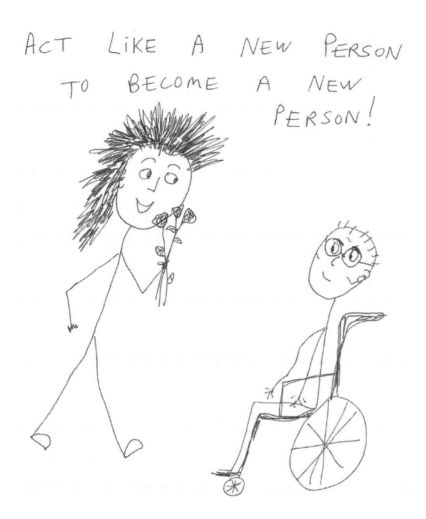

ACT LIKE A NEW PERSON TO BECOME A NEW PERSON!

If you want something different for your health (or wealth, or relationships, etc.) then guess what? **You have to become someone different!** I'm not saying that there's anything "wrong" with you... because there isn't... and/but... if you want something different, then you have to *become someone different.* It's kind of like that old joke where they say that the definition of insanity is doing the same thing over and over but expecting a different result! So, think about the person who you want to be. What does that person do? How does that person behave? And then when you are going through your day, keep asking yourself... ***what would that person do?*** When you're thinking about drinking water, or exercising, or what to eat, or when you go to bed or when to wake up, or how to treat other people... ***what would that person do?*** It's simple! (I didn't say it was easy...) Do what that person - hypothetical future you - would do, and eventually, you really will become that person!

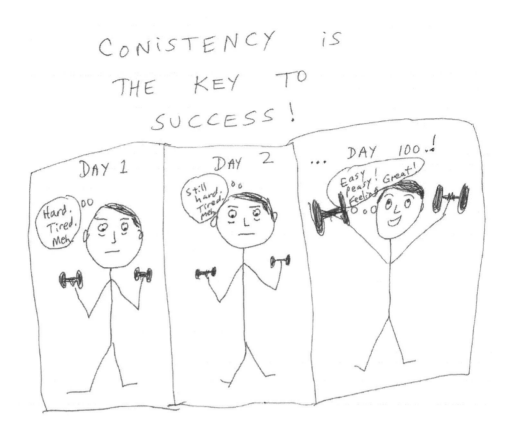

This one goes for health, business, success, or really anything big that you want to achieve.
It's all about **consistency.**
Big changes and achievements don't happen overnight or in one shot or in 2 or 3 or 10 shots!
Everything takes time, repetition and **consistency.**
But look at us here, on Daily Nugget #341!!!
How's your health been this year, after absorbing just one little nugget a day?
Probably a pretty good year?
Yes?
Well, it's been a pretty good year for me!
I didn't feel very accomplished when I wrote my first few nuggets.
But after being consistent with just this one thing every day for a year, I'm feeling darn good.
So, don't worry about trying to be consistent with "everything."
That's not possible.
Pick something that you really care about, and then make sure that you're consistent with that!

YOUR BODY IS YOUR ONLY CAR!

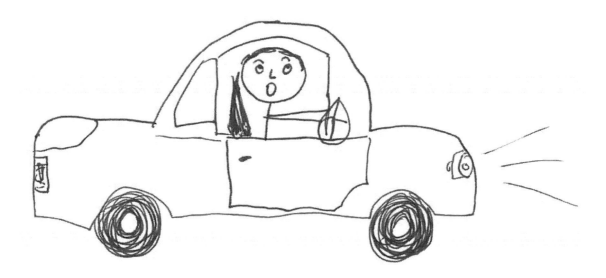

What if, on the day you were born, you were given a car? (Yeah, yeah, I know, you couldn't drive it for years and years, but stay with me here!) In this world, everyone is given a car at birth! And most of the time, it's a darn good car. However, there's just one catch... It's the **only** car you will **ever** be given. In fact, it's the only car you will *ever* be allowed to have! You couldn't even buy a new one if you had the money. One person gets just one car, and that car needs to last their entire life! That sounds like a dumb world. And kind of a lame story. But you know what??? **Your body is that car!** Your body is your only car! Think about it... If it were a car... would you take care of that car? How much care would you take? Would you change the oil on time like you're supposed to? Would you be mindful of how hard you ran the engine? Would you pay attention to the warning lights when they came on? If you treat your body like it's the only car you'll ever get for your whole life, then you will get a lot more mileage out of it, and a lot nicer of a ride, too.

PUT TOGETHER A PUZZLE!

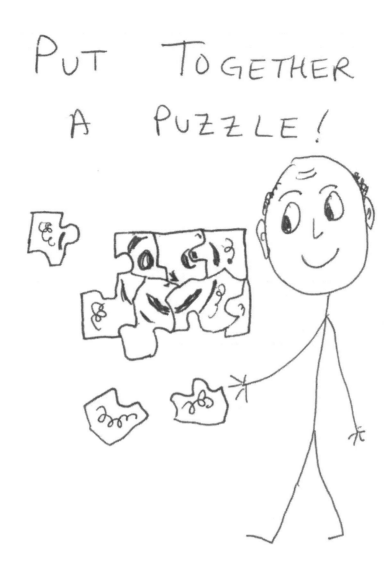

Puzzles might not seem like tools of health, but they are good for your health in at least 2 ways and probably more!

First of all, they involve quiet, technology-free time that gives your brain a rest.

Even though you may be staring at a complicated image, it doesn't overload your brain in the way that doom-scrolling, answering e-mails, etc. can!

And yet, puzzles also give your brain some healthy exercise in the areas of problem solving and spatial relations.

This helps to keep your brain sharp!

Some people even use puzzles as a group activity, with a designated "puzzle table" in a common area of the home. This can be a nice non-competitive activity that can foster quiet social time and bonding within the household.

LEARN NEW WAYS TO COOK HEALTHY THINGS

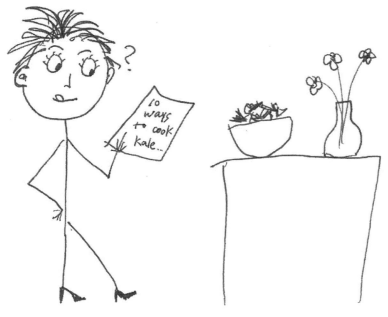

If you're a terrible cook (like me) then it seems hard to learn even one way to cook a healthy thing! And then you keep cooking that one way... and you get bored... and you fall off the wagon. Womp womp. So what's a bad cook to do? You dust yourself off, and go to the Googles (or wherever) and look up new ways to cook the thing, try something out, and stop yourself from getting bored! Let's just pick an easy one. Kale. Kale is supposed to be healthy, right? I don't use a lot of kale, but when I do, I stuff it into a blender and make a smoothie, or sometimes I cook it up with some eggs. Mostly I just cook it in olive oil and eat it with salt because I don't know what else to do with it! Well, to be a good sport and take my own advice, I just Googled "10 ways to cook kale." You know, I never even thought about putting it into soup! But there you have it. Just pick a healthy food item that you only know 1 or 2 (or zero) ways to prepare and ask your computer for 10 ways. You might get inspired!

LET FOOD BE YOUR MEDICINE, AND MEDICINE BE YOUR FOOD.

— Hippocrates

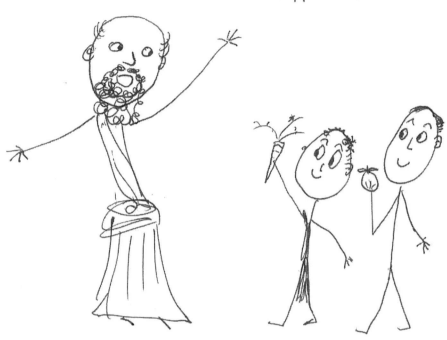

Today's Nugget is a quote from Hippocrates, aka The Father of Medicine. What amazes me about this quote is that he said it about 2400 years ago! 😲

And it's still so relevant today.

Some of the cynics out there would say, yeah, well, he didn't have access to modern medicine back then so of course he's going to use food.

To which I say, yeah, well, modern medicine sometimes has no answers to things that food can heal!

What brought this up today is that I saw my brother yesterday for the first time in about a year. It had been a horrific year for him in the health department.

Not only were the old auto-immune issues, fibromyalgia, etc. in high gear, but he had started having major epileptic seizures and was unable to work!

Modern medicine didn't have anything to offer him aside from lifetime medication and possible brain surgery!

His wife encouraged him to try one more thing: The Medical Medium.

Well, he did it.

And guess what???

Everything got better.

The seizures stopped, the fibromyalgia disappeared, the autoimmune symptoms (IBS, joint pain, skin issues, etc.) all went away!

And what, exactly, was the treatment?

Yes, there was a specific protocol, but in a nutshell, it was really just **food.**

Taking out all possible harmful foods and adding lots of specifically healthy foods.

His story almost sounds like BS - too good to be true - but he is my brother, and I know what he's been going through for many years!

And I saw with my own eyes that he's healthy and about to start a new job after spending almost a year unable to work due to the seizures.

Wow.

So, don't underestimate the power of **food** as **medicine!**

And if you want to check out my brother's Facebook group that he set up as a healing support community, it's called Raphael's Road.

Let's say it again for those in the back!

Let food be your medicine, and medicine be your food!

(that's a good mantra / affirmation, too!)

SWEET POTATO POWER

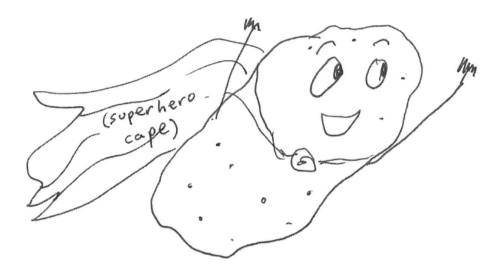

(superhero cape)

Wow - how did we get this far without mentioning the amazing sweet potato?!

The humble sweet potato is one of the most nutrient-dense foods there is.

It's rich in antioxidants, vitamins C, A, and E, minerals like potassium, manganese and iron - plus it's high in fiber and can be a low glycemic index food.

With sweet potatoes, how they are prepared makes a big difference re: how hard it can hit your blood sugar!

The best way to prepare them (for a low glycemic score) is to boil them for a long time.

(Boiled for 30 minutes brings the it down to 46, whereas boiling for 8 minutes brings it down to 61.)

Anything under 55 is considered "low glycemic."

Unfortunately, the most delicious method - peeled and baked - brings it way up to 94!

Here is an article on how cooking affects its place on the glycemic index.

Not everyone needs to be super mindful of glycemic index, so don't freak out about how to cook your sweet potatoes!

Just add it to your nuggets of health knowledge and enjoy some sweet potatoes!

(And don't forget that eating them with the skin on adds a good source of fiber!)

GET SOME GOOD LAUGHS!

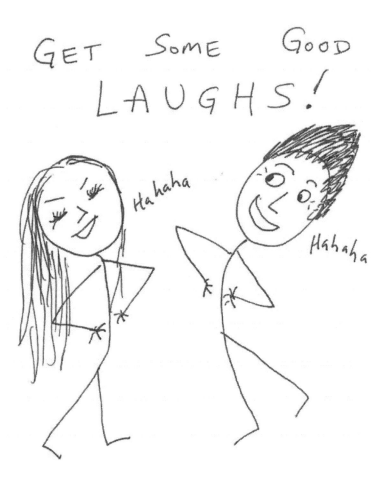

They say, "laughter is the best medicine." Well, it is some darn powerful medicine! Some people recommend watching comedy shows, listening to comedy or reading funny things. Any of those things will work if they really make you laugh! "I am amused" doesn't pack the same healing punch as a good hard belly laugh, though! (Lookin' at you, fellow fives!) But can "forced laughter" work? Yep! This is the case with "laughter yoga," where you deliberately make yourself laugh even if there is nothing "funny" going on. It becomes fun / funny, and your body reacts accordingly! You can look up some 5-minute laughter yoga workouts on YouTube. Just follow along and laugh when they laugh, even if you feel ridiculous! (Even if you have to wait until you're alone in the house. 😵) Laughter creates the exact opposite body chemistry as stress, so it's the ultimate antidote to stress!

When's the last time you had a good hard belly laugh?

(I'm pretty juvenile in the humor department, so I probably did it when a friend farted at an inopportune moment!)

PARSLEY FOR KIDNEY HEALTH

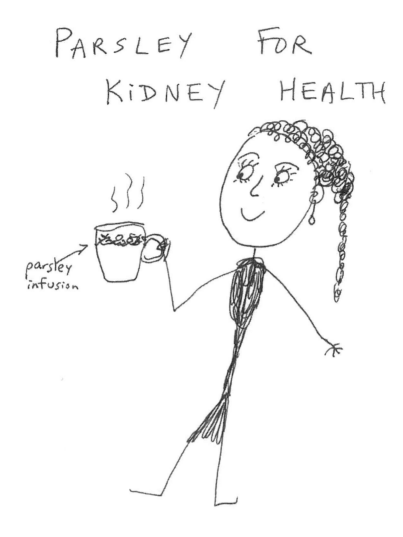

parsley infusion

Most people know that drinking plenty of water is good for your kidneys.

But did you know that parsley is also good for your kidneys?

It is one of the healthiest foods that can support kidney health!

You can add it to your salads and smoothies, or just make a nice warm infusion and drink it on a daily basis.

To make a basic parsley infusion, just add about a tablespoon of freshly crushed parsley to a cup of hot water and let it steep for about 5-7 minutes.

Then, strain it and you have a nice parsley infusion!

(or don't strain it, and get the added benefit of consuming the fiber!)

The Home Run Formula

2nd — Toxicity

1st — Emotions

3rd

Nutrition

Pitcher's mound

Home Base — Structure

HOME BASE

I could have sworn I've already done a Daily Nugget on the Home Run Formula, but... looks like I didn't!

The Home Run Formula is a model developed by Drs. Scott and Deb Walker to describe the model of health embraced in NET world.

It's a baseball diamond analogy, which I have to say because not all of us are sporty people. 😵 👾

The idea is that the problems and solutions of health can be found on 4 bases: structural, emotional, toxicity and nutrition.

You put your problem in the center - on the pitcher's mound - and then surround the bases to find your solutions.

If you cover all the bases, you'll get a home run!

This is a handy concept to keep in mind, because sometimes we can get fixated on a certain kind of solution for a certain kind of problem, and then completely forget that the solution might be on one of the other bases!

A very common example of this is mysterious hip pain.

The pain feels very "structural" - and it might even respond to structural treatments such as massage, chiropractic, etc. - but the relief never lasts more than a few hours, and then it's back. However, it can often be tied to wheat consumption (usually too much bread).

In these cases, elimination of wheat also eliminates the hip pain.

My personal version of this bread hip pain is bread low back pain!

If I start to eat too much bread, then my low back starts to hurt.

Even though it happens often, I never put 2-and-2 together until after a couple of weeks!

And then sure enough, I cut way back on the bread - or cut it out entirely - and then my low back settles down and feels good again!

But if your problem is "non-structural," such as anxiety, could there be a "structural" solution? Oddly enough, YES!

I once treated a young man whose depression and brain fog turned out to be caused by a badly subluxated cranial bone.

Once this part of his skull - his sphenoid bone - was released, the brain fog cleared up and his mood lifted.

I will admit, that's very rare compared to structural problems that need nutritional solutions, but it still happens!

Also, as a reminder, the difference between toxicity and nutrition is that toxicity means that something is inside of the body that shouldn't be there, and nutrition is focused on things that should be in the body but may not be there in the right amounts.

MAKE YOUR OWN ELECTROLYTES

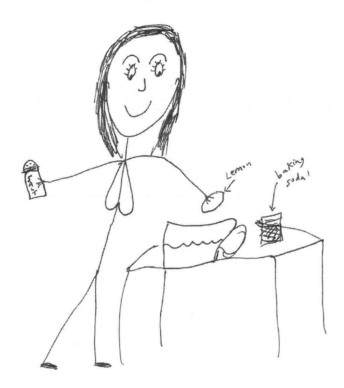

Electrolytes are minerals in your body that carry an electrical charge. They are important for maintaining your levels of hydration! Drinking extra electrolytes can be very helpful before and after a sweaty workout, on a hot day, during or after an illness, after a night of drinking, and if you have challenges with low blood pressure.

A lot of the commercial electrolytes out there have too much sugar in them.

So, it's a good thing that it's so easy to make your own!

Here is a very basic recipe:
1/2 teaspoon of pure unrefined sea salt
1/4 teaspoon baking soda
1/3 cup lemon juice
1 tablespoon lime juice

Remember, electrolytes go a long way to helping prevent sore muscles and hangovers!

HEALTH IS A JOURNEY (not a destination)

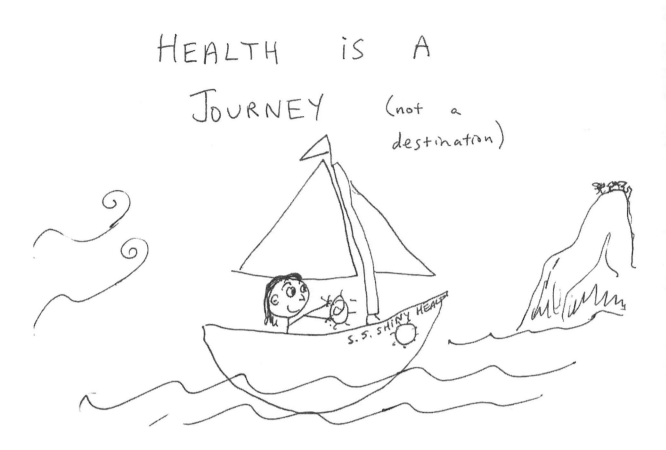

I know you've heard this before (because I know I've said it):

Health is a journey - not a destination.

It's annoying, but it's true.

There's no "there" there - even though you always need to aim in a particular direction!

You will reach destinations, and sometimes it will feel so great that you think you'll stay there forever!

But nothing really lasts forever, and remember, life is motion!

We're always moving and changing.

We have different needs for different seasons and conditions.

Sometimes it's annoying, but it's OK!

Celebrate when you reach your goals, and don't beat yourself up when a new goal appears.

It's all part of the game.

Enjoy the journey!

PEOPLE ARE (BASICALLY) DOING THEIR BEST

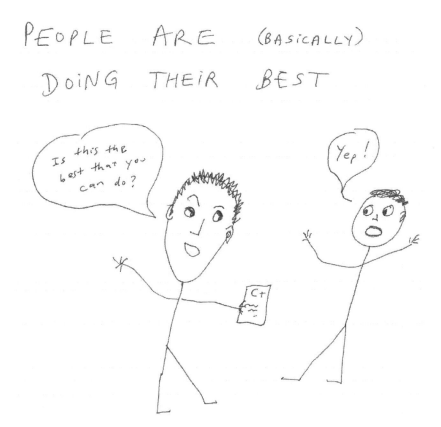

Are people really doing their best? Really??? 😑 Basically... yes! 🐵
Given their particular circumstances and conditions, most people really are doing the best they can. Think about it. Nobody wants to be a loser or a loveless jackass. So they do the best they can. I know, I know... it sure doesn't look like that from the outside! And that is a big cause of stress and strife. It also leads to a decrease in compassion. One of the mindset shifts that can lead to a decrease in cortisol - that most annoying of stress hormones! - is to accept that for the most part, people are doing the best they can. We can't know what's really happening internally for anyone but ourselves!

So, yes, that crappy driver in front of you?

They're doing the best they can.

That weirdo who voted for the maniac?

They're doing the best they can.

The maniac???

Doing the best they can.

You can always work for the positive changes you want to see in your life and in the world! But when it comes to feeling and judgements about other individual people, remember: they're doing the best they can.

USE THE RIGHT TOOL FOR THE JOB!

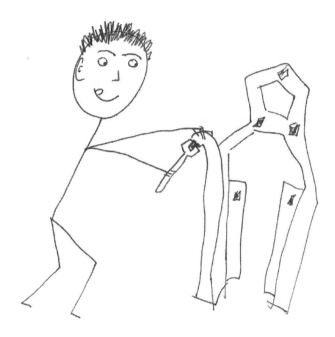

This is really an injury-prevention nugget.

Use the right tool for the job!

People come in all the time with injuries that wouldn't have happened if only they had used the right tool for the job!

Sometimes it's a sprained hand from trying to unscrew a stuck garden hose fitting when the right wrench would have made that job much easier!

Sometimes it's a strained neck from painting a ceiling with a short-handled roller when a much longer one could have allowed for a mostly neutral neck during the process!

Sometimes it's a strained back from hauling heavy items without using a cart or other moving tools. You get the idea! (Although, it also kind of sounds like the moral of the story is to pay someone younger and stronger to do these things for you.)

We live in a world where there are special tools to help make physically difficult tasks easier. If you're about to do something that could lead to an injury - even "just" a strained muscle - ask yourself, is there a tool that could make this easier or safer?

(And if you can't think of one, just ask AI!)

AVOID CHARRED MEATS !

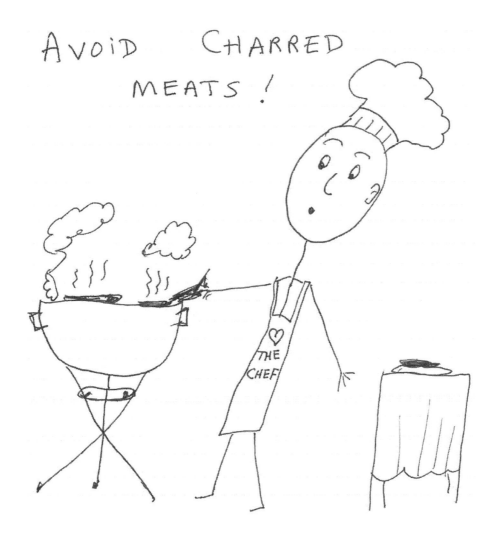

As much as it pains me to say this... *it's good to avoid charred meats.*
Unfortunately, there is a lot of evidence that charred meats contain cancer-causing compounds! This is especially sad because the char can be so tasty!
sigh
But, it is what it is. Since grilling is a big part of American culture, it's safe to say that you will still encounter grilled meats once in a while unless you are a vegetarian! So aside from avoiding the temptation or opting for smaller portions, don't forget that you can help to neutralize those cancer-causing compounds by taking in a lot more cancer *fighting* compounds (antioxidants), which you will find in abundance in vegetables! ***Especially those dark leafy green vegetables!*** So make sure to eat plenty of vegetables if you opt for meat at that BBQ, and avoid over-cooked and blackened meats!

RECORD A
PERSONAL AFFIRMATION

Affirmations can be a powerful tool for shifting your mindset, which can then shift your choices and then your **actions!** (And that is where the real treasure lies!) Some people recommend writing out affirmations and sticking them to your mirror, or putting them in your wallet, or some other place where you will see them and be reminded to say or think them on a daily basis. Like all mindset-shifting practices, affirmations require lots of *repetition.* And if something needs to be repeated in order to be effective, then you have to make it *convenient to access!* And what is the most convenient way to access something these days? For most of us, it's going to be something that's on your phone! So, record your affirmation(s) on your phone and make it easy to access. You can listen to your recording while commuting or while tidying up or while exercising. Listening to your affirmation first thing in the morning or right before you go to bed can help to program it deeper into your subconscious. Coming up with a good personal affirmation can be daunting and time-consuming, so, sometimes it can help to just borrow someone else's in the meantime! I really love author Mike Kim's personal affirmation, which is pretty long and can be found on his You Are the Brand podcast (episode 360). To be honest, I have downloaded that episode and use it for myself sometimes! Remember, an affirmation is just a simple statement of something that you wish to be true and that you really want to embed into your personal belief system and universe.

390

SET AN ALARM!

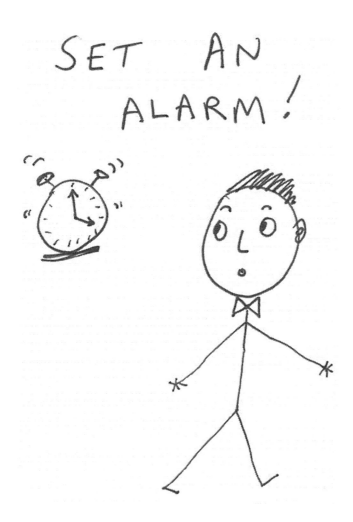

Many nuggets ago, we talked about setting an alarm for bedtime. So, what's this generic alarm setting about? It's about using alarms to help manage your time! This is mostly for those of you (read: us) who are easily distracted and can fall down time-consuming rabbit holes or forget all about what you were "going to do." You can set alarms to limit the amount of time you work before getting up to walk around the block for some fresh air! Or set an alarm to make sure you drink your water. Or set an alarm to let you know when it's time to stop doom-scrolling on your favorite depressing app! Or set an alarm to let you know when it's time to end a conversation with a long-winded friend or relative. And with all of our readily available silent alarm technology, people don't even have to notice your alarms! Remember, stress is one of the biggest killers of health, and feeling stressed out is all about feeling overwhelmed. The more you can take off of your mental plate - even something as small as remembering when to start or stop certain tasks - the more energy you will have available and the less overwhelm you will experience.

USE THE LIBRARY

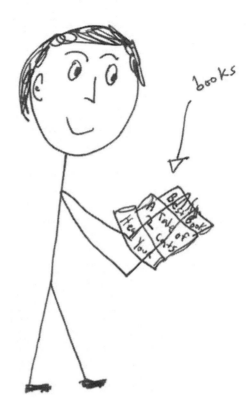

books

Libraries seem so old-fashioned. And now that so much information is available for free online, why even go there? Lots of reasons! For one thing, good old-fashioned books give your eyes a rest from staring at electronic screens. And by borrowing a book from your library, you are supporting your community while also saving some money (and avoiding new clutter) by not purchasing the book yourself! If you know the exact book that you are looking for, you can often reserve the book online and get a notification when it's ready for you to pick up! Or you can browse the shelves and discover other books on similar topics that you may have never even heard of! Going to the library forces you to slow down. We all know that we "should" slow down, but it's hard to do! So why not choose to do something positive that forces us to slow down at the same time? You can use some of the book money that you save on buying high-quality supplements!

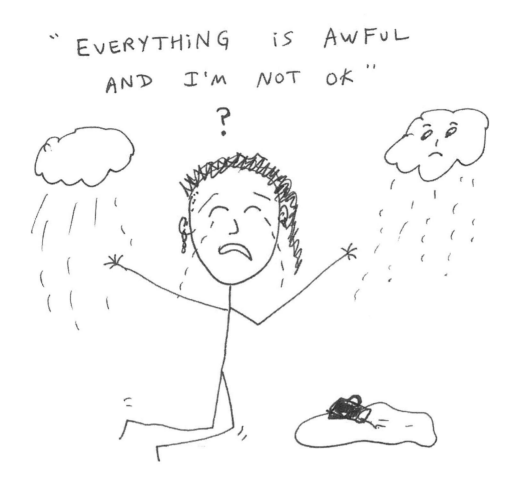

Have you heard of the "Everything is Awful and I'm Not Okay" sheet? The subtitle is **questions to ask before giving up.** I first encountered it posted on a door on a big nerd cruise earlier this year. I took a copy so that I could share it, but I also wanted to say that the author has given permission to customize the document and share it with others! All that they ask is that if you do so, that you attribute their Tumblr page where it was originally posted: **https://eponis.tumblr.com/post/113798088670/everything-is-awful-and-im-not-okay-questions-to**

So here it is.

Everything is Awful and I'm Not Okay: questions to ask before giving up:

Are you hydrated? If not, have a glass of water.

Have you eaten in the past three hours? If not, get some food — something with protein, not just simple carbs. Perhaps some nuts or hummus?

Have you showered in the past day? If not, take a shower right now.

If daytime: are you dressed? If not, put on clean clothes that aren't pajamas. Give yourself permission to wear something special, whether it's a funny t-shirt or a pretty dress.

If nighttime: are you sleepy and fatigued but resisting going to sleep? Put on pajamas, make yourself cozy in bed with a teddy bear and the sound of falling rain, and close your eyes for fifteen minutes — no electronic screens allowed. If you're still awake after that, you can get up again; no pressure.

Have you stretched your legs in the past day? If not, do so right now. If you don't have the spoons for a run or trip to the gym, just walk around the block, then keep walking as long as you please. If the weather's crap, drive to a big box store (e.g. Target) and go on a brisk walk through the aisles you normally skip.

Have you said something nice to someone in the past day? Do so, whether online or in person. Make it genuine; wait until you see something really wonderful about someone, and tell them about it.

Have you moved your body to music in the past day? If not, do so — jog for the length of an EDM song at your favorite BPM, or just dance around the room for the length of an upbeat song.

Have you cuddled a living being in the past two days? If not, do so. Don't be afraid to ask for hugs from friends or friends' pets. Most of them will enjoy the cuddles too; you're not imposing on them.

Do you feel ineffective? Pause right now and get something small completed, whether it's responding to an e-mail, loading up the dishwasher, or packing your gym bag for your next trip. Good job!

Do you feel unattractive? Take a goddamn selfie. Your friends will remind you how great you look, and you'll fight society's restrictions on what beauty can look like.

Do you feel paralyzed by indecision? Give yourself ten minutes to sit back and figure out a game plan for the day. If a particular decision or problem is still being a roadblock, simply set it aside for now, and pick something else that seems doable. Right now, the important part is to break through that stasis, even if it means doing something trivial.

Have you seen a therapist in the past few days? If not, hang on until your next therapy visit and talk through things then.

Have you been over-exerting yourself lately — physically, emotionally, socially, or intellectually? That can take a toll that lingers for days. Give yourself a break in that area, whether it's physical rest, taking time alone, or relaxing with some silly entertainment.

Have you changed any of your medications in the past couple of weeks, including skipped doses or a change in generic prescription brand? That may be screwing with your head. Give things a few days, then talk to your doctor if it doesn't settle down.

Have you waited a week? Sometimes our perception of life is skewed, and we can't even tell that we're not thinking clearly, and there's no obvious external cause. It happens. Keep yourself going for a full week, whatever it takes, and see if you still feel the same way then. You've made it this far, and you will make it through. **You are stronger than you think.**

Go Back To Basics!

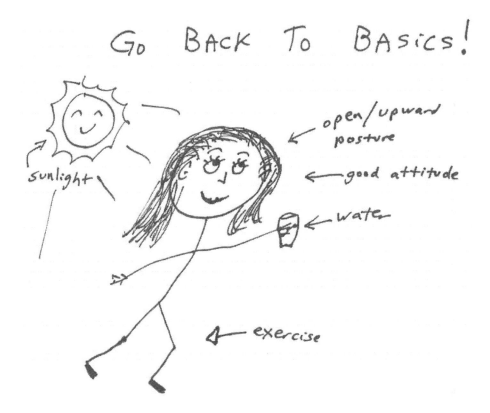

When you can't think of what to do, just remember: ***the basics are the basics for a reason!***
When things are going downhill, it's usually because the basics are out.

* Drinking enough water
* Getting enough clean fresh air and some nice vitamin-D-generating sunlight
* Moving your body and working up a sweat
* Breathing slowly and deeply
* Resting when you need a rest
* Being a friend to someone
* Eating mindfully
* Eating real food
* Going to bed at a consistent and decent hour

...

You get the idea! I intended for all 366 of the Daily Nuggets to be "basic," but they are not all
the basics. So, don't worry - you don't have to do *everything* you've been learning! When
you're feeling overwhelmed and something's not right, just take a deep breath and think
about the basics and start right there.

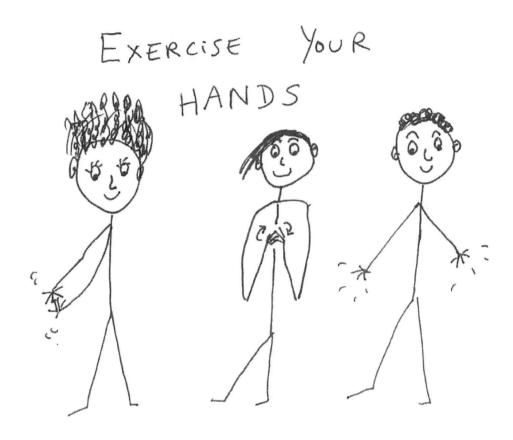

When we use a muscle all the time - like our hands - we tend to forget that they could benefit from some exercises! Aren't they already exercising all day?? Sort of... but depending on what you do, they are likely getting too much of some kinds of movement and too little of others! I found some handy hand exercises on a knitting website, and after doing them, my hands felt so much better! (And I'm not even a knitter!) I'm so glad that they have great animations on their site, because stick figure hands don't really cut it, but here are some descriptions of the exercises anyway:

1) Prayer Time: Interlace your fingers together like you're about to start praying (or begging for your life) and rotate your hands in a clockwise direction 10 times, and then switch directions for another 10.

2) Hocus Pocus: Open and stretch out your fingers with force for 10 seconds. Then, close and tighten your fingers for another 10 seconds.

3) The One Ring: Pull each finger gently (twice) and then gently rotate each one in a clockwise direction 4 times.

Check out the cool animations at: https://blog.weareknitters.com/knitters-life/hand-exercises-for-knitters/

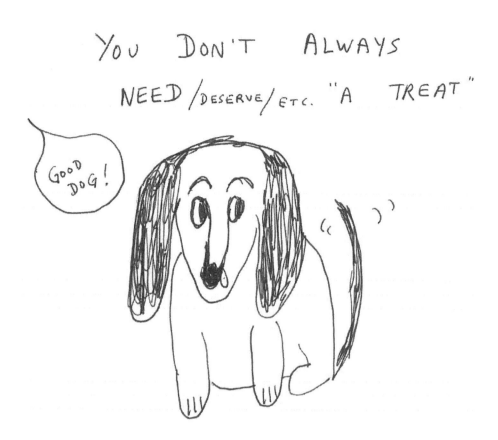

YOU DON'T ALWAYS NEED /DESERVE/ ETC. "A TREAT"

Do you ever do something that you know is bad for your health and then justify it with something like, **"I deserve a treat!"** Yeah, yeah, we all deserve a break or a treat or whatever sometimes, but... honestly... how many times (a day) have you used this one? I've certainly been there! I ate a whole plate of vegetables. So, I deserve a treat! I worked hard today. So, I deserve a treat! I was nice to that jerk. So, I deserve a treat! I'm stressed. So, I deserve a treat! Those "treats" can really add up, and they usually cause more harm than good! Remember, we're animals. And we can be trained and conditioned like animals, too. And "treats" can be a powerful trainer! Many years ago, when I had a dog, we were training her to pee on the puppy pads. She got a treat every time she did it. Eventually, she got wise to this and started peeing just a little bit - to get a treat. And then just a little bit again - to get another treat. You can see where this is going. It got ridiculous. But when it's **us** controlling the handing out of the treats (whatever it may be) to **ourselves**, then, there's no voice of reason to cut it out! So, when you find yourself saying, "I deserve a treat!" for every little grown-up thing you do, ask yourself, 'What am I, a good dog??" It's OK to just do good, hard or boring things and then just get on with it and continue on your journey! You're not "depriving" yourself of anything if you don't give yourself a "treat." Feeling good and having the energy and health to live your life is the best treat of all!

EAT QUALITY PROTEIN BEFORE WORKING OUT

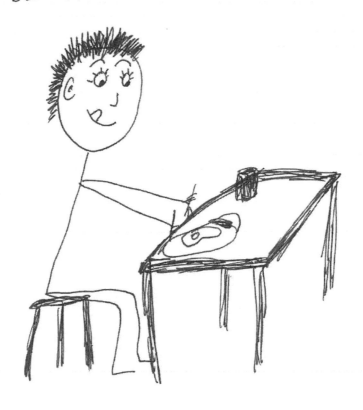

Good quality protein is especially important on workout days! You will notice a big difference in your workouts - especially strength training - if you eat a good quality protein meal on the day of your workout! Ideally, this means at least a few hours before working out. If you don't believe me, then all you have to do is compare how you feel while working out after a quality protein meal compared to working out after a carb-heavy meal. You can also compare different kinds of proteins. You will notice that your body has a preference!

I discovered that my body feels strongest if I work out after having some kind of lean meat in my meal earlier in the day. I feel less strong if my protein only came from eggs, and I feel very wimpy if my meal was mostly carbs. If you're going to work out, then make the most of it by making sure that you ate quality protein earlier in the day! (I keep saying "quality protein" instead of "meat" because if I say "meat" then some sassy vegan beast will reply and show me their muscle pics. Yeah, yeah, I know it's possible... but it ain't easy!)

GET READY TO GET OLD

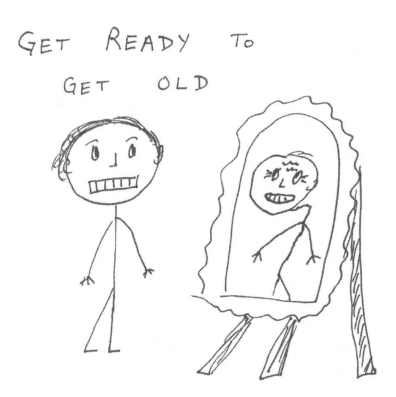

I know, I know, this one looks and sounds depressing... and didn't we already have a nugget on "get ready to die?" Isn't that kind of the same idea? No, it's not the same idea! As people get older (at least in America), a lot of "healthy living" is sold as old-avoidance - as if we can really avoid getting old! The "anti-aging" movement reminds me of this. It's considered "giving up" if you think too hard on what it means to get older! But the thing is... the human condition is the human condition. Every age has its characteristics and its challenges! Sure, there are always outliers and exceptions to the rule. But every age and season of life has its common features. Our youth-oriented culture means that a lot of people enter old age without really preparing for any of it. And "preparing" means more than "saving for retirement." It means being OK when your skin is thinner or looser than it used it to be. (Sure, you can - and should - moisturize and sunscreen and take care of it - but if you live long enough, it's going to be pretty different from what it was when you were young!)

It means looking ahead and knowing that at some point, you're just not going to want to deal with a bunch of stairs in your home. It means being OK with eventually needing (and wanting) less or different food, less or different levels of socializing, perhaps earlier bedtime (I'm already there!). It even means being OK with a certain level of aches and pains. There's nothing sad or bad or wrong with normal changes of life. It's just that season of life! As long as you're alive, you may as well keep taking care of yourself. But don't fall into feeling like a failure because you got old anyway!

It's just human life! 😑 🗿

EXERCISE OR SLEEP?

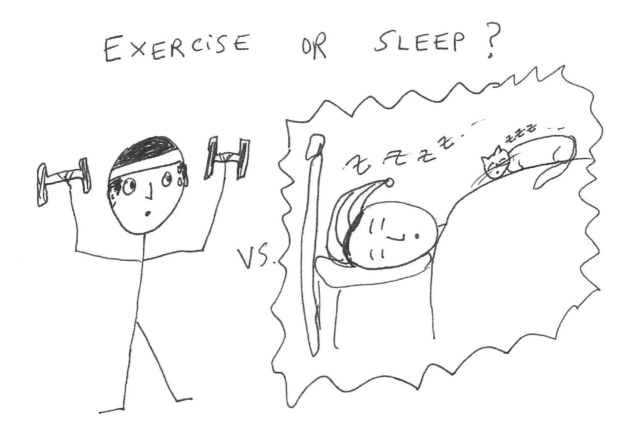

Exercise is important. Sleep is important. But... Everyone is busy!

Have you ever been **so busy** that you found yourself thinking, "Should I sleep, or should I exercise? I don't have time for both!"

Maybe you "compromise" and do some exercise and just cut your sleep short.

That's better than nothing, right? **Maybe not!**

A 10-year study showed that while exercise helps to keep the brain healthy, these benefits are lost if the exercisers were getting less than 6 hours of sleep a night!

Those "low sleepers" ended up with the same risks as the people who didn't exercise at all!

It makes sense.

We've all heard about those extremely fit people who sometimes just drop dead.

But when's the last time you heard of someone known for being incredibly well-rested who just dropped dead? 😳 🐒

So, in a perfect world, make sure to exercise **and** to get about 7-8 hours of sleep per night!

But if you have to pick just one... get the 7-8 hours of sleep!

The Awkward Nugget of Humanity...

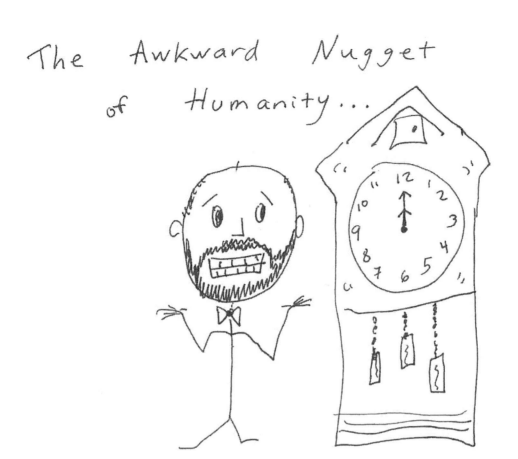

Well, that's it!

That's all my nuggets!

Yesterday was Daily Nugget #366,

which means that if it's a leap year, then we've spent exactly 1 year together!

And if it's any other year then we got a bonus day.

The Nugget of Shame was something that nobody was ever meant to see.

I had it loaded and ready to go if I ever failed to launch a nugget e-mail one day or left town without pre-loading enough nuggets! The idea was to let you know that I hadn't forgotten you and/but that I'm only human!

Thankfully, nobody ever woke up to The Nugget of Shame! 😄

But I thought you might enjoy seeing the picture anyway.

ARE YOU SITTING ON A NUGGET?

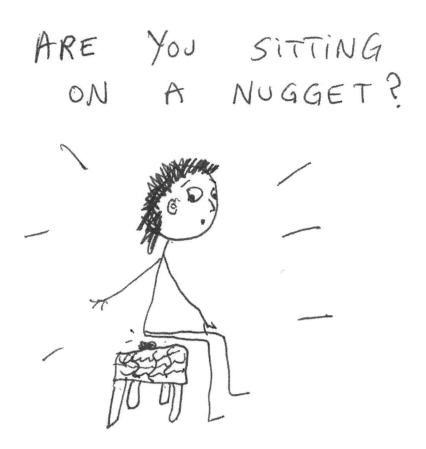

My original goal was to create 366 Daily Health Nuggets so that I could eventually compile them into a book. Well, here we are! It was a struggle to come up with 366, but there's always more to know! Some nuggets are better than others, and I want to continually evolve and replace the less-helpful ones with better ones.

So, if **you** have a simple health gem that you think should be included in the Daily Nugget e-mails or a future edition of the book, let me know!

You can contact me through my website: www.drkimsf.com

Thanks for your support! 🖤🙏

The Duds

Sometimes, a nugget turns out to be a dud... 😳 🫣

Here are the ones that (so far) just didn't make the cut!

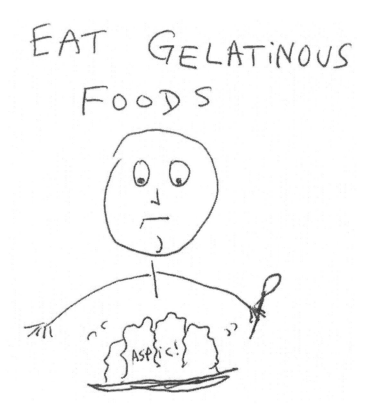

OK, this one didn't even make it past the picture phase! No one's going to eat this aspic abomination. I forgot all about it until I was moving picture files on my computer!

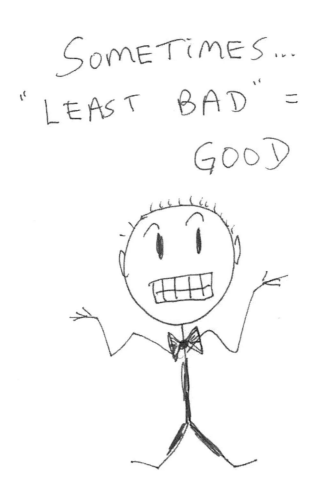

SOMETIMES...
" LEAST BAD " =
GOOD

This sounds like pretty reasonable advice! But I don't remember what I was going to say about it, and I'm pretty sure that whatever I was aiming for ended up being covered in a different nugget. Again, the picture was found during the file transfer process!

Hmmm... 🫨

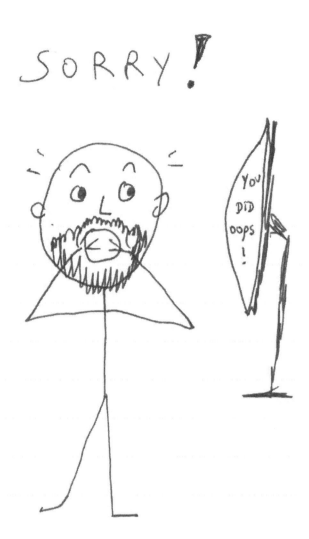

I can't remember if this was supposed to go with a nugget about saying **you're** sorry, or if it was a nugget about **me** apologizing to **you** about something! (It might have been a precursor to the Nugget of Shame. Because that sure does looks like me...)

2 - INGREDIENT "HEALTHY" COOKIES!

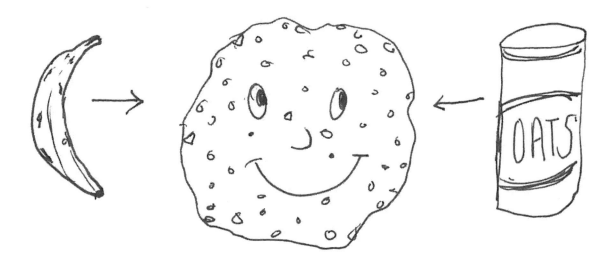

> Oh, and **this** dud did make it out to about 120 unsuspecting Nuggeteers before I pulled it! It sounded so good and reasonable that I didn't think I even needed to test it ahead of time! FAIL! This was the worst "cookie" I've ever eaten. And I've eaten a **lot** of questionable cookies. So... try this at your own peril. Maybe it's all about what kind of oats or how old the banana... I dunno. But I hereby wash my hands of this one!

Can cookies really be "healthy?"

I suppose it's debatable... but... we're not here to debate!

As far as we're concerned, some cookies can be deemed "close enough!"

In our overly-processed world, one healthy sign is a very short ingredient list.

And it doesn't get much shorter than 2 ingredients!

To make these "healthy cookies," you just need 2 things" 1 over-ripe banana and about 1/2 a cup of rolled oats ("quick cooking" is OK but not "instant").

You just mash that old banana in a bowl and mix in the oats until it's totally mixed in.

Then scoop out little balls of the mixture onto a parchment lined baking sheet (or a silicone mat), flatten them into cookie looking discs, and bake at 350 for about 15 minutes.

And that's it!

If you want to make more, then use 2 big over ripe bananas and 1 cup of oats.

Simple is beautiful! 😎

Bonus Material

Ear Chart for Acupressure, Auriculotherapy, etc. (from the "Pull My Ear" nugget)

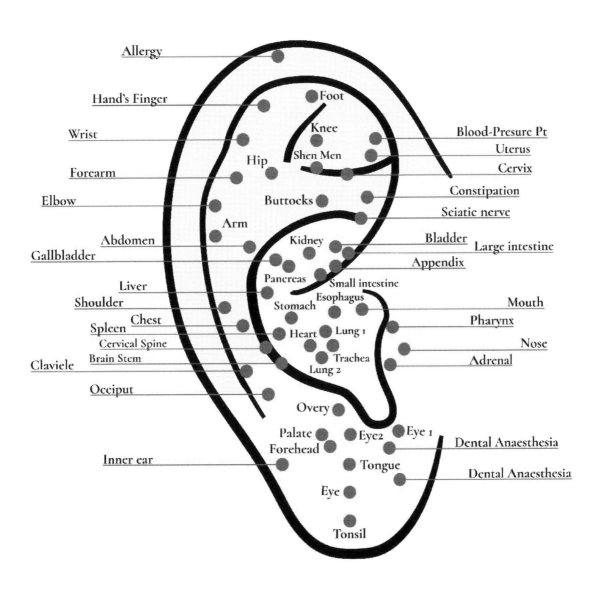

Diagram of the back of the ear, with acupressure and auriculotherapy points.

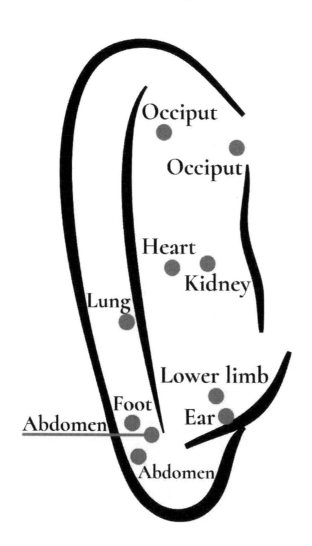

Occiput

Occiput

Heart

Kidney

Lung

Lower limb

Foot

Abdomen

Ear

Abdomen

FOOT REFLEXOLOGY CHART

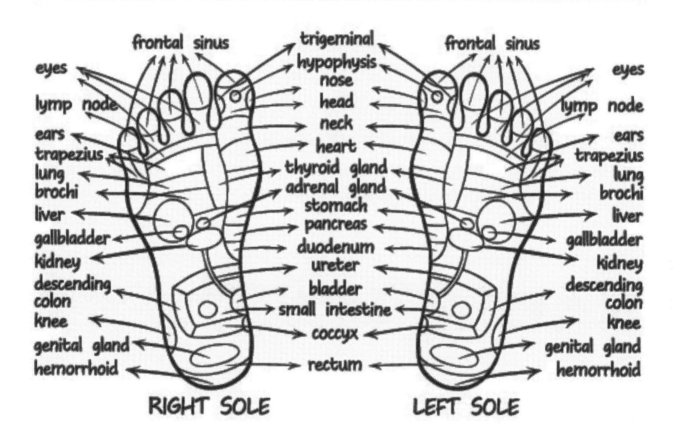

frontal sinus
eyes
lymp node
ears
trapezius
lung
brochi
liver
gallbladder
kidney
descending colon
knee
genital gland
hemorrhoid

trigeminal
hypophysis
nose
head
neck
heart
thyroid gland
adrenal gland
stomach
pancreas
duodenum
ureter
bladder
small intestine
coccyx
rectum

frontal sinus
eyes
lymp node
ears
trapezius
lung
brochi
liver
gallbladder
kidney
descending colon
knee
genital gland
hemorrhoid

RIGHT SOLE

LEFT SOLE

Quickie Enneagram Test

The Enneagram is an elegant system with tremendous nuance. Although there are only 9 basic "types," the system allows for hundreds of subtypes when you take into consideration wings and subtypes! The first step in determining where you land is to figure out your basic type. Most Enneagram typing quizzes are very long. And even then, the results are not always clear. This short quiz is based on the QUEST (Quick and Easy Enneagram Sorting Test) which can be found in The Wisdom of the Enneagram, by Don Richard Riso and Russ Hudson.

For the Quickie Enneagram Test to work best, keep these guidelines in mind. **Don't overthink it!** Go with the answer that *feels* right for you, even if you don't agree with it 100% and even if you disagree with some of the elements. Of the choices presented, one of the paragraphs in each group will probably resonate with you more than the other two, You should agree with the general vibe of the paragraph, even though you might disagree with specific elements within it.

Go with your gut, and just make the choice that you seem to be drawn to.

You will be presented with 2 groups of 3 paragraphs. In each group, choose just 1 paragraph which you seem to resonate with.

Choose the answer that reflects the way that you have generally been throughout your life.

If you really can't choose just 1, then it's OK to choose 2 answers within one group. We can still figure out your type from there! (But you can't pick 2 answers from each group.) For example, you could pick A from group X and 1 and 3 from group Y.

Group X

A.   I don't like to draw attention to myself, and I'm basically a quiet person. I'm used to being on my own, and I'm comfortable without having to be active all the time. I'm not competitive and I'm uncomfortable taking the lead. My imagination is where I am most excited, and that makes me seem like a bit of a dreamer.

B.   I'm a person who usually knows what I want. I work hard, play hard and when I want something I go for it. I'm pretty independent, set my own goals, get involved and make things happen. I want to have an impact, and I don't like sitting around. I'm not looking for a fight, but I don't let people push me around, either. Life works best when you can look it in the eye and meet it head on.

C.   I am a hard worker and do what needs to be done. I honor my commitments and I feel terrible if I fall short of the mark. I am dedicated and extremely responsible. I make personal sacrifices for the good of others and I want them to know that I am there for them. I do what I believe is right for the group. People are often unaware of the sacrifices that I have made. I won't rest and relax for myself unless there is time left after my responsibilities!

Circle your choice from **Group** X: A   B   C

Group Y

1. I am a "glass half full" kind of person. I feel that things will usually work out for the best, and I generally have a positive outlook on life. I usually keep myself busy and enjoy helping other people to be happy. I enjoy sharing my well-being with others, and I can always find something to be enthusiastic about! When I'm feeling down, I don't like to show it to anyone. Sometimes I put off dealing with my own problems for too long because I'm always trying to stay positive!

2. I have strong feelings about things. People can tell when I'm unhappy. When I'm upset, I want people to respond and feel as passionately as I do. I'm more sensitive than I let on, and I can be guarded with people. It's pretty clear where people stand with me, but I also want to know where I stand with them. I don't like being told what to do. I know the rules, but I want to decide for myself.

3. I am logical, self-controlled and efficient. I am uncomfortable dealing with feelings. I prefer working on my own and can be a bit of a perfectionist. I avoid bringing my feelings into problems and personal conflicts. I may seem cool and detached, but I just don't want my emotions to get in the way. When others try to "get to me," I usually don't show my reactions.

Circle your choice from **Group** Y: 1   2   3

Interpreting the Quickie Enneagram Test			
	Results	*Type*	*Type Name and Key Characteristics*
Your answers will give you a two-character code. For example, choosing paragraph B in group X, and paragraph 2 in group Y produces the two-character code B2.	**A1**	9	The Peacemaker: *Just wants everyone to get along*
	A2	4	The Individualist: *Feels special, yet fundamentally flawed*
	A3	5	The Investigator: *Wants to KNOW everything, be the expert*
	B1	7	The Enthusiast: *Doesn't want to miss out on ANYTHING*
	B2	8	The Challenger: *Wants to be the boss, take control*
	B3	3	The Achiever: *Wants to be #1 – the best!*
To find out which basic Enneagram type is indicated by the Quickie Test, look to the column on the right.	**C1**	2	The Helper: *Just wants to help!*
	C2	6	The Loyalist: *Loyal, responsible, craves stability*
	C3	1	The Perfectionist: *Wants everything done RIGHT*

411

Pain Tapping Body Maps – illustrations by Anne Lauder

Tap the face points (located on (page 323) based on where the pain is located based on these body maps!

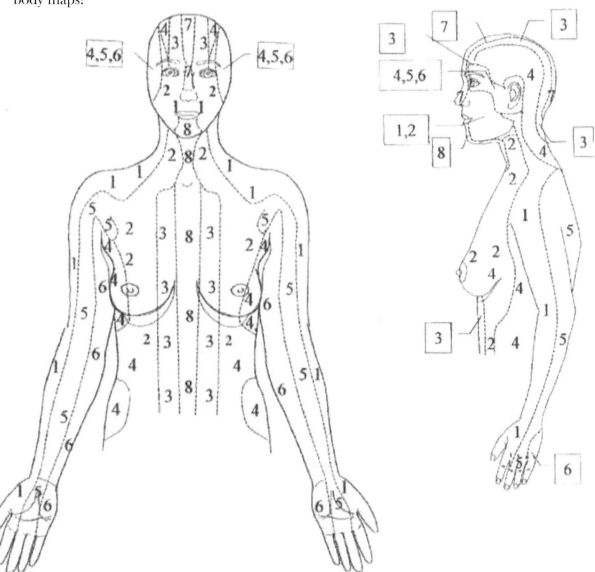

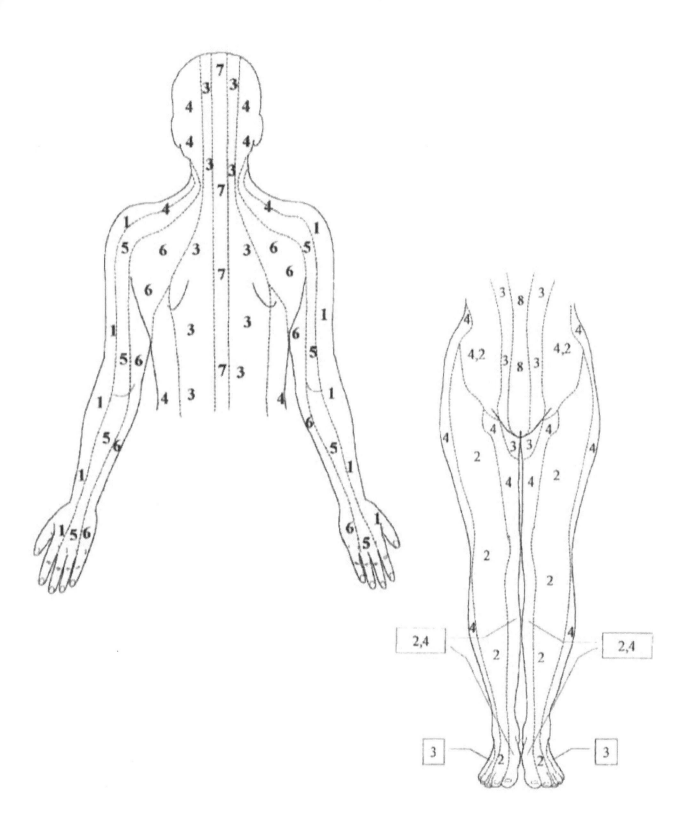

413

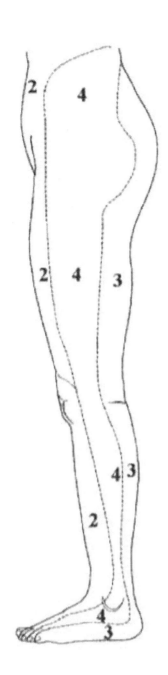

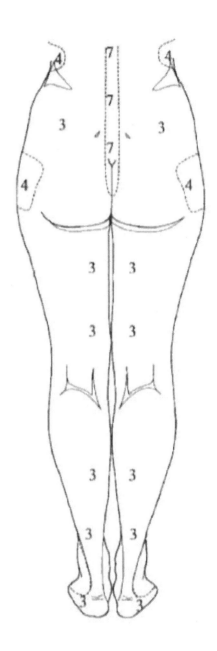

414

Index

416

Made in the USA
Monee, IL
22 January 2024

51597290R00240